T0384979

# Neuroscience and Media

This volume explores how advances in the fields of evolutionary neuroscience and cognitive psychology are informing media studies with a better understanding of how humans perceive, think, and experience emotion within mediated environments. The book highlights interdisciplinary and transdisciplinary approaches to the production and reception of cinema, television, the Internet, and other forms of mediated communication that take into account new understandings of how the embodied brain senses and interacts with its symbolic environment. Moreover, as popular media shape perceptions of the promises and limits of brain science, contributors also examine the representation of neuroscience and cognitive psychology within mediated culture.

**Michael Grabowski**, PhD, is an associate professor of communication at Manhattan College. His work explores how different forms of mediated communication shape the way people think and act within their symbolic environments. He has won two Emmy Awards and has worked on documentaries, feature films, commercials, music videos, and news.

# Routledge Research in Cultural and Media Studies

*For a full list of titles in this series, please visit www.routledge.com*

# Neuroscience and Media

New Understandings and Representations

**Edited by**
**Michael Grabowski**

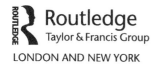

Routledge
Taylor & Francis Group

LONDON AND NEW YORK

First published 2015
by Routledge

2 Park Square, Milton Park, Abingdon, Oxfordshire OX14 4RN
711 Third Avenue, New York, NY 10017

*Routledge is an imprint of the Taylor & Francis Group, an informa business*

First issued in paperback 2018

*Library of Congress Cataloging-in-Publication Data*
CIP data has been applied for.

ISBN: 978-1-138-81150-8 (hbk)
ISBN: 978-1-138-54847-3 (pbk)


Typeset in Sabon
by Apex CoVantage, LLC

# Contents

# Figures and Tables

## FIGURES

## TABLES

# Acknowledgments

The idea for this collection began in 2011 at the National Communication Association Annual Convention in New Orleans. I thank everyone who provided me with valuable feedback there and encouraged me to pursue this project. Members of the Media Ecology Association and the Society for the Cognitive Studies of the Moving Image also have been generous in their support. I thank Mary Rothschild for ensuring the inclusion of media and the developing brain. My colleagues in the Department of Communication at Manhattan College, and especially chairperson Thom Gencarelli, have been incredibly supportive during this process, and I value not only their expertise but also their friendship. Charles R. Tropp has been invaluable for his tremendous formatting and proofreading skills and has helped turn a collection of essays into a book. I am grateful to my editor Felisa Salvago-Keyes, Katie Laurentiev, and everyone at Routledge who have made the process of publishing this book a positive one. Of course, there would be no collection without its contributors, all of whom have selflessly given their time and energy to bring these essays to you. Lastly, thank you to my family, Ethan, Maya, Gillian, and Laura, who have endured my disappearance while assembling this work. All this would not have been possible without your love.

# Introduction

*By Michael Grabowski*

The brain is the medium of the mind, the physical substance that gathers, stores, recalls, and generates perceptions, information, ideas, and emotions. Despite its central role in understanding our environment, how the brain functions had long remained a mystery.[1]

Over the last twenty years, however, new tools have allowed researchers to peer inside the brain while it works. Most notably, functional magnetic resonance imaging (fMRI) tied to computational techniques has provided a non-invasive technique to monitor brain activity down in real time to the resolution of less than a cubic millimeter.[2] Older technologies like EEG have improved their resolution, and patients waiting for brain surgery have volunteered to have specific neurons stimulated or monitored without harm for the purpose of research.[3] Scientists have a much more nuanced understanding of the role of neurochemistry in brain function,[4] and genetic engineering has allowed researchers to modify the blueprint used to build the brain in some animals.[5] Most recently, the *New York Times* reported on the Human Connectome Project, an effort to map the neural pathways of the brain.[6] More advances likely are to come quickly, as President Obama proposed early in 2013 a $100 million initiative dedicated to mapping the human brain. Comparing the endeavor to the development of the microchip and the Internet, the President said, ". . . we still haven't unlocked the mystery of the three pounds of matter that sits between our ears."[7]

Accompanying these advances, stories about how our brains operate have infused popular culture and disciplines beyond neuroscience. New articles, blogs posts, and books regularly appear that explore the way brain science contributes to other areas of study. Headlines about how brain chemistry influences one's taste in music, social relationships, career choices, and ethical decisions are pervasive throughout popular media. Moreover, fields as diverse as philosophy, education, political science, economics, sociology, history, literature studies, and the fine arts are all incorporating new knowledge about the brain within their disciplines. The brain itself has become an iconic fixture in advertising, selling everything from digital televisions and smart phones to cereal, vacuum cleaners, and toothpaste. Brain structure and function, once a subject of conversation limited to scientists, is now publicly discussed in general interest publications such as *Time*: "The Brain: A User's Guide," "Secrets of the Teen Brain," and "How to Sharpen Your Mind" are a few sample cover stories. Television programs, such as Discovery's *The Big Brain Theory* and Charlie Rose's *The Brain Series*, disseminate information and promote researchers through interviews and visualizations of the brain. The brain, once the domain of neurosurgeons and research scientists, is now becoming more accessible and a subject of study to those outside these specific fields.

As these stories take root in culture, they become part of a general narrative about the twenty-first century as an era of the brain.[8] How do media shape this narrative, and how can the study of media itself benefit from these new insights? These questions have prompted the writing of this book.

*Neuroscience and Media: New Understandings and Representations* explores how advances in the fields of evolutionary neuroscience, neurochemistry, brain imaging, and cognitive psychology are informing media studies with a better understanding of how humans perceive, think, and feel within mediated environments. The contributors to this book work in backgrounds as varied as pediatrics, neuroscience, anthropology, cinema studies, and communication, but they all have in common an interest in working across disciplines to address these questions. Just as advances in brain science can illuminate media studies, theories of communication can clarify the rhetoric concerning brain structure, function, and development. Although a tremendous amount of progress has been made in understanding the brain, the application of neuroscience as a utopian solution to cultural problems presents new challenges. This book takes a critical approach to examining how mediated communication shapes metaphors and concepts about the brain.

Part I, "The Brain on Media," considers how theory and discovery in brain structure and functions can help to support, explain, or revise theories and issues in the field of communication. The first chapter lays out a theory of communication based on an understanding of the brain that is embodied and extended through media. Finding common ground in the work of Marshall McLuhan and Danish film scholar Torben Grodal, it seeks to establish a foundation of mediated communication rooted in cognitive and emotive brain function. Annie Lang has likened the field of communication to a Kuhnian state of crisis and has called for ". . . understand[ing] communication as a fundamental, dynamic, natural aspect of human adaptation to the environment."[9] An ecological model of the brain and media can be a path forward, joining the theoretical foundations of media ecology with empirical evidence of how the embodied brain perceives and reacts to its environment.

The next chapter, "Nurturing the Developing Brains of Digital Natives," examines how an environment of ubiquitous digital media influences the building and organization of neural pathways. As the director of the Center on Media and Child Health at Boston Children's Hospital, Dr. Michael

Rich advises pediatricians and families on healthy media use that promotes child health and development. In this chapter, he and his graduate student Farah Qureshi note that between birth and the age of two, the human brain triples in volume, and billions of synaptic connections are formed. They cite research that shows the limited interactivity of digital media is not neurologically optimal for the developing brain. They argue that a digital media culture harms children in at least two ways: occupying children's time with these media limit exposure to face-to-face interaction and manipulation of the physical world, and parents and caregivers distracted by demanding digital devices spend less time interacting with children, creating a model of a screen-focused rather than human-centered environment. As the plasticity of the brain prunes unused neural connections while strengthening those reinforced by screen exposure, television and other screen-based digital media promise to transform the brains of future generations in ways we are only beginning to understand.

The third chapter, "Neurobiology of Teen Brain Development and the Digital Age," focuses on the development of the frontal lobe and its role in impulse control and decision making. Jennifer T. Sneider and Marisa M. Silveri are neuroscientists at Harvard Medical School who use fMRI to study physical addiction in teens and adults, but they turn their attention here to the controversial topic of media addiction. They cite evidence that addictive behaviors are more likely to occur during the teen years, before the frontal lobe of the cerebral cortex has matured. The frontal lobe has been shown to inhibit more emotional, less thoughtful outbursts and balance the sensitivity to reward from the ventral striatum, while aiding in memory and the learning of new skills. As teens engage in gaming, social media, and other digital technologies that reinforce reward pathways, these media effectively override the frontal lobe, and addictive behavior becomes more prevalent. Studies show that pathologies like Internet addiction disorder are associated with functional and structural brain abnormalities that resemble substance-related addictions. While not conclusive, these studies certainly demand more study in how the stimuli and rewards that digital media provide alter the development of the teen brain.

After surveying the developing brain in new media environments, the book turns its attention to how we perceive those environments. Using brain research to counter the traditional view that the experience of watching a movie requires only our senses of sight and sound, Luis Rocha Antunes's "Neural Correlates of the Multisensory Film Experience" argues that mediated experience engages senses less explored, such as proprioception, thermoception, and the vestibular. Most study of film assume the properties of the medium, light and sound, have a one-to-one correspondence with our senses, but Antunes shows that perception is multisensory and multimodal, employing several mechanisms of feedback that shape the model of the environment that is perceived. In particular, the hypothalamus and the superior colliculus work to integrate senses and engage responses that change the perception of stimuli. Using Kubrick's *2001: A Space Odyssey* as an example, Antunes shows how our experience of a film engages the propriceptive sense, resulting in motor actions that in turn influence what we see. Though the discussion in this chapter concentrates on film, its conclusions bear numerous consequences for our understanding of perception and experience across all media that engage our senses.

Building on the multisensory perception of media, Dana Coestor explores how narratives are constructed from bits of perceptual data into an experience network to create meaningful, contextualized experiences. "The Reverberatory Narrative: Toward Story as a Multisensory Network" recounts how Coestor's 1998 multimedia documentary *Pretty* employed the transparency of memory as described by Anderson's activation theory of memory.[10] Experimenting with fragmented narratives in both art and journalism, Coestor constructed a story using interactive art installations, print media, film, and digital content. These narrative singularities pulled in disparate stories, words, images, and content along strings of context. The leaps in associative content allow for new narratives to emerge, as Antonio Damasio describes unified perceptions that can emerge from fragmented data in the process of making a memory.[11] With the use of digital applications like Storify and the proliferation of social media, Coestor argues that we are entering an age of immersive, contextualized, data-driven experiences. She proposes a new kind of journalism that is more aligned with how the brain produces memory and operates as narrative networks rather than narrative sequences.

In "Embodied Protonarratives Embedded in Systems of Contexts: A Neurocinematic Approach," Pia Tikka and Mauri Kaipainen examine how recent advances in neuroscience, in general, and neurocinematics, in particular, allow an explanatory grounding for narrative comprehension based on the embodied mind approach. The chapter discusses the efficiency of cinematic narratives to communicate social situations and how the associated neural processes rely on underlying prototypical, schematic structures. They define protonarratives as a set of relatively universal behavioral patterns that are a part of the brain's functional networks and are shaped by the physical engagement with the surrounding world. However, narratives cannot be fully understood by their protonarratives, as the context in which they are presented changes how they are perceived. They suggest that the neural processes of mentalizing and mirroring are two fundamental, complementary processes of contextualization. The chapter concludes that dynamically evolving narrative perspectives may explain the variation of experiences among viewers of mediated content and contribute to understanding how we interpret cinematic simulations of life situations against socio-cultural contexts.

One contextual element of narrative construction may be the properties of the medium in which narratives are constructed. The next chapter examines this possibility in the case of print media. "Seeing In, and Out, to the

Extended Mind through an EEG Analysis of Page and Screen Reading" takes on the question of whether digital e-reading devices, such as Amazon's Kindle and Apple's iPad, produce a medium-specific difference in perception as opposed to reading from the printed page. Examining other research that attempts to isolate visual perception and cognition, as well as conducting EEG experiments with screen and page reading, Robert MacDougall concludes that, while media may be a contributing factor in perception, they exist within a context of many other environmental factors, including the past reading experiences of participants, level of reading comprehension, and the use of stimulant, anti-anxiety, and anti-depression drugs. Thus, media habitation and habituation become central questions when examining the perception of media, leading to the conclusion that media themselves are not deterministic in their effects but, as extensions of human perception, integrate within an ecology of perception and cognition.

In the final chapter in part I, award-winning journalist Bob Schapiro teams up with anthropologist Stanley H. Ambrose to recast propaganda as a socially evolved trait that helps to establish identity and social cohesion. They claim that the propaganda emerged as the organization of human groups grew beyond those linked by genetic kinship and toward ones connected by shared ideas and beliefs. "On the Origins of Propaganda: Bio-Cultural and Evolutionary Perspectives on Social Cohesion" argues that, by generating cognitive dissonance, propaganda builds upon a reliance on identity systems. They cite experiments that examine the neurotransmitters oyxtocin, vasopressin, and serotonin to establish a physiological explanation for the effects of propaganda. By clarifying the definition of propaganda as a form of communication that affects or utilizes an identity system, this chapter hopes to illuminate its use in constructive memory formation, altruistic punishment, recursion, diplomatic speech, advertising, and many other forms of socialization.

Part II of the book, "Media on the Brain," examines the representation of neuroscience and cognitive psychology within mediated culture. As popular media shape perceptions of the promises and limits of brain science, it is worthy to take a step back and ask what messages are amplified, repeated, or suppressed. How do publics conform new discoveries about the brain with what they already believe to be true, and how are these findings (mis) represented? For example, Steven Gibson's "Mind Control in Hollywood" looks at how television shows and movies have represented various forms of mind control and shows how these representations rely on different philosophies of the mind. As scenes of mind control and brainwashing are used for entertainment purposes to drive plot, they also help to build assumptions about how the mind works, and those assumptions, as reflected in television programs, have changed over time from the mind as an individualized, mechanistic device to a more collective conception of the self.

Emilia Musumeci shows how neuroscience has been used in news media and courtrooms as a way to explain or condemn criminal behavior. In " 'My

Brain Made Me Do It!' Neuroscience, Criminal Justice, and Media," she documents the pairing of the terms neuroscience and law in recent years and shows the transition of testimony in courtrooms from the more ambiguous field psychology to the data-driven and seemingly less fallible neurosciences. News articles about crime use neuroscience to connote a voyeuristic peering into the minds of psychopaths and killers, and behavioral genetics provides a basis for courts to question the agency of criminals who may be victims of "bad genes." These cultural developments lead Musumeci to conclude that the transfer of power from psychology to neuroscience has resulted in the perception of neuroscientists as the mythical experts of human behavior.

The following two chapters examine how old and new media represent collaboration between neuroscience and traditional methods of manipulating the mind. Jenell Johnson writes in "The Golden Voice of Neuroscience: Fact Finding in Western Buddhist Media" that when writing for a Western Buddhist audience, authors must negotiate the epistemological tension between traditional and scientific authority. Despite claims of collaboration and interdisciplinary pursuit, these articles often present neuroscience as the ultimate authority on matters of the mind and, like other popular science writing, tend toward reductionism, essentialism, and bolstered claims of certainty. New, collaborative media present other challenges, as noted by Andrée E.C. Betancourt and Elise E. Labbé in "Mindful Media: Representations of the Effects of Mindfulness on the Brain in YouTube Videos." As they explore a selection of videos tagged with the words "meditation," "mindfulness," "brain," and "effect," they discover that a majority of videos have been created to market corporations, nonprofit organizations, or individuals. Few comments referenced the relationship between the brain and meditation, despite its established physiological benefits. They conclude that online communities are still largely segregated, and that ethnographic approaches may elicit more insight into the everyday practices of these communities.

Using popular concepts from neuroscience to advertise products and services certainly extends beyond mindfulness. Celia Andreu-Sánchez and Miguel Ángel Martín-Pascual document how ad campaigns use images of the brain and neuroscientific terms to lend credibility to products and services. Their chapter, "Selling the Brain: Representation of Neuroscience in Advertising," demonstrates that the brain often is used to connote creativity, intelligent decision making, and reason. Some ads use a hemispheric model of the brain to suggest that products are both useful and fun, while others show arrangements of products to produce the shape of a brain. The authors conclude that brain images often serve as a substitute for the logical presentation of a product's attributes, paradoxically using science to support claims that cannot be tested.

The final chapter, "Braining Your Life and Living Your Brain: The Cyborg Gaze and Brain-Images," examines the use of brain imaging as an artifact of power that reifies norms of gender, illness, and aging. Alexander I. Stingl exposes the mechanization behind the popular use of medical imaging, which mimics an unconditional visuality despite often displaying a translation of non-visual data. Once the image becomes reified, power is transferred from the gazer to the producers of the image. Male and female brains solidify gender categories despite individual and cultural variation, and the aged brain constructs ageing as a medicalized, chronic illness rather than a natural life process. Questioning the epistemological authority of medial imaging is not to deny the usefulness of these images but merely recognizes the persuasive power these images hold.

These chapters are by no means a comprehensive survey of the areas of research that can benefit from a transdisciplinary collaboration, nor should this book be taken as a definitive statement that neuroscience is the only proper lens through which to focus on these issues. However, the examples put forward in this book present templates for collaboration between scholars in the sciences, social sciences, and humanities to provide a multimodal description of how we use media and how media change how we communicate, understand, and act. Certainly many more examples exist, and it is the hope of these contributors that this volume encourages more exchanges of ideas that provide a fruitful way forward for communication research.

## NOTES

1. Stanley Finger provides a thorough history of brain science in *Origins of Neuroscience: A History of Explorations into Brain Function* (New York: Oxford University Press, 1994).
2. Frederico A. C. Azevedo et al., "Equal Numbers of Neuronal and Nonneuronal Cells Make the Human Brain an Isometrically Scaled-up Primate Brain," *Journal of Comparative Neurology* 513, no. 5 (2009): 532–41, doi:10.1002/cne.21974; Lise Lyck et al., "An Empirical Analysis of the Precision of Estimating the Numbers of Neurons and Glia in Human Neocortex Using a Fractionator-Design with Sub-Sampling," *Journal of Neuroscience Methods* 182, no. 2 (2009): 143–56, doi:10.1016/j.jneumeth.2009.06.003.
3. Amy Standen, "Epilepsy Patients Help Decode the Brain's Hidden Signals," NPR, http://www.npr.org/blogs/health/2013/12/09/248999497/epilepsy-patients-help-decode-the-brains-hidden-signals.
4. Scott T. Brady et al., *Basic Neurochemistry: Principles of Molecular, Cellular, and Medical Neurobiology*, 8th ed. (Boston: Elsevier/Academic Press, 2012).
5. Dana M. Santos, *Genetic Engineering: Recent Developments in Applications* (Oakville, ON: Apple Academic Press, 2011).
6. James Gorman, "The Brain, in Exquisite Detail," *New York Times*, January 6, 2014, http://www.nytimes.com/2014/01/07/science/the-brain-in-exquisite-detail.html.
7. Scott Wilson, "Obama Outlines Human Brain-Mapping Initiative," *Washington Post*, April 3, 2013, http://www.washingtonpost.com/politics/obama-outlines-human-brain-mapping-initiative/2013/04/02/4fc460b2–9b9a-11e2–9a79-eb5280c81c63_story.html.
8. Vaughan Bell, "Changing Brains: Why Neuroscience Is Ending the Prozac Era," *The Guardian*, September 21, 2013, http://www.theguardian.com/science/

2013/sep/22/brains-neuroscience-prozac-psychiatric-drugs; Cathy N. David-son, *Now You See It: How Technology and Brain Science Will Transform Schools and Business for the 21st Century* (New York: Penguin Books, 2012); Matthew Knight, "Mapping out a New Era in Brain Research," *CNN*, May 9, 2012, http://www.cnn.com/2012/03/01/tech/innovation/brain-map-connecto me/index.html.

9. Annie Lang, "Discipline in Crisis? The Shifting Paradigm of Mass Commu-nication Research: Discipline in Crisis," *Communication Theory* 23, no. 1 (2013): 23, doi:10.1111/comt.12000.

10. John R. Anderson, "A Spreading Activation Theory of Memory," *Journal of Verbal Learning and Verbal Behavior* 22, no. 3 (1983): 261–95, doi:10.1016/ S0022-5371(83)90201-3.

11. Antonio R. Damasio, *Self Comes to Mind: Constructing the Conscious Brain* (New York: Vintage Books, 2012).

Part I

# The Brain on Media

# 1 Neuromediation

## An Ecological Model of Mediated Communication

*Michael Grabowski*

Understanding mediated communication involves building a model that conforms to the observed environment and correctly predicts its influence upon that environment. Oftentimes, these models are limited by the questions that are asked: How efficient is a channel of communication? What information is transmitted? What meanings are generated? How do people use media? How do media shape culture? Each model is embedded with political, economic, and social assumptions. The words sender, user, player, actor, spectator, audience, viewer, and participant each presuppose how people interact with media. The metaphors we use to describe media bring with them associations that may obscure instead of clarify understanding. Messages do not flow through a pipe (unless the sender is using pneumatic tubes), we do not "hand off" a message electronically, and our brains do not fill up with information poured into it, although it may feel like that at times.

Of course, no model, by definition, can exactly reproduce the environment it represents. Models need only be good enough to address the questions concerning those who use them. As a journalist who saw firsthand the efforts of propaganda crafters during World War I, Walter Lippmann sought a means to use mass media in order to influence public consent of governmental policies.[1] Likewise, Harold Lasswell analyzed the effectiveness of wartime propaganda,[2] and he established a widely used model of propaganda that served as a precursor to a systematic study of communication.[3] His model (Figure 1.1a) incorporated a sender, channel, and receiver but also included the effect of any communicated message, consistent with his study of the effectiveness of propaganda. Claude Shannon and Warren Weaver's transmission model of communication (Figure 1.1b) served engineers well as they sought to explain the capacity of a channel for transmitting signals.[4] Concerned with the ability of electromagnetic systems to successfully preserve information despite the introduction of noise into a signal, these mathematicians reduced communication to the sending and receiving of messages. Norbert Wiener's contribution to the model completed the loop, confirming transmissions are successful by providing feedback to the sender. By reducing communicators to senders and receivers of

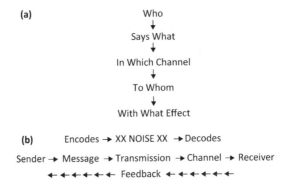

*Figure 1.1*   Traditional Models of Communication: (a) Lasswell's Model and (b) Shannon-Weaver-Wiener Transmission Model

information, early communication theorists could work on the problem of channel capacity for telephony and radio communication. The efficiency and accuracy of messages became the focus of communication theory.[5]

Theorizing communication as information transmission and reception became a framework for several branches of communication studies, including the dominant field of effects research.[6] Some theories, like political economy, gatekeeping, framing, and agenda setting, focused on the senders of messages. Content analysis examined the messages themselves, and uses and gratifications, audience analysis, and cultivation theory concerned themselves with receivers. Debates centered on (and continue to be argued over) issues like the efficiencies of message transmission, the limited effects of communicated messages,[7] concentrated power over communication channels,[8] or the power of audiences to construct the messages they receive.[9]

However, the transmission model fails to address other uses of communication. For instance, people often engage in forms of communication not to send information unknown to the receiver, but as part of a ritual that reinforces group identity and confirms a worldview. Media critic James Carey argued that communication exists within a context of "social processes wherein symbolic forms are created, apprehended, and used."[10] His ritual model asks qualitative questions about the symbolic systems employed to comprehend and understand definitions of reality. Arising out of his concern of how the juxtaposition of mass media and traditional human communication form a democratic culture, Carey's model is a culmination of critical theory and cultural studies, which both question the assumptions behind the traditional transmission model.

As effects researchers focused their attention on the messages communicated across channels of communication, another theorist asked how the channels themselves acted upon cultures. Marshall McLuhan's aphorism "the medium is the message" may suggest that his theory fits squarely within the channel portion of the transmission model, but that would misrepresent both McLuhan's concerns and the model he constructed to address them. Rather, he argued that messages themselves were largely irrelevant in the shaping of culture. For McLuhan, messages were ". . . like the juicy piece of meat carried by the burglar to distract the watchdog of the mind."[11] Instead, the dominant media cultures use to communicate structure that culture around specific sense ratios. McLuhan relied upon Harold Innis[12] to show that media possess different biases as they extend in space and time. Just as other technologies extend and amplify parts of the human body (a hammer extends the fist, an automobile extends the legs), media act as extensions of the human perceptual nervous system, according to McLuhan. A photograph extends the eye, and radio extends the ear.

Critics of McLuhan wrongly saw his work as an embrace of electronic media and an attack on intellectual culture[13] or a form of technological determinism that discounted human intervention.[14] Yet, McLuhan asserted that media technologies are not deterministic in and of themselves. Rather, they have deterministic effects because their users are unaware of those effects. McLuhan referred to the myth of Narcissus to illustrate this point. Narcissus did not fall in love with himself, but with a reflection of himself, which he saw as another being. Narcissus was unaware that the object of his love was his own construction. McLuhan characterized this condition as a form of narcosis, an autoamputation of senses to which a person is oblivious.[15]

McLuhan observed that a new medium changes the entire sensory environment into which it is introduced. Media change sense ratios, altering the perception of one's environment. One of his students, Neil Postman, popularized McLuhan's ecology of media ecology. Postman defined media ecology as

> . . . the study of information environments. It is concerned to understand how technologies and techniques of communication control the form, quantity, speed, distribution and direction of information; and how, in turn, such information configurations or biases affect people's perceptions, values, and attitudes.[16]

Unlike previous models discussed earlier, media ecology maintains that changes in the media environment are not additive but ecological. A new medium changes not only the messages sent through it but the entire symbolic system in which it exists. Like the physical ecology of a biome, the symbolic ecology of an information environment reacts to the interaction of media within that environment.[17]

Media ecology addresses the question of how media extend our perception, but how do our senses perceive our mediated environment? Since McLuhan wrote *Understanding Media*, neuroscience has moved beyond a hemispherical model of the brain to map out several regions with specialized functions. Tools like electroencephalography (EEG), positron emission tomography (PET), functional magnetic resonance imaging (fMRI), and magnetoencephalography (MEG) have allowed researchers to observe brain function in real time and with increasing resolution.[18] Cognitive psychologists began to work with systems neuroscience and brain imaging to link perception and behavior to biological and neurological responses. With this new understanding, any theory of mediated communication should take into account how the brain processes symbolic forms. Media ecology serves as a good starting point for this inquiry.

If we think of the brain as a medium through which we process information about our environment, a media ecological analysis would ask in what manner its properties influence *how* that information is processed. Like a body of water that bends the light which passes through it, the structures of the brain shape and process perceptions according to the neural networks they have formed. Mediated communication has tapped into these perceptual systems and exploits the characteristics of those systems. I have chosen to call this process *neuromediation*.

Like other models of communication, neuromediation addresses specific questions: How does each medium engage with our perceptions? What internal brain structures generate meaning from perceived mediated symbols? Which regions of the brain attend to different symbolic forms? How do the physical forms of symbols (what semioticians would call signifiers) and their context influence how they are processed? What information does the brain ignore when attending to media? In its essence, neuromediation concerns itself with the relationship between media and the brain.

This model relies on several advancements in brain research. First, it takes into account the fact that the brain is made up of a complex of suborganal structures. Advances in brain mapping have moved beyond the function of gross structures (brain stem, cerebrum, cerebellum) to a complex network of brain regions, such as the amygdala, basal ganglia, hippocampus, hypothalamus, thalamus, and cortical areas. The cerebral cortex consists of frontal, parietal temporal, and occipital lobes, each of which is further divided into regions that serve specialized functions. Localized structures correlate with specific activities, like the fusiform face area, which is involved in facial recognition and object categorization; Broca's and Wernicke's areas, related to language recognition and speech production; the hippocampus, used in the formation of memories of novel events; and the nucleus amygdalae, which process and regulate emotions like fear and pleasure.[19] In addition, researchers better understand paths of neural activity, like auditory processing from the cochlear nucleus to the superior olivary nuclei to the inferior colliculus through the medial geniculate nucleus to the primary auditory cortex. Sound perception, in fact, takes two pathways: a ventral stream helps in identifying sounds, while the dorsal stream helps to locate the origin of sounds. Visual information travels along the optic nerve through the optic chiasm to the lateral geniculate body to the visual cortex in the occipital lobe.[20] Moreover, researchers have mapped out the V1 area of the visual cortex and demonstrated a retinaltopic relationship. Computational brain imaging has devised a method for reading neural activity in this area and reproducing an approximation of what that area "sees."[21] Although neuroscience is far from mapping every neural network, enough is already known to inform communication theory and provide a more detailed model of the interaction between the brain and media.

Second, the model adopts the hypothesis that the brain is embodied. Several neuroscientists, including Antonio Damasio[22] and Joseph LeDoux,[23] have argued that cognition, emotion, and the body function together to create a sense of the self. A long philosophical tradition of embodiment has linked brain and culture with some debate.[24] More conservatively, this model refers to the extension of the brain through the sensory and motor nervous system and the endocrine system, which secretes neurotransmitters like dopamine, somatostatin, oxytocin, and vasopressin. Changes in these systems are reciprocal: motor action is perceived by the vestibular, proprioceptive, and haptic senses, and secretions of some hormones lead to neural activity that triggers other neurotransmitters. Some processing of sensory information occurs outside of the brain; many are familiar with reflex actions, which are processed in the spinal cord.[25] In addition, retinal cells engage in parallel processing of visual data before information is sent through the optic nerve.[26] Recently, medical researchers have found that the microbial environment communicates with the developing brain and can alter cognitive and behavioral functions.[27] These observations demonstrate that the brain is not an isolated organ separate from the body but integrated throughout the organism and into its environment.

Third, any holistic model of the brain must reconcile that it is bounded by genetics and epigenetics but retains a plasticity that is modified by new experiences in both physical and symbolic forms. The human brain has evolved from earlier mammalian ancestors, and many primate species have similar brain structures.[28] Genetic mutations may alter brain development, but humans share an anatomy that is consistent across the species. Thus, we are not blank slates upon which our experiences are written. However, recent research in epigenetics demonstrates that the genes encoded in DNA are not the only determiners of brain structure and function. Rather, mitochondrial RNA and the formation of specific proteins can pass traits on to subsequent generations. Furthermore, experiences themselves can lead to epigenetic changes like memory capacity, anxiety, and fear conditioning.[29] Despite these bounds, brain plasticity accounts for individual and cultural differentiation. As an individual engages in new interpersonal and mediated experiences, neural pathways are created, strengthened, or eradicated. Research in neurological disorders and brain trauma shows how brain structures take on new functions with a change in sensory or motor operation.[30]

Finally, the model incorporates the fact that media technologies extend the limits of human perception. One early genre of motion pictures was the travelogue, which showed exotic locales that audiences would be unlikely to visit.[31] Portrait photographs provide a window back in time to long departed relatives. Stroboscopic slow-motion cinematography and microscopic and telescopic imaging reveal processes normally concealed from view. These extensions create an observed environment different from the natural world in which the human brain evolved. Neuromediation explores how the tension between fixed brain structures and brain plasticity cope with a culturally and technologically evolving environment.

The process of neuromediation functions in two reciprocal ways. Our mediated environment, in a sense, extends our embodied brains beyond our bodies. As individuals change the ecology of their symbolic environment, their experiences and available perceptions within that environment change. At the same time, the structures and functions of our neural networks influence how we perceive and act upon our symbolic environment. Just as each medium of communication biases content, our sensory systems themselves attend to some perceptions, while discarding others. In a way, our neural networks mediate our symbolic environment.

I have delimited neuromediation to the perception of mediated communication to distinguish the role of media in shaping communication in ways that interpersonal forms do not. A large body of biological and psychological research has explored how the brain processes oral communication, narrative, and perceptions of the natural world.[32] This research certainly is related to and can inform the study of media. However, media change the scale and character of communication much more rapidly than interpersonal forms. In less than two centuries, telegraphy first separated communication from transportation, radio engendered a mass audience, television has redefined the relationship between news and entertainment, and the Internet has both connected and retribalized societies into a global village, all faster than human perception could evolve. How these media interact with a human sensory system adapted for small group cultures living on the savannah is what this essay, and the ones that follow, attempt to address.

Indeed, communication scholars already have argued for a cognitive approach to media. Annie Lang and her colleagues study the psychophysiological changes that occur over time when interacting with media technologies.[33] Lang has asked whether the paradigm of mass communication research is in crisis and offers a way forward by redefining ". . . media in terms of human-centric variables."[34] Cognitive theory has informed studies in media literacy[35] and the psychology of mass media.[36] This is a field ready for the transdisciplinary study of how particular media, bounded culturally and historically, interact with the brain.

Media studies also can turn to cognitive film theorists for guidance on joining cognitive psychology and neuroscience with theories of communication. Turning away from the approaches of psychoanalytic film theory, David Bordwell asked how filmmakers tap into the mental processes of audiences with the publication of *Narration in the Fiction Film*.[37] Together with Noël Carroll and Joseph and Barbara Anderson, these scholars established a cognitive approach to film studies.[38] They looked to the pioneering but forgotten work of psychologist Hugo Münsterberg, who used an empirical approach to studying the psychological effects of the motion picture.[39] Today, the field has grown and includes contributions from those who have written about the interdependence of emotion and cognition in film,[40] a cognitive philosophy of film,[41] evolutionary film theory,[42] and psychological and neuroscientific perspectives of film.[43] Uri Hasson established the field of neurocinematics as an empirical analysis of film viewing using fMRI imaging,[44] and Jeffrey M. Zacks has examined the brain as it sorts out events in narrative cinema.[45]

One contributor is particularly useful for the model of film aesthetics he has proposed. Torben Grodal proposed the PECMA flow model in 1997 (Figure 1.2), based on the functioning of the human nervous system, with the publication of *Moving Pictures*.[46] Warning against a mechanical understanding of information flow, Grodal described the brain as an organ process, as axon and dendrite branches, the connections between brain cells, continuously grow and retreat between neurons. According to the model, perceptions from sense organs flow into emotional and cognitive centers of the brain, generating arousals and associations that activate premotor and motor areas. Though his model suggests a directional flow from perception to emotion to cognition and motor action, Grodal is careful to note that the relationship between these systems are complex and interconnected and that bottom-up flows occur simultaneously with top-down flows.[47]

The implication of this complex flow reinforces an understanding of the brain not as a single organ but as an ecological system of several sub-organ structures and functions that extend beyond the brain itself. Perception is not a passive activity, merely receiving stimuli acting upon it, but an active process that shapes and constructs a perceived environment rather than faithfully reproducing it. Part of that perception involves emotions, as neuroscientists have documented direct neural paths from sense organs to the nucleus amygdalae, meaning that emotions resulting from a stimulus occur before someone is conscious of the stimulus.[48] Only a small portion of perceived stimuli are passed on to cognitive centers, including the prefrontal cortex, meaning that humans are usually not aware of the environment they

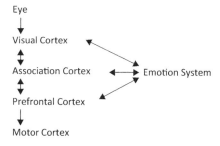

*Figure 1.2*  The PECMA Flow Model

are perceiving, as so amply documented by the work of cognitive psychologists Christopher Chabris and Daniel Simons.[49] However, some perceived data pass directly to the motor action system, allowing individuals to react to a stimulus without being aware of it. The bidirectional flow is illustrated by the fact that the same neural networks in the fusiform face area are activated when we see someone we recognize or when we simply picture the person in the mind. Likewise, neurons in the premotor cortex activate when we perform a specific action or perceive someone else performing that same action.

This perspective is highly compatible with and provides a physiological model for cultural semiotics. The associations between signifiers and various referents can be understood as interconnected neural networks that are bounded by evolutionary genetics but are formed as new experiences create new connections between already established patterns. A Kindle is like a book but also like a computer. An iPad can be like a magazine, but only if one has experienced a magazine.[50] As experiences are repeated and reinforced within a cultural structure, networks are strengthened and begin to bypass the prefrontal cortex, building habits and emotions of which we become unaware. Experience becomes environmental and patterns ideology.

The PECMA flow model can be a starting point for understanding the interaction of media and perception. However, one limitation of the cognitive film approach is the atomization of its study. Much writing in this area is concerned with the interaction of a film "text" and a generalized "viewer." This is understandable, as researchers seek to decipher the universal human perceptual functions that motion pictures utilize. However, one must be careful to attend to cultural experiences and other shared environmental factors, including exposure to language, rituals, and other cultural practices. Meanings vary across individuals and cultures, as past experience molds associations, memories, and emotional responses to texts. They are neither arbitrary nor fixed but bounded by brain structure and neural connections (Figure 1.3).

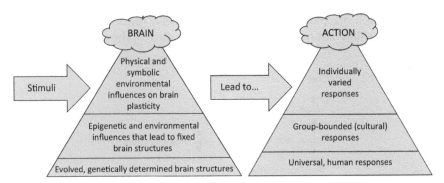

*Figure 1.3*   Brain as Medium: Messages Both Generate Meaning and Condition the Brain

In addition, all mediated content is shaped by the medium used to carry that content. Sometimes, like in the case of broadcasting live entertainment program on television, the bias of a medium enhances the content. Other times, like a continuing courtroom trial broadcast on television, the bias interferes with the purpose of the content.[51] Some media, like radio, engage a single sense, whereas others have the potential to adjust sense ratios. In other words, media are not transparent conveyers of messages but become a conditioning force upon them. Like Narcissus, we often are unaware of those effects, as well as the biases of our own perceptual systems, as we consume mediated content.

Neuromediation is not a fixed model but one in process. As researchers work to map out neural pathways in greater detail, they are likely to reveal new understandings about how the brain attends to mediated communication. Collaboration with cognitive psychology, psychophysiology, and neuroscience can provide and popularize a model of the brain in media studies that is associational, ecological, and embodied. Foundational concepts in media ecology and cognitive film studies can help to speed the advance of this understanding. Students and scholars of communication should embrace what John Brockman has called "the third culture,"[52] a joining of science, social science, and humanities in pursuit of answers that are fleeting to individual disciplines. By communicating across disciplines, researchers can further explore how humans sense, feel, think, and act upon and within their mediated environment.

## NOTES

1. Walter Lippmann, *Public Opinion* (New York: Free Press, 1997).
2. Harold D. Lasswell, *Propaganda Technique in World War I* (Cambridge, MA: MIT Press, 1971).
3. Harold D. Lasswell, "The Structure and Function of Communication in Society," in *The Communication of Ideas*, ed. Lyman Bryson, 37–51 (New York: Institute for Religious and Social Studies, 1948).
4. Claude Elwood Shannon and Warren Weaver, *The Mathematical Theory of Communication* (Urbana: University of Illinois Press, 1949).
5. Jeremy Campbell, *Grammatical Man: Information, Entropy, Language, and Life* (New York: Simon and Schuster, 1982).
6. For an overview of media effects research, as well as a countervailing view, see Robin L. Nabi and Mary Beth Oliver, eds., *The Sage Handbook of Media Processes and Effects* (Thousand Oaks, CA: Sage, 2009). A sampling of current research in media effects is provided in Jennings Bryant and Mary Beth Oliver, eds., *Media Effects: Advances in Theory and Research*, 3rd ed. (New York: Routledge, 2009).
7. Elihu Katz and Paul Lazarsfeld, *Personal Influence: The Part Played by People in the Flow of Mass Communications*, 2nd ed. (New Brunswick, NJ: Transaction, 2006).
8. Ben H. Bagdikian, *The Media Monopoly*, 6th ed. (Boston: Beacon Press, 2000); Edward S. Herman, *Manufacturing Consent: The Political Economy of the Mass Media* (New York: Pantheon Books, 2002).

9. Stewart Hall, "Encoding/Decoding," in *Culture Media Language*, ed. Stewart Hall et al., 128–38 (London: Hutchinson, 1980); Tamar Liebes and Elihu Katz, *The Export of Meaning: Cross-Cultural Readings of Dallas* (Cambridge: Polity Press, 1993); David Morley, *The Nationwide Audience: Structure and Decoding* (London: British Film Institute, 1980).
10. James W. Carey, *Communication as Culture: Essays on Media and Society* (New York: Routledge, 1992), 30.
11. Marshall McLuhan, *Understanding Media: The Extensions of Man*, 1st MIT Press ed. (Cambridge, MA: MIT Press, 1994), 18.
12. Harold Adams Innis, *The Bias of Communication* (Toronto: University of Toronto Press, 1951).
13. Dudley Young, "Are the Days of McLuhanacy Numbered?," review of *McLuhan: Pro and Con*, ed. Raymond Rosenthal, *New York Times*, September 8, 1968, Sunday Book Review, http://www.nytimes.com/books/97/11/02/home/mcluhan-mcluhan.html.
14. Williams writes, "If the effect of the medium is the same, whoever controls or uses it, and whatever apparent content he may try to insert, then we can forget ordinary political and cultural argument and let the technology run itself." Raymond Williams, *Television: Technology and Cultural Form* (London: Routledge, 2003), 131.
15. McLuhan, *Understanding Media*, 41–42. For a defense of McLuhan against charges of technological determinism, see Lance Strate, "Studying Media as Media: McLuhan and the Media Ecology Approach," *MediaTropes eJournal* 1 (2008): 127–42.
16. Neil Postman, *Teaching as a Conserving Activity* (New York: Delacorte Press, 1979), 186.
17. For an overview of the media ecology tradition, see Casey Man Kong Lum, *Perspectives on Culture, Technology, and Communication: The Media Ecology Tradition* (Cresskill, NJ: Hampton Press, 2006).
18. Marcus E. Raichle, "A Brief History of Human Brain Mapping," *Trends in Neurosciences* 32, no. 2 (2009): 118–26, doi:10.1016/j.tins.2008.11.001.
19. For an overview of brain structures and common neural pathways, see Thomas A. Woolsey, *The Brain Atlas: A Visual Guide to the Human Central Nervous System*, 3rd ed. (Hoboken, NJ: John Wiley, 2008).
20. An introductory but thorough description of sensory neural pathways can be found in E. Bruce Goldstein, *Sensation and Perception*, 9th ed. (Belmont, CA: Wadsworth, Cengage Learning, 2014).
21. Yoichi Miyawaki et al., "Visual Image Reconstruction from Human Brain Activity Using a Combination of Multiscale Local Image Decoders," *Neuron* 60, no. 5 (2008): 915–29, doi:10.1016/j.neuron.2008.11.004.
22. Antonio R. Damasio, *The Feeling of What Happens: Body and Emotion in the Making of Consciousness* (New York: Harcourt, 2000); Antonio R. Damasio, *Descartes' Error: Emotion, Reason, and the Human Brain* (London: Penguin, 2005); Antonio R. Damasio, *Self Comes to Mind: Constructing the Conscious Brain* (New York: Vintage Books, 2012).
23. Joseph E. LeDoux, *The Emotional Brain: The Mysterious Underpinnings of Emotional Life* (New York: Simon and Schuster, 1996); LeDoux, *Synaptic Self: How Our Brains Become Who We Are* (New York: Penguin Books, 2003).
24. Linguist George Lakoff explored the relationship between metaphors and cognition in *Metaphors We Live By* (Chicago: University of Chicago Press, 2003). He juxtaposes these concepts against traditional Western philosophy in George Lakoff and Mark Johnson, *Philosophy in the Flesh: The Embodied Mind and Its Challenge to Western Thought* (New York: Basic Books, 1999). Current research in this area is presented in John Michael Krois, ed., *Embodiment in*

*Cognition and Culture*, Advances in Consciousness Research 71 (Amsterdam: John Benjamins, 2007).

25. Eric R. Kandel, ed., *Principles of Neural Science*, 5th ed (New York: McGraw-Hill, 2013), 790.
26. Jeffrey S. Diamond and William N. Grimes, "Distributed Parallel Processing in Retinal Amacrine Cells," in *The Computing Dendrite: From Structure to Function*, ed. Herman Cuntz, 191–204 (New York: Springer, 2013).
27. Martha Douglas-Escobar, Elizabeth Elliott, and Josef Neu, "Effect of Intestinal Microbial Ecology on the Developing Brain," *JAMA Pediatrics* 167, no. 4 (2013): 374, doi:10.1001/jamapediatrics.2013.497.
28. Dean Falk and Kathleen Rita Gibson, *Evolutionary Anatomy of the Primate Cerebral Cortex* (Cambridge: Cambridge University Press, 2008).
29. J. David Sweatt, "Experience-Dependent Epigenetic Modifications in the Central Nervous System," *Biological Psychiatry* 65, no. 3 (2009): 191–97, doi:10.1016/j.biopsych.2008.09.002.
30. Peter R. Huttenlocher, *Neural Plasticity: The Effects of Environment on the Development of the Cerebral Cortex* (Cambridge, MA: Harvard University Press, 2002); Ford F. Ebner, ed., *Neural Plasticity in Adult Somatic Sensory-Motor Systems* (Boca Raton, FL: Taylor and Francis, 2005).
31. Jennifer Lynn Peterson, *Education in the School of Dreams: Travelogues and Early Nonfiction Film* (Durham, NC: Duke University Press, 2013).
32. A summary of interpersonal communication research can be found in Kory Floyd and Tamara D. Afifi, "Biological and Psychological Perspectives on Interpersonal Communication," in *The Sage Handbook of Interpersonal Communication*, 4th ed., ed. Mark L. Knapp and John A. Daly, 87–130 (Thousand Oaks, CA: Sage, 2011). Interestingly, because fMRI research requires participants to remain alone and immobile in an enclosed environment, experiments require mediated communication using headphones and a reflected video screen. This mediation usually is discounted in the writing up of interpersonal communication research.
33. Annie Lang, Robert F. Potter, and Paul Bolls, "Where Psychophysiology Meets the Media: Taking the Effects Out of Mass Media Research," in *Media Effects: Advances in Theory and Research*, 3rd ed., ed. Jennings Bryant and Mary Beth Oliver, 185–206 (New York: Routledge, 2009); Annie Lang, "The Limited Capacity Model of Mediated Message Processing," *Journal of Communication* 50, no. 1 (2000): 46–70, doi:10.1111/j.1460-2466.2000.tb02833.x.
34. Annie Lang, "Discipline in Crisis? The Shifting Paradigm of Mass Communication Research: Discipline in Crisis," *Communication Theory* 23, no. 1 (2013): 10–24, doi:10.1111/comt.12000.
35. W. James Potter, *Theory of Media Literacy: A Cognitive Approach* (Thousand Oaks, CA: Sage, 2004).
36. Richard Jackson Harris, *A Cognitive Psychology of Mass Communication*, 5th ed. (New York: Routledge, 2009).
37. David Bordwell, *Narration in the Fiction Film* (Madison: University of Wisconsin Press, 1985).
38. Noël Carroll, *Theorizing the Moving Image* (Cambridge: Cambridge University Press, 1996); Carroll, *The Philosophy of Motion Pictures*, rev. ed. (Oxford: Blackwell, 2007); Joseph Anderson and Barbara Fisher Anderson, *Moving Image Theory Ecological Considerations* (Carbondale: Southern Illinois University Press, 2005); Joseph D Anderson, *The Reality of Illusion: An Ecological Approach to Cognitive Film Theory* (Carbondale: Southern Illinois University Press, 1998).
39. Hugo Münsterberg, *The Photoplay: A Psychological Study* (New York: D. Appleton, 1916).

40. Carl R. Plantinga and Greg M. Smith, eds., *Passionate Views: Film, Cognition, and Emotion* (Baltimore: Johns Hopkins University Press, 1999); Carl R. Plantinga, *Moving Viewers: American Film and the Spectator's Experience* (Berkeley: University of California Press, 2009).
41. Richard Allen and Murray Smith, *Film Theory and Philosophy* (Oxford: Oxford University Press, 1999).
42. Torben Kragh Grodal, *Embodied Visions: Evolution, Emotion, Culture, and Film* (Oxford: Oxford University Press, 2009).
43. For a current sampling of research in this field, see Arthur P. Shimamura, ed., *Psychocinematics: Exploring Cognition at the Movies* (Oxford: Oxford University Press, 2013); Ted Nannicelli and Paul Taberham, eds., *Cognitive Media Theory* (New York: Routledge, 2014). Of particular note are James Cutting and Tim Smith, who have engaged in detailed shot analyses and eye tracking of film audiences.
44. Uri Hasson et al., "Neurocinematics: The Neuroscience of Film," *Projections* 2, no. 1 (2008): 1–26, doi:10.3167/proj.2008.020102.
45. Jeffrey M. Zacks, "The Brain's Cutting-Room Floor: Segmentation of Narrative Cinema," *Frontiers in Human Neuroscience* 4 (2010), doi:10.3389/fnhum.2010.00168.
46. Torben Kragh Grodal, *Moving Pictures: A New Theory of Film Genres, Feelings, and Cognition* (Oxford: Oxford University Press, 1997).
47. Grodal, *Embodied Visions*, 152.
48. Leonard Mlodinow, *Subliminal: How Your Unconscious Mind Rules Your Behavior* (New York: Vintage Books, 2013).
49. Christopher F. Chabris and Daniel J. Simons, *The Invisible Gorilla: And Other Ways Our Intuitions Deceive Us* (New York: Broadway Paperbacks, 2010).
50. For a brilliant demonstration of the inversion of this concept, see "A Magazine Is an iPad That Does Not Work," YouTube video, 1:25, posted by "UserExperiencesWorks," October 6, 2011, http://www.youtube.com/watch?v=aXV-yaFmQNk.
51. For a discourse on the biases of the television medium, see Neil Postman, *Amusing Ourselves to Death: Public Discourse in the Age of Show Business*, 20th anniversary ed. (New York: Penguin Books, 2006).
52. John Brockman, *The Third Culture* (New York: Simon and Schuster, 1996).

# 2 Nurturing the Developing Brains of Digital Natives

*Michael Rich and Farah Qureshi*

Human beings develop the most sophisticated and complex brain in the animal kingdom in part because they are born with a brain that is underdeveloped. All other major organ systems are small but function as they will in adulthood. In comparison, the brain is embryonic. Most other animals are born capable of independent survival, their brains prewired with reflexes to seek food, water, and shelter. Indeed, many animal parents abandon their young at or before birth. In contrast, human infants cannot keep themselves warm, feed, avoid threats, or care for themselves. Without nurture, they will die.

How is this an advantage? At birth, the human brain has all of the neurons it will ever have. With few prewired instincts or abilities, the human brain builds itself in response to stimuli and challenges from the environment in which it will function. Responding to demand confers a huge advantage of resilience and ultimate complexity over organisms that have survival circuitry already in place. A baby's brain triples in volume during the first two years of life as it makes synaptic connections, reinforces those circuits that are used, and, as importantly, prunes away those circuits that are not used. In a rich environment with healthy stimuli, pruning serves to improve the signal-to-noise ratio, helping the growing child focus on important stimuli and filter out the unimportant. In an impoverished environment, as we have learned from the tragedy of institutionalized Romanian orphans,[1] essential brain circuitry does not get stimulated, is not reinforced, and can get pruned away. As electronic screen media are introduced and used at younger and younger ages, we need to understand the nature and quality of stimuli they provide and how those stimuli may influence the developing brain.

## THEORETICAL PERSPECTIVES ON COGNITIVE DEVELOPMENT

To comprehend how today's complex digital landscape affects human brain development, one must first take a step back and broadly consider how a growing child's environment influences her development. Children and adolescents do not simply grow up within their immediate physical surroundings, but rather within the context of their constantly evolving interactions with the numerous structural and social environments in which they live. These dynamic relationships characterize what Bronfenbrenner termed "the ecology of human development."[2] According to his ecological systems theory, young people are influenced by "the relations between [their] settings, and by the larger contexts in which the settings are embedded."[2] With the advent of the Internet, the settings and contexts in which children are growing up have become more complicated and more fluid. The twenty-first-century world comprises both physical spaces and virtual spaces, which can take on equally important roles for young people, whose "online" and "offline" lives are increasingly indistinguishable. Indeed, technology and media have created another context—a digital context—in which children grow and develop.

Our current concept of how children come to understand themselves and the world in which they live has been guided strongly by the work of Jean Piaget. Piaget's proposed stages of cognitive development describe the process by which children make sense of the world around them through their perceptions and sensory experiences.[3] As children progress through developmental stages, they evolve from having an egocentric perspective[4] rooted in concrete thought to a broader view of the world and the capability for abstract thinking.[5]

Piagetian theory has played an important role in shaping developmental psychology. Though Piaget acknowledges that experience plays a role in influencing this process,[3] his model of cognitive development is largely theoretical and fails to incorporate an ecological understanding of development as a process that occurs within the nested environments that make up a child's world. Furthermore, it does not address the fact that aspects of healthy development occur as a natural consequence of evolution (the ability to visually differentiate colors and shapes, for instance), whereas other aspects are driven predominantly by experience.

More recently, a new approach has emerged to advance our understanding of brain plasticity by differentiating cognitive development processes as either experience expectant or experience dependent.[6] Experience expectant processes are defined as "designed to utilize the sort of environmental information that is ubiquitous and has been so throughout much of the evolutionary history of the species."[6] It is these experiences that are associated with the overproduction of synapses that occurs early in life, as well as sensitive or critical periods of development. Conversely, experience-dependent processes are those that "involve the storage of information that is unique to the individual" and are typically associated with the creation of new synaptic connections when a child is exposed to new and repeated experiences.[6] Building off of this new understanding of development, an emerging body of research in developmental cognitive neuroscience has sought to connect neurobiology and psychology to explain the cognitive and behavioral changes that occur across childhood and adolescence.[7] Although there is still much to understand with respect to the biology of behavior and cognition, this approach has provided a basic scaffold upon which research on media effects has been based.

## WHAT WE KNOW ABOUT MEDIA EFFECTS ON BRAIN DEVELOPMENT AND EARLY LEARNING

Although no theories have been proposed to explain how different forms of media specifically influence the developing brain, considerable research has been dedicated to understanding media effects broadly, particularly as they relate to socialization.[8] For children and youth, this approach captures many key cognitive milestones, such as language acquisition, learning, and social and emotional development. Because most research has focused on behavioral effects, empirical studies are generally not driven by developmental theory but rather rely on general principles of social learning and media psychology.[8]

Among the most commonly cited theories to explain media effects is Bandura's Social Learning Theory, and particularly, the notion of observational learning.[9] Observational learning is essentially the process by which children witness an action and internalize the subsequent reinforcements they observe.[10] It is believed that children are more likely to imitate a behavior if it is portrayed positively and received well and less likely if it is punished.[10] In Bandura's early Bobo Doll experiments, he found that children who viewed a film in which an individual treated the doll violently were more likely to act aggressively toward the doll themselves compared to children who did not view the film.[11,12] In response to critiques that his theory was too focused on behavior, Bandura revised and rebranded it as Social Cognitive Theory as a way to address the cognitive processes that explain why, in the face of the same exposure, some children will imitate the modeled behavior, while others will not.[9]

Another prominent theory in media psychology is Cultivation Theory,[13] which proposes that the more individuals are exposed to media, the more likely they are to be influenced by it. From this theoretical perspective, it is believed that "media-based content creates memories, reinforces engrained memories, and makes existing memories more readily available for use."[8] Similarly, Script Theory proposes that media provides youth with behavioral scripts about how to feel, react, or behave in different situations.[8] As behavioral scripts become further cognitively embedded, "children and adolescents seek out environments that are consistent with their script-linked beliefs."[8] Thus, media can serve to both establish new scripts and reinforce existing ones.[8]

Lastly, researchers have also employed cognitive priming to explain the effects of media on children.[14] Priming occurs when environmental experiences create linked cognitive networks, and "the more often a network is used, the greater the likelihood that it will be activated in the future."[8] With the growing presence of media in the lives of children, these priming processes can result in cognitive networks that are perpetually active and that ultimately "bias an individual's available thoughts, emotions, and concepts."[8] Cognitive priming, Script Theory, Cultivation Theory, and Social Learning Theory are all called upon often in research focusing on the behavioral and cognitive effects of media exposure, including the positive impact of prosocial media in childhood and the negative effects of violent media across the life course.

More recently, attempts have been made to integrate these different perspectives into a single, comprehensive media effects theory. It was with that in mind that Valkenburg and Peter[15] developed the differential susceptibility to media model, which takes into account both media-related and non-media-related variables, such as individual differences and social contexts. At the heart of this model is the notion that the effects of media exposure on an individual are conditional on the individual's disposition, development, and social factors.[15] Unlike previous theoretical perspectives that suggest that the effects of media exposure are experienced uniformly, this approach proposes a more flexible explanation that takes into account the fact that not all individuals who are exposed to violent media, for example, become aggressive.

Although recent efforts to integrate existing knowledge on media effects have been promising, this area of study still suffers from a lack of a firm conceptual understanding of how these processes play out across development. As children grow, not only do they undergo significant physical, cognitive, and social changes, but their relationship with media changes as well. Adopting a life course approach to tackling these issues would enable researchers to better understand and study sensitive periods and differential effects of media exposure by age. By focusing specifically on brain development, it could further existing efforts to bridge our understanding of how environments and experience influence biology and cognition, and how together they shape the ways young people develop an understanding of the world and how they engage with it. Although we are just beginning to investigate the effects of media exposure on the developing brain, we can explore avenues of inquiry by examining the findings of media effects research in relation to hallmarks of cognitive development through childhood.

## Infancy and Toddlerhood

The first twenty-four months of a child's life marks a period of tremendous physical growth and neurodevelopment. Although the most dramatic period of brain development occurs while a child is in utero, by age two, the brain reaches approximately 80 percent of its adult weight[16] due, in part, to synapse overproduction.[17] Developmentally, this translates to a period of tremendous learning and skill acquisition. Learning that occurs in the context of media exposure relies predominantly on children's representational capacity, which allows them to "decode symbolically presented material in order to process the content."[18] Imitation is considered the most salient means by which this occurs, and the theoretical basis of its study was spearheaded by Albert Bandura's work on Social Learning Theory. Over the years, imitative learning concepts have been applied to Theory of Mind research to help explain how infants acquire knowledge about how individuals think and feel.[18] In addition to imitation, which is an enactive representational skill, children also learn through iconic and symbolic representational skills, including learning through memories of information related to certain stimuli and learning from understandable dialogue that directs children's attention to content of which they are able to make sense.[18] As infants transition to toddlerhood (up to age three), they begin to develop a sense of self-awareness, but their cognitive processes are still "constrained by limited memory abilities, a lack of logic, and a difficulty distinguishing what is real and what is fantasy."[19]

Past research on media effects early in life focused predominantly on imitative learning from television and video. In 1999, the American Academy of Pediatrics formally recommended that infants and toddlers under the age of two years not be exposed to any forms of screen media.[20] Although this advice was based on no empirical evidence, subsequent research on how media exposure influences early childhood development has since supported such a recommendation, including a number of longitudinal studies that implicated exposure to television with poor cognitive outcomes.[21,22,23] Most notably, a study by Zimmerman and Christakis[22] discovered that each additional hour of television viewed early in life was associated with poorer test scores in reading and math at age six, even after controlling for parent cognitive stimulation and a number of potentially confounding demographic variables.

A substantial body of research has also found evidence of a "video deficit effect,"[24] in which children younger than three years of age appear to learn better from live action than through actions presented on video.[23] This impairment is evidenced by the delay children experience in imitating actions that are portrayed through video compared to in person[25] and is attributed to young children's inability to fully comprehend what they view on screen.[26] In a study involving object retrieval tasks, it was found that young children who were shown where an object was on video were less competent in retrieving the object compared to those who were shown where the object was through a window.[18,27] Children who were three years old appeared to complete this task quite well compared to two-and-a-half-year-olds, who completed it with mixed results, and two-year-olds, who completed it poorly.[27] The comparatively poorer ability of children younger than two years to learn from video has also been attributed to infants' and toddlers' inability to cognitively translate what they observe two-dimensionally on a screen into the three-dimensional physical world.[23]

At the same time, however, the negative impact of early exposures to screen media can also be explained by the substitute role it often takes in the place of child playtime and parent interaction, both of which are critical to children's cognitive development. Research has shown that young children's playtime tends to be interrupted by the presence of background television.[18,28] However, because children of this age are typically exposed to media developed specifically for young audiences, it is more likely that children's playtime and television viewing occur simultaneously.[29] With respect to parent-child engagement, however, studies have found that parents are less likely to interact with their child in the presence of television.[30,31] When parents viewed infant-directed television programming with their child, it was found that children whose parents were more engaged and provided "scaffolding" (asking questions or providing descriptions related to the program content) paid more attention to the television program and were more responsive to it.[32] However, considering what is known about children's impaired learning from video compared to live interactions and from children's distractibility from play with background television, it can be argued that parents of infants and toddlers should spend their time interacting and engaging with their children free of screen media.[33]

Although learning is often assessed early in life by children's ability to imitate what they observe, a number of studies have also sought to determine how media exposure influences speech acquisition and language development. Studies that have examined the effect of baby-directed media (such as Baby Einstein DVDs) have typically found no association with educational gains[33] and that children learned "virtually no words from the video."[34,35] In fact, research seems to provide further support of a video deficit with respect to language learning, as it has been discovered that although children are indeed capable of learning language skills through video,[36] speech acquisition is more effective when it occurs through live models rather than televised ones.[33]

Ultimately, however, it has been found that duration of exposure may be less important than the nature of the content to which the children are exposed. In fact, a two-year longitudinal study of developmentally appropriate content suited to a toddler's cognitive needs (interactive shows like *Blue's Clues* or *Dora the Explorer* that encourage kids to talk to the television) are associated with improved expressive language skills and vocabularies at age thirty months compared to children who watched shows that were not developmentally suited to their age group (*Sesame Street*) or did not include intelligible language modeling (*Teletubbies*).[37] The importance of content applies to other cognitive outcomes as well, as evidenced in a study by Barr and colleagues,[38] which found that among one-year-olds, high levels of adult television exposure were associated with poorer executive functioning (namely, attention and working memory) at age four, whereas exposure to educational programming did not have this association.

Perhaps the most important but difficult questions to answer regarding media exposure during this critical period of rapid growth and development are yet to be answered:

1. At what point is a child able to decode the two-dimensional pattern of color, light, and darkness on a screen into an analog of the three-dimensional physical world in which he or she lives?
2. How do the activities and experiences displaced by an infant's or toddler's screen use compare to that screen use in terms of stimulating optimal brain development, reinforcing useful neural circuits, and avoiding disuse of important circuitry?
3. Will children who have been entertained, educated, and pacified by electronic screens since they were infants and toddlers grow up to think, behave, learn, and imagine differently, and what kind of society will they create?

## Early Childhood

Between the ages of three and five, the overproduction of synapses that characterizes brain development during a child's first years of life reaches a plateau as experience-expectant synaptic pruning begins. Cognitively, children begin to exhibit directed attention but still have a difficult time thinking in abstract terms.[19] With respect to psychological development, children begin to develop Theory of Mind, which is "a multi-faceted construct that captures the capacity to make inferences about others' mental states, such as intentions, emotions, desires, and beliefs."[39] In short, they learn that an individual's mental state is not always readily apparent or directly observable to another. Children also begin to identify emotions more concretely, because the "frontal neocortex matures and becomes interconnected in order to aid in more accurate emotional appraisal and emotional self-regulatory functions."[18] In fact, learning what emotions mean and how to control them are key features of this time in development. As children begin to gain self-regulation skills, they also begin to "reflect on [their] actions, delay gratification, tolerate frustration, and adjust or inhibit [their] behaviors to suit particular situational demands."[19] Taken together in the context of children's expanding social networks, these burgeoning skills contribute to an emerging sense of social competence.[18] Indeed, socioemotional competencies constitute an important foundation upon which both children's future relationships and cognitive development are built.[33]

When considering the impact of childhood media exposure on learning outcomes, it has been found that television programming that is not targeted to a child's stage of development, such as adult-directed content, is associated with poorer cognitive outcomes.[38] However, no such association was observed with child-directed media.[38] In fact, evaluations of television shows like *Sesame Street*—which was developed to reduce disparities in school readiness[33,40]—have demonstrated associations with improved learning outcomes.[41] Beyond *Sesame Street*, preschoolers' exposure to other forms of educational television content, particularly shows that encourage viewer interaction, are associated with improved attention and greater problem-solving skills.[33,42,43]

A considerable amount of research has been dedicated to studying the prosocial effects of television on children, particularly as it relates to programs like *Sesame Street, Mr. Rogers' Neighborhood*, and *Barney & Friends*. Since it's inception more than forty years ago, one of *Sesame Street*'s main objectives has been to "teach children about emotional coping."[33] In addition to modeling emotional coping strategies, shows like *Mr. Rogers' Neighborhood* and *Barney & Friends* also aimed to teach children about positive ways to engage socially with their peers and have been associated with more positive peer interactions[44] and better manners.[45] Conceptually, both Social Cognitive Theory and Script Theory provide strong explanations for the effects of prosocial content as an imitative learning phenomenon.[33] However, at the same time, these outcomes can also be explained by Moral Development Theory,[33] which posits that children's ability to comprehend the motivations and actions of fictional characters improve as they develop morally, and this improved skill allows them to apply the lessons they learn from screen media to their own lives.[46]

## Middle Childhood

Development processes that begin in the preschool years—including those involving directed attention and higher level cognition—continue through the ages of six to twelve, when children begin to think more abstractly and develop a self concept. However, the most notable changes children experience during this period are not cognitive, but social, as their peer networks expand beyond their immediate family and grow in both size and influence. Indeed, a defining feature of middle childhood is social development and the establishment of highly valued friendships, relationships that will eventually become as or more important than those with the immediate family.[19] These years provide a rich stage for the reception, establishment, and transmission of social norms. One such norm that has received a disproportionate amount of attention with respect to media effects research is that of violence, as it relates to both film and television portrayals, as well as interactive engagement through video and computer games. It was concern for the effect of television on this "impressionable" age group that led the U.S. Congress to draw public attention to the influence of violent screen content on juvenile delinquency, a quaint concept now but of real concern in the early 1950s.[47] While the Congressional inquiries motivated scientific investigation of media effects over ensuing decades, representatives of the media industries noted that there was no evidence of effects at that time, skillfully framing the issue as a difference of value systems and invoking First Amendment rights to freedom of expression. The values-driven debate over "good" versus "bad" media persists to this day, obfuscating serious discourse and stalemating public understanding and response.

Links between violent media exposure in childhood and aggressive behavior are widely substantiated in the literature[48,49,50] and hotly contested in the public sphere.[51,52] Albert Bandura's Bobo Doll experiments of the 1960s were among the first empirical studies to observe a link between media violence and subsequent aggressive behaviors and have since been replicated.[53] However, lab-based approaches to studying this association have been highly criticized due to inherent methodological weaknesses,[33] including the use of poor measures for aggression and contrived viewing arrangements.[54] Consequently, research shifted toward more field experiments,[55,56] which also substantiated the association, and correlational studies,[33,57] which further supported proposed links while also controlling for possible confounding factors, such as parent education, socioeconomic status, and school achievement. Furthermore, seminal longitudinal studies conducted by Eron and colleagues in the 1970s[58,59,60] proved to be highly influential in establishing causality. In these studies, the authors followed a cohort of children for twenty-two years and found that, particularly among boys, exposure to violent television programming in the third grade was strongly associated with aggressive behavior ten years later. A subsequent follow-up of the participants at age thirty further supported the observed association.[61] More recently, a longitudinal study with a fifteen-year follow-up by Huesmann and colleagues also found evidence of a positive association between exposure to television violence and long-term aggressive behaviors.[62,63] Despite overwhelming evidence to the contrary, these links are often called into question by concerns about reverse causation, meaning that young people who have an aggressive disposition actively seek out violent media rather than violent media priming individuals to be more aggressive. Ultimately, however, the majority of researchers have concluded that the association between exposure to violent media and subsequent aggressive thoughts and behaviors is indeed valid. However, the relationship between media exposure and aggression is likely reciprocal,[59] in that they are "mutually reinforcing over time."[33,64] Indeed, research on desensitization effects has found evidence of it with respect to both psychophysiology and behavior.[65,66] In the long term, this can manifest in the form of lower empathy.[67,68,69]

## CONCLUSION

Although significant correlations have been established between certain types of screen media content and subsequent skills, attitudes, and behaviors, many of the associations found have been cross-sectional in nature and among adolescents or adults. Much work still needs to be done to build the strength of these associations and the mechanisms by which they work to have confidence in their contributions, among others, to outcomes of concern. Initial research with interactive media indicates that it is likely a more powerful teacher and rehearser of behavioral scripts for older children compared to receptive screen media, like television and films. However, we do not know when and how very young children are able to decode what they see on a screen and translate it into an understanding of the world on which they can act.

With tablets, smartphones, and other mobile devices with easy interfaces being marketed to younger and younger children, and with more and more parents using these devices to distract and pacify very young children, we are conducting a vast uncontrolled experiment in human development. Although investigation of the effects of media exposure on children continues, over the course of the next several decades we will discover, with or without research, the effects of the screen media choices we are making for children.

## REFERENCES

1. Nelson, Charles, A. *Romania's Abandoned Children: Deprivation, Brain Development, and the Struggle for Recovery.* Cambridge, MA: Harvard University Press, 2014.
2. Bronfenbrenner, Urie. *The Ecology of Human Development: Experiments by Nature and Design.* Cambridge, MA: Harvard University Press, 1979.
3. Piaget, Jean. "Development and Learning." *Journal of Research in Science Teaching* 2 (1964): 176–86.
4. Piaget, Jean. *The Language and Thought of the Child.* New York: Harcourt Brace, 1959.
5. Piaget, Jean. *Play, Dreams, and Imitation in Childhood.* New York: W. W. Norton, 1951.
6. Greenough, William T., Black, James E., and Wallace, Christopher, S. "Experience and Brain Development." *Child Development* 58 (1987): 539–59.
7. Nelson, Charles A. *Neuroscience of Cognitive Development: The Role of Experience and the Developing Brain.* Hoboken, NJ: John Wiley, 2006.
8. Kirsh, Steven J. *Media and Youth: A Developmental Perspective.* Malden, MA: John Wiley, 2010.
9. Bandura, Albert. *Social Foundations of Thought and Action: A Social Cognitive Theory.* Englewood Cliffs, NJ: Prentice Hall, 1986.
10. Bandura, Albert. "Influence of Models' Reinforcement Contingencies on the Acquisition of Imitative Response." *Journal of Personality and Social Psychology* 1 (1965): 589–95.
11. Bandura, Albert, Ross, Dorothea, and Ross, Sheila A. "Various Reinforcement and Imitative Learning." *Journal of Abnormal and Social Psychology* 67 (1963): 601–7.
12. Bandura, Albert, Ross, Dorothea, and Ross, Sheila A. "Imitation of Film-mediated Aggressive Models." *Journal of Abnormal and Social Psychology* 66 (1963): 3–11.

13. Gerbner, George, Gross, Larry, Morgan, Michael, and Signorelli, Nancy. "Growing Up with Television: The Cultivation Perspective." In *Media Effects*, edited by Jennings Bryant and Dolf Zillmann. Hillsdale, NJ: Lawrence Erlbaum, 1994.
14. Roskos-Ewoldsen, David R., Roskos-Ewoldsen, Beverly, and Dillman Carpentier, Francesca R. "Media Priming: An Updated Synthesis." In *Media Effects: Advances in Theory and Research*, edited by Jennings Bryant and Mary Beth Oliver. New York: Routledge, 2009.
15. Valkenburg, Patti M., and Peter, Jochen. "The Differential Susceptibility to Media Effects Model." *Journal of Communication* 63 (2013): 221–43.
16. Kretschmann, H. J., Kammradt, G., Krauthausen, I., Sauer, B., and Wingert, F. "Brain Growth in Man." *Biblioteca Anatomica* 28 (1986): 1–26.
17. Casey, B. J., Giedd, Jay N., and Thomas, Kathleen M. "Structural and Functional Brain Development and Its Relation to Cognitive Development." *Biological Psychology* 54 (2000): 241–57.
18. McCartney, Kathleen, and Phillips, Deborah, eds. *Blackwell Handbook of Early Childhood Development.* Malden, MA: Blackwell, 2008.
19. Gentile, Douglas A., and Sesma, Arturo. "Developmental Approaches to Understanding Media Effects on Individuals." In *Media Violence and Children: A Complete Guide for Parents and Professionals*, edited by Douglas A. Gentile (Westport, CT: Praeger, 2003).
20. American Academy of Pediatrics, Committee on Public Education. "Media Education." *Pediatrics* 104 (1999): 341–42.
21. Tomopoulos, Suzy, Dreyer, Bernard P., Berkule, Samantha, Fierman, Arthur H., Brockmeyer, Carolyn, and Mendelsohn, Alan L. "Infant Media Exposure and Toddler Development." *Archives of Pediatric and Adolescent Medicine* 164 (2010): 1105–11.
22. Zimmerman, Frederick J., and Christakis, Dmitri A. "Children's Television Viewing and Cognitive Outcomes." *Archives of Pediatric and Adolescent Medicine* 159 (2005): 619–25.
23. Barr, Rachel. "Transfer of Learning between 2D and 3D Sources during Infancy: Informing Theory and Practice." *Developmental Review* 30 (2010): 128–54.
24. Anderson, Daniel R., and Pempek, Tiffany A. "Television and Very Young Children." *American Behavioral Scientist* 48 (2005): 505–22.
25. Barr, Rachel, and Hayne, Harlene. "Developmental Changes in Imitation from Television during Infancy." *Child Development* 70 (1999): 1067–81.
26. Troseth, G. L., and Deloache, J. "The Medium Can Obscure the Message: Young Children's Understanding of Video." *Child Development* 69 (1998): 950–65.
27. Schmitt, Kelly L., and Anderson, Daniel R. "Television and Reality: Toddlers' Use of Visual Information from Video to Guide Behavior." *Media Psychology* 4 (2002): 51–76.
28. Schmidt, Marie E., Pempek, Tiffany A., Kirkorian, Heather L., Lund, Anne F., and Anderson, Daniel R. "The Effect of Background Television on the Toy Play Behavior of Very Young Children." *Child Development* 79 (2008): 1137–51.
29. Huston, Aletha C., Wright, John C., Marquis, Janet, and Green, Samuel B. "How Young Children Spend Their Time: Television and Other Activities." *Developmental Psychology* 35 (1999): 912–25.
30. Christakis, Dmitri A., Gilkerson, Jill, Richards, Jeffrey A., Zimmerman, Frederick J., Garrison, Michelle M., Xu, Dongxin, Gray, Sharmistha, and Yapanel, U. "Audible Television and Decreased Adult Words, Infant Vocalizations, and

Conversational Turns: A Population-Based Study." *Archives of Pediatrics and Adolescent Medicine* 163 (2001): 554–58.

31. Kirkorian, Heather L., Pempek, Tiffany A., Murphy, Lauren A., Schmidt, Marie E., and Anderson, Daniel R. "The Impact of Background Television on Parent-Child Interaction." *Child Development* 80 (2009): 1350–59.

32. Barr, Rachel, Zack, Elizabeth, Garcia, Amaya, and Muentener, Paul. "Infants' Attention and Responsiveness to Television Increases with Prior Exposure and Parental Interaction." *Infancy* 13 (2008): 30–56.

33. Strasburger, Victor C., Wilson, Barbara, J., and Jordan, Amy B. *Children, Adolescents, and the Media.* Thousand Oaks, CA: Sage, 2014.

34. DeLoache, Judy S., Chiong, Cynthia, Sherman, Kathleen, Islam, Nadia, Vanderborght, Mieke, Troseth, Georgene L., Strouse, Gabrielle A., and O'Doherty, Katherine. "Do Babies Learn from Baby Media?" *Psychological Science* 21 (2010): 1570–74.

35. Krcmar, Marina. "Word Learning in Very Young Children from Infant-Directed DVDs." *Journal of Communication* 61 (2011): 780–94.

36. Rice, Mabel L., Huston, Aletha C., Turglio, Rosemarie, and Wright, John C. "Words from *Sesame Street*: Learning Vocabulary While Viewing." *Developmental Psychology* 26 (1990): 421–28.

37. Linebarger, Deborah L., and Walker, Dale. "Infants' and Toddlers' Television Viewing and Language Outcomes." *American Behavioral Scientist* 48 (2005): 624–45.

38. Barr, Rachel, Lauricella, Alexis, Zack, Elizabeth, and Calvert, Sandra L. "Infant and Early Childhood Exposure to Adult-Directed and Child-Directed Television Programming: Relations with Cognitive Skills at Age Four." *Merill-Palmer Quarterly* 56 (2010): 21–48.

39. Barr, Rachel. "Developing Social Understanding in a Social Context." In *Blackwell Handbook of Early Childhood Development*, edited by Kathleen McCartney and Deborah Phillips Malden, MA: Blackwell, 2008.

40. Fisch, Shalom, and Truglio, Rosemarie, eds. *"G" Is for Growing.* Mahwah, NJ: Lawrence Erlbaum, 2001.

41. Fisch, Shalom, Truglio, Rosemary, and Cole, Charlotte F. "The Impact of *Sesame Street* on Preschool Children: A Review and Synthesis of 30 Years' Research." *Media Psychology* 1 (1999): 165–90.

42. Crawley, Alisha M., Anderson, Daniel R., Wilder, Alice, Williams, Marsha, and Santomero, Angela. "Effects of Repeated Exposures to a Single Episode of the Television Program *Blue's Clues* on the Viewing Behaviors and Comprehension of Preschool Children." *Journal of Educational Psychology* 91 (1999): 630–37.

43. Crawley, Alisha M., Anderson, Daniel R., Santomero, Angela, Wilder, Alice, Williams, Marsha, Evans, Marie K., and Bryant, Jennings. "Do Children Learn How to Watch Television? The Impact of Extensive Experience with *Blue's Clues* on Preschool Children's Television Watching Behavior." *Journal of Communication* 52 (2002): 264–79.

44. Friedrich-Cofer, Lynette K., Huston-Stein, Aletha, McBride Kipnis, Dorothy, Susman, Elizabeth J., and Clewett, Ann S. "Environmental Enhancement of Prosocial Television Content: Effects on Interpersonal Behavior, Imaginative Play, and Self-Regulation in a Natural Setting." *Developmental Psychology* 15 (1979): 637–46.

45. Singer, Jerome L., and Singer, Dorothy G., *"Barney & Friends* as Entertainment and Education: Evaluating the Quality of Effectiveness of a Television Series for Preschool Children." In *Research Paradigms, Television, and Social Behavior*, edited by Joy K. Asamen and Gordon L. Berry. Beverly Hills, CA: Sage, 1998.

46. Glover, R. J., Garmon, L. C., and Hull, D. M. "Media's Moral Messages: Assessing Perceptions of Moral Content in Television Programming." *Journal of Moral Education* 40 (2011): 89–104.
47. Senate Committee on the Judiciary. *Interim Report on Television and Juvenile Delinquency* (1955).
48. Anderson, Craig A., Shibuya, Akiko, Ihori, Nobuko, Swing, Edward L., Bushman, Brad J., Sakamoto, Akira, Rothstein, Hannah R., and Saleem, Muniba. "Violent Video Game Effects on Aggression, Empathy, and Prosocial Behavior in Eastern and Western Countries: A Meta-Analytic Review." *Psychological Bulletin* 136 (2010): 151–73.
49. Anderson, Craig A. "An Update on the Effects of Playing Violent Video Games." *Journal of Adolescence* 27 (2004): 113–22.
50. Bushman, Brad J., and Anderson, Craig A. "Media Violence and the American Public: Scientific Facts versus Media Misinformation." *American Psychologist* 56 (2001): 477–89.
51. Ferguson, Christopher J., and Kilburn, John. "Much Ado about Nothing: The Misestimation and Overinterpretation of Violent Video Game Effects in Eastern and Western Nations: Comment on Anderson et al. (2010)." *Psychological Bulletin* 136 (2010): 174–78.
52. Ferguson, Christopher J. "The Good, the Bad and the Ugly: A Meta-Analytic Review of Positive and Negative Effects of Violent Video Games." *Psychiatric Quarterly* 78 (2007): 309–16.
53. Coyne, Sarah M., Nelson, David A., Lawton, Frances, Haslam, Shelly, Rooney, Lucy, Titterington, Leigh, Trainor, Hannah, Remnant, Jack, and Ogunlaja, Leah. "The Effects of Viewing Physical and Relational Aggression in the Media: Evidence for a Cross-over Effect." *Journal of Experimental Psychology* 44 (2008): 1551–54.
54. Fowles, Jib. *The Case for Television Violence*. Thousand Oaks, CA: Sage, 1999.
55. Steuer, Faye B., Applefield, James M., and Smith, Rodney. "Televised Aggression and Interpersonal Aggression of Preschool Children." *Journal of Experimental Child Psychology* 11 (1971): 442–47.
56. Boyatzis, Chris J., Matillo, Gina M., and Nesbitt, Kristen M. "Effects of the *Mighty Morphin Power Rangers* on Children's Aggression with Peers." *Child Study Journal* 25 (1995): 45–55.
57. Ybarra, Michele L., Diener-West, Marie, Markow, Dana, Leaf, Philip J., Hamburger, Merle, and Boxer, Paul. "Linkages between Internet and Other Media Violence with Seriously Violent Behavior by Youth." *Pediatrics* 122 (2008): 929–37.
58. Eron, Leonard D., Huesmann, L. Rowell, Lefkowitz, Monroe M., and Walder, Leopold O. "Does Television Violence Cause Aggression?" *American Psychologist* 27 (1972): 253–63.
59. Huesmann, L. Rowell. "Psychological Processes Promoting the Relation between Exposure to Media Violence and Aggressive Behavior by the Viewer." *Journal of Social Issues* 42 (1986): 125–39.
60. Huesmann, L. Rowell, Eron, Leonard D., Lefkowitz, Monroe M., and Walder, Leopold O. "Stability of Aggression over Time and Generations." *Developmental Psychology* 20 (1984): 1120–34.
61. Huesmann, L. R., and Miller, L. S. "Long-Term Effects of Repeated Exposure to Media Violence in Childhood." In *Aggressive Behavior: Current Perspectives*, edited by L. R. Huesman. New York: Plenum, 1994.
62. Huesmann, L. Rowell, Moise-Titus, Jessica, Podolski, Cheryl-Lynn, and Eron, Leonard D. "Longitudinal Relations between Children's Exposure to TV Violence and Their Aggressive and Violent Behavior in Young Adulthood: 1977–1992." *Developmental Psychology* 39 (2003): 2001–21.

63. Johnson, Jeffrey G., Cohen, Patricia, Smailes, Elizabeth M., Kasen, Stephanie, and Brook, Judith S. "Television Viewing and Aggressive Behavior during Adolescence and Adulthood." *Science* 295 (2002): 2468–71.
64. Slater, Michael D. "Alienation, Aggression, and Sensation Seeking as Predictors of Adolescent Use of Violent Film, Computer, and Website Content." *Journal of Communication* 53 (2003): 105–21.
65. Englehart, Christopher R., Bartholow, Bruce D., Kerr, Geoffrey T., and Bushman, Brad J. "This Is Your Brain on Video Games: Neural Desensitization to Violence Predicts Increased Aggression Following Violent Video Game Exposure." *Journal of Experimental Social Psychology* 47 (2011): 1033–36.
66. Bushman, Brad J., and Anderson, Craig A. "Comfortably Numb: Desensitizing Effects of Violent Media on Helping Others." *Psychological Science* 20 (2009): 273–77.
67. Funk, Jeanne B., Buchman, Debra D., Jenks, Jennifer, and Bechtoldt, Heidi. "Playing Violent Video Games, Desensitization, and Moral Evaluation in Children." *Journal of Applied Developmental Psychology* 24 (2003): 413–36.
68. Krahe, Barbara, and Moller, Ingrid. "Longitudinal Effects of Media Violence on Aggression and Empathy among German Adolescents." *Journal of Applied Developmental Psychology* 31 (2010): 401–9.
69. Krahe, Barbara, Moller, Ingrid, Huesmann, L. Rowell, Kirwil, Lucyna, Felber, Juliane, and Berger, Anja. "Desensitization to Media Violence: Links with Habitual Media Violence Exposure, Aggressive Cognitions, and Aggressive Behavior." *Journal of Personality and Social Psychology* 100 (2011): 630–46.

# 3  Neurobiology of Teen Brain Development and the Digital Age

*Jennifer T. Sneider and Marisa M. Silveri*

The evolution of digital media is dramatically changing the environment in which we learn about the world, and particularly the way adolescents socialize and interact with their peers, and develop self-identify and independence. Adolescents spend an average of eight and a half hours per day interacting with digital devices, with more than one electronic device simultaneously being used 30 percent of the time.[1] Given the notable average exposure of total media device time during adolescence, an age span well characterized as involving significant brain and cognitive maturation, it is necessary to consider the impact of the media evolution on the adolescent brain, and whether the emergence and increasing use of electronics influences brain development, for better or for worse, or perhaps both.

## WINDOW INTO THE ADOLESCENT BRAIN

Over the past two decades, much like digital evolution, there have been significant advances in brain imaging technologies that provide a non-invasive window into the dynamic developmental sculpting of the adolescent brain.[2] Studies using magnetic resonance imaging (MRI) technology have helped us to identify important structural and functional milestones in brain development, in ways that have increased our knowledge beyond what has been learned through studies of brain-injured patients and postmortem brain tissue.[3] For instance, by age five or six, overall brain size generally reaches a plateau, however, significant developmental brain reorganization begins around the onset of adolescence (about ten years of age) and continues in rapid fashion into the early twenties.[4] Consistent with physiological maturation from adolescence through emerging adulthood (the span lasting from roughly age eighteen to age twenty-two),[5] brain MRI studies have generally revealed a linear increase in white matter tissue and a non-linear decrease in gray matter tissue during childhood and adolescence. Changes in white matter are thought to reflect myelination of axons, which leads to improvements in communication between brain cells. Alterations in gray matter are attributed to pruning and elimination of brain cells, or neurons, with less efficient brain cells being pruned away in an effort to increase overall brain efficiency.[6] While significant changes have been observed over a ten-year span lasting from adolescence to emerging adulthood,[7] significant developmental brain changes have been detected in as little as a seven-month span within adolescence, suggesting that structural changes are incredibly dynamic, occurring in very rapid fashion.[8]

While such reorganization occurs across many regions of the brain during childhood and adolescence, the majority of reconstruction (myelination and neuronal pruning) occurs toward the latter half of adolescence and predominantly in the frontal lobe.[9] Thus, the frontal lobe is the last region of the brain to undergo major maturational changes, which is necessary for the development of higher order cognitive abilities; for example, executive functions, which include planning, organization, impulse control, and decision making.[10] These essential brain changes therefore have important relevance for understanding vulnerabilities associated with the critical period of adolescent brain reorganization, which is a time associated with an age-appropriate need for optimal decision making to overcome increased impulsiveness and risk taking (e.g., including but not limited to alcohol and drug use and other risky behaviors).[11]

The increased propensity to seek out novel stimulation and engage in risk-taking behaviors during adolescence is thought to be related to immature cognitive and behavioral response inhibition abilities.[12] Accordingly, functional magnetic resonance imaging (fMRI), used to measure brain activation during the performance of cognitive tasks, demonstrates significant functional changes in the magnitude of frontal lobe activity during executive function tasks.[13] These studies highlight the importance of maturation of regions of the frontal lobe, such as the prefrontal cortex, including anterior cingulate cortex and dorsal lateral prefrontal cortex subregions, in contributing to age-related improvements in self-regulatory control.[14] Consistent with evidence of immature structural and functional aspects of cognitive control is the finding that levels of the important inhibitory neurochemical, γ-amino butyric acid (GABA), are also lower in the frontal lobe of adolescents compared to young adults. Lower GABA levels significantly predicted worse accuracy on a cognitive control task (Go No Go task) in adolescents.[15] To add another level of complexity to the development of the adolescent brain, the immature frontal lobe neural circuitry associated with suboptimal, yet rapidly improving, cognitive control is simultaneously in competition with the brain's reward system (including but not limited to the ventral striatum), which reaches functionally maturity early in adolescence.[16] Thus, to make optimal decisions that lead to positive outcomes, such as preparing for a test in school or avoiding risks such as alcohol use, an adolescent not only needs to have the knowledge of which decision will lead to the better outcome but needs to simultaneously inhibit suboptimal or poor choices, which in the face of something rewarding (e.g., peer approval) can be even more difficult. The development of this complex process relies on the healthy maturation of the adolescent frontal lobe and associated improvements in decision making.

Several important structures in the brain undergo developmental changes that are involved in improvements in cognitive performance during adolescence. However, unlike the late developing frontal lobe, other brain regions reach functional maturity earlier in life. The amygdala is a region of brain that is necessary for rapid responding, which under some circumstances promotes survival of the organism.[17] For instance, rapid behavioral responding to stimuli such as fearful or threatening faces without the need for more complex integration of multiple brain regions permits the mobilization necessary for a quick escape. Using fMRI, functional amygdala responses to fearful faces have been observed in children as young as eight years of age, a pattern that does not change throughout the rest of adolescence.[18] The amygdala also responds to other survival-related stimuli such as food. In a study where adolescents and adults passively viewed images of food, stimuli that are both related to survival and are rewarding, both age groups exhibited significant activation of the amygdala, whereas adults showed activation of the frontal lobe in addition to amygdala responses.[19] Results from this study suggest that while adolescents and adults are viewing the same images, brain activation in response to those images differ with age, but not in a manner that is better or worse.

While the frontal cortex undergoes the most substantial structural and functional changes during adolescence, significant developmental changes also occur in the hippocampus,[20] a region of the brain that mediates learning and memory.[21] Although fewer efforts have focused on healthy development of the hippocampus using brain imaging, developmental changes in this region have been reported during adolescence[22] that are strongly influenced by sex differences.[23] Importantly, learning and memory are crucial functions that are necessary for adolescents to learn and to retain the information that will help them make good decisions, succeed in school, and ultimately become independent. The hippocampus is notably more vulnerable to a host of insults during adolescence as compared to adulthood, including the impact of alcohol effects on learning and memory.[24] Thus, the goals of adolescent brain development include (1) improved brain efficiency, via the removal of inefficient neurons and improved communication, or myelination, between remaining neurons; (2) maturation of frontal lobe circuitry to inhibit more rapid, less thought out responding, driven in part by the early maturation of the amygdala, and to overcome competition from the ventral striatum, governing an increased sensitivity to reward; and (3) ongoing collection and retention of information into long-term storage via the hippocampus, which permits not only the acquisition of new skills but also the development of new strategies to perform cognitive tasks (leading to academic, among other, successes) and to apply new information to improve decision making; for example, learning from success as well as mistakes.

## SOCIAL AND EMOTIONAL DEVELOPMENT

Maturation of the neural circuitry associated with social and emotional development also occurs in a rapid fashion during adolescence. Age-specific patterns of brain activation, including the prefrontal cortex and amygdala, are observed during the viewing of fearful facial affect in adolescents, which correlates with measures of emotional intelligence and levels of anxiety.[25] Emotional intelligence (EI, or EQ) is considered to be an array of functional abilities that include the capacity to understand and communicate one's emotions, understand and appreciate the feelings of others, and have flexibility in dealing with everyday problems.[26] Anxiety levels, as well as EI, are likely to reflect reactivity to emotional events,[27] which can influence the ability to read emotional cues and utilize emotion to guide decision making and behavior.

EI and anxiety appear to have important utility as indicators of academic adaptation during adolescence.[28] For instance, higher EI has been positively correlated with teacher ratings of academic adaptation.[29] Hunt and colleagues have also reported that in adults, higher EI is associated with fewer trauma-related psychological symptoms.[30] Adults with higher EI tended to use a monitoring strategy (processing) for coping, whereas those with lower EI tended to use a blunting strategy (avoidance). In contrast, low EI has been linked with risk for early onset of substance use[31] and externalizing behaviors[32] during adolescence, which are even more prevalent in at-risk youth (e.g., youth with a positive family history of alcohol or drug abuse).[33] Indeed, higher negative emotionality, such as higher stress reactivity, alienation, and aggression, are also related to an earlier onset of substance use.[34] In terms of anxiety levels, anxiety at clinically relevant levels has been associated with poorer school performance,[35] whereas elevated anxiety levels within the normal range serve to enhance academic performance,[36] perhaps consistent with the Yerkes-Dodson law,[37] indicating a U-shaped relationship between anxiety and academic performance. Thus, as frontal lobe circuitry is developing and becoming integrated with the limbic system (emotional regulation circuitry, including the amygdala and hippocampus), inhibition of emotional responding provided by the frontal lobe is an important contribution to the development and refinements of healthy decision-making abilities, particularly in the face of stress and anxiety that often accompanies adolescence.[38]

Because social and emotional development is simultaneously occurring as teens improve their decision-making skills, social media provides an avenue for some of this emotional growth in a manner that provides immediate gratification and feeds the increased sensitivity to rewards during this age span. Interestingly, with regard to the asynchronous development of cognitive control relative to reward-seeking during adolescence, greater activation of reward-related brain areas (e.g., ventral striatum and orbitofrontal cortex) is observed in teens compared to adults, which is further enhanced when peers are believed to be observing their performance.[39] In other words, it is already difficult for the adolescent frontal lobe to guide decision making that works against something rewarding; however, when a peer is present, this difficultly is even more enhanced. Given that social media provides infinite access to the presence of peers, immature cognitive control during the emotional storminess of adolescence can be a dangerous combination that needs to be regulated by adults. This natural developmental process of improved self-regulation, as it overlaps with the growth and availability of digital media, can therefore have serious consequences for adolescents, as decision making, both good and bad, is frequently being captured by social media, for example, Facebook or MySpace, in ways that have never existed before now. Thus, poor decision making in particular is easily broadcasted on social media sites for the entire virtual world to see. Indeed, it is plausible that access to social media could improve emotional development via increased opportunities for social interaction that may otherwise be difficult in adolescents that tend toward shyness or have clinical levels of anxiety. Thus, while speculative, there are potential treatment interventions via digital media (e.g., Internet) that might have increased efficacy because of being more amenable to adolescent populations, which is currently a growing area of research investigation.[40]

## ADOLESCENT BRAIN AND VULNERABILITY FOR ADDICTION

While rapid improvements in the decision-making machinery, seated chiefly in the developing frontal lobe, help modulate more emotional, less thoughtful responses and manage increased sensitivity to reward, this also makes the adolescent notably more vulnerable to developing addictive behaviors. That is, a suboptimal, yet rapidly improving, cognitive control system makes it more difficult to inhibit behaviors such as initiating or continuing alcohol or drug consumption, even in the face of real or potential negative outcomes associated with use (parental disapproval, academic consequences, hangover, injury, traffic accidents, assaults, etc.). Indeed, epidemiological data demonstrate that the younger the onset of substance use, the greater the likelihood of developing a substance abuse disorder later in life.[41] While investigations of the neurobiology underlying this heightened vulnerability of adolescents to alcohol and drug addiction are under way, a common neural circuitry has been implicated across many forms of addiction beyond alcohol and drug abuse, food and gambling addictions, and addictions to digital media; that is, pathological/problematic Internet use (PIU) or Internet addiction disorder (IAD).[42] The prevalence of IAD has been significantly increasing in adolescent populations, leading to growing debates on the pros and cons of digital media technology, which include the use of cell phones, laptops, gaming devices, and the Internet; often these devices are used simultaneously. To date, however, there is a paucity of data available examining relationships between the developing brain, digital media, and cognitive processing. However, given the growing concern that abnormal social behaviors may lead to addictive media use and vice versa, there is clearly a critical need for understanding the impact of digital media on the adolescent brain. The issue may not lie in the technology itself but in the context of use and how other activities are affected in adolescents; that is, decreases in physical playtime or impacts on creativity.[43] Again, these types of studies are likely under way, and within the next several years, data from brain imaging studies will, it is hoped, shed light on the influence of digital media on the adolescent brain. There has been an accumulation of brain imaging studies investigating structural and functional brain changes associated with excessive Internet use, which can develop into a behavioral addiction or IAD, with online gaming producing significant social, emotional, and neurobiological consequences.[44] Recent studies are emerging that highlight functional and structural brain abnormalities in individuals with IAD, similar to those observed in individuals with substance-related addictions,[45] often in the brain circuitry that is undergoing important developmental changes during adolescents.

Alterations in the thickness of cortical tissue (predominantly gray matter) have been reported in adolescents ages seventeen to twenty-two with Internet gaming addiction (IGA).[46] Brain imaging demonstrates decreased thickness in some brain areas, left lateral orbitofrontal cortex, insula cortex, and entorhinal cortex, whereas other brain areas have increased thickness, left precentral gyrus, precuneus, and middle temporal cortex. Not only are structural brain alterations evident in those with an online gaming addiction, altered cortical thickness is significantly correlated with poorer performance on a task measuring cognitive control in an online addiction gaming group. Whether brain alterations precede the development of the gaming addiction, or whether brain alterations are a consequence of gaming remains an important question to be addressed in future studies. Nonetheless, important relationships between brain structure and function and addictive behaviors provide important insight regarding the increased vulnerability of the adolescence brain to addiction, in this case associated with addiction to digital media.

Functional activation changes associated with gaming addiction have also been reported. Emerging adults aged eighteen to twenty-three years underwent a brain scan while viewing images from the *World of Warcraft* game.[47] Compared to a non-gaming group, significantly greater brain activation was evident in bilateral inferior frontal gyrus, cingulate gyrus, and right inferior parietal lobule of game addicts, which was positively correlated with craving scores. The results suggest cue (game stimuli)-induced craving in young adult gaming addicts, in brain areas implicated in memory, attention, and emotion.[48] In a study using a different type of fMRI that measures brain activity at rest (resting-state fMRI), adolescents with IGA disorders had increased functional connectivity (more connections between brain regions) in the bilateral cerebellum posterior lobe and middle temporal gyrus, whereas the bilateral inferior parietal lobule and right inferior temporal gyrus displayed less connections between regions, as compared to an age-matched control group.[49] Alterations in functional connectivity, for example, interconnectedness between brain regions necessary for efficient neuronal communication, across these brain regions were significantly associated with higher scores on the Chen Internet Addiction Scale. In addition, adolescents with IGA as compared to non-IGA adolescents demonstrated significantly altered blood flow (providing delivery of necessary oxygen and nutrients for neurons to function) in multiple brain regions, including higher blood flow in regions of the frontal lobe, amygdala, and hippocampus and lower blood flow in the temporal and occipital lobes, as well as in the cingulate gyrus region of the frontal lobe.[50] Taken together, these significant brain alterations associated with IGA in adolescents are similar to abnormalities exhibited by patients with substance addiction, supporting an overlap in the neurobiological underpinnings across addictive disorders.[51]

## DIGITAL MEDIA AND BRAIN FUNCTION

While there is a growing number of brain imaging studies on Internet or gaming addictions, there are very few studies examining the impact of other types of digital media on brain function. Of the limited data available, a recent study using fMRI to examine brain activation while viewing the social media website, Facebook,[52] reported significant relationships between the way the brain processes self-relevant gains in reputation and degree of Facebook use and brain activation in the nucleus accumbens of adults. More specifically, greater reward-related activity observed in the left nucleus accumbens predicted Facebook use when subjects were responding to gains in reputation related to the self, but not gains for others or monetary related activity. The ventral striatum, which includes the nucleus accumbens, has been implicated in the processing of rewards important for motivation of human behavior such as food or money.[53] This is one of the first studies to measure the response of the brain to rewarding nature of self-relevant gains in reputation achieved via Facebook.[54] In another fMRI study examining brain activation associated with peer interactions and social feedback, adult participants not only evaluated themselves with more desirable feedback but also demonstrated significant activity in the bilateral ventral striatum and in the anterior cingulate and medial prefrontal areas of the frontal lobe in the rewarding component.[55] Given the unique developmental differences between adolescent and adult brain structure and function, it is plausible that rewards associated with self-relevant gains may not only be greater in adolescents but driven by a different neural circuitry that, at an early development stage, could lead to alterations in the way the system matures. Clearly similar studies investigating neural substrates associated with social media use are warranted in adolescent populations.

Affective reactivity from late childhood to early adolescence has been examined in relation to brain activation associated with engagement in risky behaviors or resistance to peer influence.[56] Thirty-eight participants underwent two fMRI scanning sessions, at age ten and thirteen years, while viewing affective facial stimuli. The findings demonstrated a significant correlation between increased ventral striatum response to affective facial displays and increased resistance to peer influence from late childhood to early adolescence. Amygdala and ventral striatum responses were more negatively coupled during early adolescence when processing sad and happy than neutral faces. These findings suggest that differential circumstances affect subcortical activity, which in turn may help regulate successful emotional responses to one's environment. Thus, training in emotion regulation techniques may support resistance to peer influence and prevent risky behavior during transition to adolescence, which may have increased relevance for at-risk individuals with a vulnerability to peer pressure, particularly in light of the challenges that accompany digital media use during adolescence.[57]

Structural neural changes were also found in association with video game training in adolescent and adult populations. In a recent study using voxel-based morphometry,[58] significant increases were observed in gray matter in the right hippocampus, right dorsolateral prefrontal cortex (DLPFC), and bilateral cerebellum after two months of daily (at least thirty minutes per day) performance of a three-dimensional platformer game (*Super Mario 64*). Furthermore, gray matter increases in the hippocampus and DLPFC were correlated with the desire to play video games. These data suggest structural brain plasticity after video game training, suggesting that such use could counteract future risk factors for schizophrenia or post-traumatic stress disorder, as these disorders are associated with smaller hippocampi and prefrontal cortex. In a structural MRI study of adolescents, a positive association was observed between amount of time (hours per week) video game playing and greater cortical thickness in the left DLPFC and left frontal eye fields, regions related to executive control, strategic planning, and visuo-motor integration for execution of eye movements.[59] Moreover, a positive association was also observed between greater gray matter volume in the bilateral parahippocampus and the left occipital cortex/inferior parietal lobe and lifetime video playing time (joystick years) in adult male participants.[60] Taken together, further research is needed to more thoroughly characterize the longitudinal profile of brain changes associated with video game use as well as potentially clinical applications that could bolster brain regions that mediate visual attention and navigation.

## DIGITAL MEDIA: POTENTIAL POSITIVE AND NEGATIVE OUTCOMES

Research on digital media report that 93 percent of adolescents use the Internet, gaining access to the Web via public or personal computers or mobile phones, with 75 percent of adolescents owning a personal mobile phone.[61] Positive and negative effects of media on youth and associated changes reported at the National Institute on Media and the Family (Minneapolis, Minnesota) conference revealed that there are three areas of investigation that are of growing interest: physiological and neurological effects of media use, individual differences on media use, and media education.[62] Although it will be important to investigate differential responses to media exposure and the neural circuitry that underlies effects on emotion and attention, current advances in media education programs are already improving parental awareness and understanding. For instance, parents of two- to seventeen-year-olds with greater awareness of media effects are better able to monitor and balance their children's media use.[63] Overall, there is a clear need to maximize the benefits of new media, while minimizing potential harm or risks.[64]

One example of a positive outcome associated with digital media use is the increased opportunities for sexual education and health and self-directed learning programs to educate youth. According to a review on effective programs using new digital media for adolescent populations aged thirteen to twenty-four years for sexuality education interventions, most approaches are Web-based, whereas other approaches include mobile phone applications, social networking sites (SNS), online video bulletin board discussions, and gaming. In six of the ten studies reviewed, digital media use increased knowledge for sexual health promotion in areas related to sexually transmitted infections, HIV/AIDS, and teen pregnancy.[65] Additionally, middle school students who participated in a computer-based intervention program "It's Your Game: Keep It Real" were less likely to initiate sexual activity relative to the control group at ninth-grade follow-up.[66] Importantly, new digital media approaches can be tailored to the participants by creating personal profiles, which is important given that youth have differing levels of sexual experience and comfort in learning this important material. Furthermore, digital teaching platforms have also emerged as a new category of educational instruments to help foster learning not only for students but also for teachers, although technology-advanced school environments are still limited in number.[67] The iPad is an example of a digital teaching platform that serves as an interactive multimedia tool, permitting one-on-one educational learning between students and teachers and also allowing for customization of classroom learning. These devices provide important digital resources via educational applications (i.e., apps) that foster creativity using foundational apps (used across curriculum areas and grades) and essential apps (integrating specific curriculum material and resources into the digital classroom).[68]

In contrast, exposure of adolescents to electronic media use has also been associated with negative health-related outcomes, including obesity and overweight risk in children. For instance, Rich and colleagues have extensively investigated links between media use and obesity in young adolescents and reported that how adolescents use media and the type of media used influence obesity, as opposed to screen time duration alone.[69] Additional moderating factors include increased food consumption during advertising, altered eating behaviors during screen time, sedentary viewing behaviors during screen time, socioeconomic status, family culture, context of use (e.g., what else is happening during use), gender of viewer, and sleep. More recently, higher body mass index in adolescents was positively associated with television viewing rather than computer or video game use.[70] The authors suggest that television is the only screen medium that exposes viewers to advertisements for nutritionally poor foods, which may lead to distracted eating or increased caloric intake, thus contributing to a risk factor for obesity. Indeed, comparable studies investigating duration of social media and other digital media use are also likely under way.

## CLINICAL TREATMENT: INTERNET ADDICTION

While IAD has become widespread, less is known about the efficacy of treatments for such conditions. In a recent meta-analysis conducted by Winkler and colleagues, based on sixteen studies including 670 participants (focused on non-Western countries, e.g., East Asia), results indicate that pharmacological and psychological interventions are highly effective means to reduce symptoms, such as time spent online, depression, and anxiety. While findings are considered preliminary, statistical effect sizes were large and robust, although follow-up data were not available for pharmacological treatment studies.[71]

A recent review of twenty-nine quantitative studies on cognitions (beliefs and assumptions) and seven cognitive behavioral therapy studies revealed four major factors underlying Internet gaming disorder (IGD): beliefs about video gaming rewards; maladaptive and inflexible rules about gaming behavior; over-reliance on gaming to meet self-esteem needs; and gaming as a way of earning social acceptance.[72] It was suggested that a better understanding of maladaptive cognitions associated with IGD may help to improve and advance therapeutic interventions. Furthermore, King and Delfabbro[73] highlight the importance of assessing behavioral outcome measures following treatment such as rates of recovery and prevalence of relapse, and also, inclusion of proper comparison groups. Given that the majority of the existing treatment studies did not assess efficacy of pharmacological interventions for IGD based on follow-up measurements, the data are currently insufficient to determine potential long-term benefits of pharmacological treatments for IGD.[74]

IGD is now included in the recently released *Diagnostic and Statistical Manual of Mental Disorders*, 5th ed. (*DSM–5*), which is the gold standard in the field of clinical psychology for assessing the presence of psychiatric symptoms and conditions.[75] IGD, along with pathological gambling, falls within the "Substance-Related and Addictive Disorders" category of the *DSM–5*.[76] Such diagnostic criteria should ultimately enhance the development of individualized clinical treatment plans for the effective reduction of symptoms associated with pathological digital media use, as well as provide a detailed framework for facilitating the much needed research on underlying neurobiological mechanisms.[77]

## CONCLUSION

In summary, there has been a dramatic increase in digital media use in individuals across the life-span, but most dramatically being introduced in children and adolescents. While there are positive learning opportunities associated with the surge of digital technology use among adolescents, how this technology will affect the evolution of brain and cognition development has yet to be elucidated. Conversely, a serious risk associated with growing digital media use includes an increasing prevalence of online gaming addictions in adolescents. Data from adolescent populations reveal neurobiological alterations that are similar to those observed in other addictive disorders. Abnormalities can be widespread, including altered functional connectivity, disturbances in functional brain activation, and changes in structural brain tissue. While expansion of digital media use reflects an important evolution in technology development, during the period of critical adolescent brain development, increased exposure to digital devices can increase the risk of detrimental social and emotional consequences, such as declines in academic performance and increased risk for addictive disorders. Thus, there are many neurobiological questions that need to be answered: How might reductions in time spent manually handwriting and increases in typing and digital reading alter brain development? What are the advantages of early computer use in the classroom? What are the effects of increased processing speeds and rapid presentation of information on attention (e.g., attention deficit hyperactivity disorder, ADHD) and memory during adolescence? How might excessive digital media use affect mental health and addiction vulnerability? These questions will undoubtedly be a major focus of research on the effects of digital technology on the neurobiology of teen brain development for the next decade and beyond.

## NOTES

1. Victoria J. Rideout, Ulla G. Foehr, and Donald F. Roberts, *Generation M²: Media in the lives of 8- to 18-Year-Olds* (Menlo Park, CA: Henry J. Kaiser Family Foundation, 2010).
2. S. J. Blakemore, "Development of the Social Brain in Adolescence," *JRSM* 105, no. 3 (2012): 111–16, doi:10.1258/jrsm.2011.110221; Adriana Galván, Linda Van Leijenhorst, and Kristine M. McGlennen, "Considerations for Imaging the Adolescent Brain," *Developmental Cognitive Neuroscience* 2, no. 3 (2012): 293–302, doi:10.1016/j.dcn.2012.02.002; Jay N. Giedd, "The

Digital Revolution and Adolescent Brain Evolution," *Journal of Adolescent Health* 51, no. 2 (2012): 101–5, doi:10.1016/j.jadohealth.2012.06.002.
3. Jay N. Giedd, "The Teen Brain: Insights from Neuroimaging," *Journal of Adolescent Health* 42, no. 4 (2008): 335–43, doi:10.1016/j.jadohealth.2008.01.007.
4. Jay N. Giedd et al., "Quantitative MRI of the Temporal Lobe, Amygdala, and Hippocampus in Normal Human Development: Ages 4–18 Years," *Journal of Comparative Neurology* 366, no. 2 (1996): 223–30, doi:10.1002/(SICI)1096-9861(19960304)366:2 223::AID-CNE3 3.0.CO;2-7; N. Gogtay et al., "Dynamic Mapping of Human Cortical Development during Childhood through Early Adulthood," *Proceedings of the National Academy of Sciences* 101, no. 21 (2004): 8174–79, doi:10.1073/pnas.0402680101; Terry L. Jernigan et al., "Maturation of Human Cerebrum Observed *In Vivo* during Adolescence," *Brain* 114, no. 5 (1991): 2037–49, doi:10.1093/brain/114.5.2037; A. Pfefferbaum et al., "A Quantitative Magnetic Resonance Imaging Study of Changes in Brain Morphology from Infancy to Late Adulthood," *Archives of Neurology* 51, no. 9 (1994): 874–87, doi:10.1001/archneur.1994.00540210046012.
5. Jeffrey Jensen Arnett, "Emerging Adulthood: A Theory of Development from the Late Teens through the Twenties.," *American Psychologist* 55, no. 5 (2000): 469–80, doi:10.1037/0003-066X.55.5.469.
6. Jay N. Giedd et al, "Brain Development during Childhood and Adolescence: A Longitudinal MRI Study," *Nature Neuroscience* 2, no. 10 (1999): 861–63; Pfefferbaum et al., "Quantitative Magnetic Resonance"; Elizabeth R. Sowell et al., "Development of Cortical and Subcortical Brain Structures in Childhood and Adolescence: A Structural MRI Study," *Developmental Medicine and Child Neurology* 44, no. 1 (2007): 4–16, doi:10.1111/j.1469–8749.2002.tb00253.x.
7. Gogtay et al., "Dynamic Mapping."
8. Edith V. Sullivan et al., "Developmental Change in Regional Brain Structure over 7 Months in Early Adolescence: Comparison of Approaches for Longitudinal Atlas-Based Parcellation," *NeuroImage* 57, no. 1 (2011): 214–24, doi:10.1016/j.neuroimage.2011.04.003.
9. Gogtay et al., "Dynamic Mapping"; Tomáš Paus, "Mapping Brain Maturation and Cognitive Development during Adolescence," *Trends in Cognitive Sciences* 9, no. 2 (2005): 60–68, doi:10.1016/j.tics.2004.12.008.
10. Vicki Anderson, "Assessing Executive Functions in Children: Biological, Psychological, and Developmental Considerations," *Pediatric Rehabilitation* 4, no. 3 (2001): 119–36, doi:10.1080/13638490110091347; Brent A. Vogt, David M. Finch, and Carl R. Olson, "Functional Heterogeneity in Cingulate Cortex: The Anterior Executive and Posterior Evaluative Regions," *Cerebral Cortex* 2, no. 6 (1992): 435–43, doi:10.1093/cercor/2.6.435-a.
11. J. Arnett, "Reckless Behavior in Adolescence: A Developmental Perspective," *Developmental Review* 12, no. 4 (1992): 339–73, doi:10.1016/0273-2297(92)90013-R; L. P. Spear, "The Adolescent Brain and Age-Related Behavioral Manifestations," *Neuroscience and Biobehavioral Reviews* 24, no. 4 (2000): 417–63, doi:10.1016/S0149-7634(00)00014-2.
12. Arnett, "Reckless Behavior"; R. M. Trimpop, J. H. Kerr, and B. Kirkcaldy, "Comparing Personality Constructs of Risk-Taking Behavior," *Personality and Individual Differences* 26, no. 2 (1998): 237–54, doi:10.1016/S0191-8869(98)00048-8.
13. B. J. Casey, Adriana Galvan, and Todd A. Hare, "Changes in Cerebral Functional Organization during Cognitive Development," *Current Opinion in*

*Neurobiology* 15, no. 2 (2005): 239–44, doi:10.1016/j.conb.2005.03.012; Katya Rubia et al., "Functional Frontalisation with Age: Mapping Neuro-developmental Trajectories with fMRI," *Neuroscience and Biobehavioral Reviews* 24, no. 1 (2000): 13–19, doi:10.1016/S0149-7634(99)00055-X; Katya Rubia et al., "Linear Age-Correlated Functional Development of Right Inferior Fronto-Striato-Cerebellar Networks during Response Inhibition and Anterior Cingulate during Error-Related Processes," *Human Brain Mapping* 28, no. 11 (2007): 1163–77, doi:10.1002/hbm.20347; Katya Rubia et al., "Progressive Increase of Frontostriatal Brain Activation from Childhood to Adulthood during Event-Related Tasks of Cognitive Control," *Human Brain Mapping* 27, no. 12 (2006): 973–93, doi:10.1002/hbm.20237; Leanne Tamm, Vinod Menon, and Allan L. Reiss, "Maturation of Brain Function Associated with Response Inhibition," *Journal of the American Academy of Child and Adolescent Psychiatry* 41, no. 10 (2002): 1231–38, doi:10.1097/00004583-200210000-00013.

14. Casey et al., "Changes in Cerebral"; B. J. Casey, Jay N. Giedd, and Kathleen M. Thomas, "Structural and Functional Brain Development and Its Relation to Cognitive Development," *Biological Psychology* 54, no. 1–3 (2000): 241–57, doi:10.1016/S0301-0511(00)00058-2; Frank N. Dempster, "The Rise and Fall of the Inhibitory Mechanism: Toward a Unified Theory of Cognitive Development and Aging," *Developmental Review* 12, no. 1 (1992): 45–75, doi:10.1016/0273-2297(92)90003-K; Sarah Durston et al., "A Shift from Diffuse to Focal Cortical Activity with Development," *Developmental Science* 9, no. 1 (2006): 1–8, doi:10.1111/j.1467-7687.2005.00454.x; Alecia D. Schweinsburg et al., "An fMRI Study of Response Inhibition in Youths with a Family History of Alcoholism," *Annals of the New York Academy of Sciences* 1021, no. 1 (2004): 391–94, doi:10.1196/annals.1308.050; Marisa M. Silveri et al., "Adolescents at Risk for Alcohol Abuse Demonstrate Altered Frontal Lobe Activation during Stroop Performance," *Alcoholism: Clinical and Experimental Research* 35, no. 2 (2011): 218–28, doi:10.1111/j.1530-0277.2010.01337.x.

15. Marisa M. Silveri et al., "Frontal Lobe γ-Aminobutyric Acid Levels during Adolescence: Associations with Impulsivity and Response Inhibition," *Biological Psychiatry* 74, no. 4 (2013): 296–304, doi:10.1016/j.biopsych.2013.01.033.

16. Laurence Steinberg, "A Dual Systems Model of Adolescent Risk-Taking," *Developmental Psychobiology* 52, no. 3 (2010): 216–24, doi:10.1002/dev.20445.

17. Joseph LeDoux, "Emotional Networks and Motor Control: A Fearful View," in *Progress in Brain Research*, vol. 107, 437–46 (New York: Elsevier, 1996), http://linkinghub.elsevier.com/retrieve/pii/S0079612308618804; Joseph LeDoux, "The Emotional Brain, Fear, and the Amygdala," *Cellular and Molecular Neurobiology* 23, no. 4–5 (2003): 727–38.

18. William D. S. Killgore, Mika Oki, and Deborah A. Yurgelun-Todd, "Sex-Specific Developmental Changes in Amygdala Responses to Affective Faces," *Neuroreport* 12, no. 2 (2001): 427–33; William D. S. Killgore and Deborah A. Yurgelun-Todd, "Neural Correlates of Emotional Intelligence in Adolescent Children," *Cognitive, Affective, and Behavioral Neuroscience* 7, no. 2 (2007): 140–51, doi:10.3758/CABN.7.2.140; Deborah A. Yurgelun-Todd and William D. S. Killgore, "Fear-Related Activity in the Prefrontal Cortex Increases with Age during Adolescence: A Preliminary fMRI Study," *Neuroscience Letters* 406, no. 3 (2006): 194–99, doi:10.1016/j.neulet.2006.07.046.

19. William D. S. Killgore and Deborah A. Yurgelun-Todd, "Developmental Changes in the Functional Brain Responses of Adolescents to Images of High

and Low-Calorie Foods," *Developmental Psychobiology* 47, no. 4 (2005): 377–97, doi:10.1002/dev.20099.

20. Giedd et al., "Quantitative MRI"; Nitin Gogtay et al., "Dynamic Mapping of Normal Human Hippocampal Development," *Hippocampus* 16, no. 8 (2006): 664–72, doi:10.1002/hipo.20193; Akiko Uematsu et al., "Developmental Trajectories of Amygdala and Hippocampus from Infancy to Early Adulthood in Healthy Individuals," ed. Frank Krueger, *PLoS ONE* 7, no. 10 (2012): e46970, doi:10.1371/journal.pone.0046970.

21. Vivien S. Chin, Candice E. Van Skike, and Douglas B. Matthews, "Effects of Ethanol on Hippocampal Function during Adolescence: A Look at the Past and Thoughts on the Future," *Alcohol* 44, no. 1 (2010): 3–14, doi:10.1016/j.alcohol.2009.10.015; Kimberly Nixon et al., "Roles of Neural Stem Cells and Adult Neurogenesis in Adolescent Alcohol Use Disorders," *Alcohol* 44, no. 1 (2010): 39–56, doi:10.1016/j.alcohol.2009.11.001.

22. Giedd et al., "Quantitative MRI"; Gogtay et al., "Dynamic Mapping"; Elizabeth R. Sowell and Terry L. Jernigan, "Further MRI Evidence of Late Brain Maturation: Limbic Volume Increases and Changing Asymmetries during Childhood and Adolescence," *Developmental Neuropsychology* 14, no. 4 (1998): 599–617, doi:10.1080/87565649809540731; M. Suzuki, "Male-Specific Volume Expansion of the Human Hippocampus during Adolescence," *Cerebral Cortex* 15, no. 2 (2004): 187–93, doi:10.1093/cercor/bhh121.

23. Jay N. Giedd et al., "Sexual Dimorphism of the Developing Human Brain," *Progress in Neuro-Psychopharmacology and Biological Psychiatry* 21, no. 8 (1997): 1185–1201, doi:10.1016/S0278-5846(97)00158-9; Killgore et al., "Sex-specific"; William D.S. Killgore and Deborah A. Yurgelun-Todd, "Sex-Related Developmental Differences in the Lateralized Activation of the Prefrontal Cortex and Amygdala during Perception of Facial Affect," *Perceptual and Motor Skills* 99, no. 2 (2004): 371–91.

24. Jun He et al., "Chronic Alcohol Exposure Reduces Hippocampal Neurogenesis and Dendritic Growth of Newborn Neurons," *European Journal of Neuroscience* 21, no. 10 (2005): 2711–20, doi:10.1111/j.1460-9568.2005.04120.x; Barbara J. Markwiese et al., "Differential Effects of Ethanol on Memory in Adolescent and Adult Rats," *Alcoholism: Clinical and Experimental Research* 22, no. 2 (1998): 416–21, doi:10.1111/j.1530-0277.1998.tb03668.x; Gery Schulteis et al., "Intermittent Binge Alcohol Exposure during the Periadolescent Period Induces Spatial Working Memory Deficits in Young Adult Rats," *Alcohol* 42, no. 6 (2008): 459–67, doi:10.1016/j.alcohol.2008.05.002; Ratna Sircar and Debashish Sircar, "Adolescent Rats Exposed to Repeated Ethanol Treatment Show Lingering Behavioral Impairments," *Alcoholism: Clinical and Experimental Research* 29, no. 8 (2005): 1402–10, doi:10.1097/01.alc.0000175012.77756.d9; H. Scott Swartzwelder et al., "Developmental Differences in the Acquisition of Tolerance to Ethanol," *Alcohol* 15, no. 4 (1998): 311–14, doi:10.1016/S0741-8329(97)00135-3; H. Scott Swartzwelder, W.A. Wilson, and M.I. Tayyeb, "Age-Dependent Inhibition of Long-Term Potentiation by Ethanol in Immature Versus Mature Hippocampus," *Alcoholism: Clinical and Experimental Research* 19, no. 6 (1995): 1480–85, doi:10.1111/j.1530-0277.1995.tb01011.x.

25. Killgore and Yurgelun-Todd, "Neural Correlates."

26. Reuven Bar-On, *BarOn Emotional Quotient Inventory: Technical Manual* (North Tonawanda, NY: MHS, 2000); Reuven Bar-On, "Exploring the Neurological Substrate of Emotional and Social Intelligence," *Brain* 126, no. 8 (2003): 1790–1800, doi:10.1093/brain/awg177.

27. Killgore and Yurgelun-Todd, "Neural Correlates."

28. Luigi Mazzone et al., "The Role of Anxiety Symptoms in School Performance in a Community Sample of Children and Adolescents," *BMC Public Health* 7, no. 1 (2007): 347, doi:10.1186/1471-2458-7-347; José M. Mestre, Rocío Guil, Paulo N. Lopes, Peter Salovey, and Paloma Gil-Olarte, "Emotional Intelligence and Social and Academic Adaptation to School," *Psicothema* 18 (2006): 112–17.
29. Mestre et al., "Emotional Intelligence."
30. Nigel Hunt and Dee Evans, "Predicting Traumatic Stress Using Emotional Intelligence," *Behaviour Research and Therapy* 42, no. 7 (2004): 791–98, doi:10.1016/j.brat.2003.07.009.
31. Irene J. Elkins et al., "Personality Traits and the Development of Nicotine, Alcohol, and Illicit Drug Disorders: Prospective Links from Adolescence to Young Adulthood," *Journal of Abnormal Psychology* 115, no. 1 (2006): 26–39, doi:10.1037/0021-843X.115.1.26; Julie B. Kaplow et al., "The Prospective Relation between Dimensions of Anxiety and the Initiation of Adolescent Alcohol Use," *Journal of Clinical Child and Adolescent Psychology* 30, no. 3 (2001): 316–26, doi:10.1207/S15374424JCCP3003_4.
32. L. Diane Santesso et al., "Frontal Electroencephalogram Activation Asymmetry, Emotional Intelligence, and Externalizing Behaviors in 10-Year-Old Children," *Child Psychiatry and Human Development* 36, no. 3 (2006): 311–28, doi:10.1007/s10578-005-0005-2.
33. Marc A. Schuckit et al., "Externalizing Disorders in the Offspring from the San Diego Prospective Study of Alcoholism," *Journal of Psychiatric Research* 42, no. 8 (2008): 644–52, doi:10.1016/j.jpsychires.2007.07.013.
34. Elkins et al., "Personality Traits."
35. Hunt and Evans, "Predicting Traumatic Stress."
36. Mazzone et al., "Role of Anxiety."
37. Robert M. Yerkes and John D. Dodson, "The Relation of Strength of Stimulus to Rapidity of Habit-Formation," *Journal of Comparative Neurology and Psychology* 18, no. 5 (1908): 459–82, doi:10.1002/cne.920180503.
38. Killgore and Yurgelun-Todd, "Neural Correlates"; Deborah Yurgelun-Todd, "Emotional and Cognitive Changes during Adolescence," *Current Opinion in Neurobiology* 17, no. 2 (2007): 251–57, doi:10.1016/j.conb.2007.03.009.
39. Jason Chein et al., "Peers Increase Adolescent Risk Taking by Enhancing Activity in the Brain's Reward Circuitry: Peer Influence on Risk Taking," *Developmental Science* 14, no. 2 (2011): F1–F10, doi:10.1111/j.1467-7687.2010.01035.x.
40. David C. Mohr et al., "Behavioral Intervention Technologies: Evidence Review and Recommendations for Future Research in Mental Health," *General Hospital Psychiatry* 35, no. 4 (2013): 332–38, doi:10.1016/j.genhosppsych.2013.03.008.
41. B. F. Grant and D. A. Dawson, "Age at Onset of Alcohol Use and Its Association with DSM-IV Alcohol Abuse and Dependence: Results from the National Longitudinal Alcohol Epidemiologic Survey," *Journal of Substance Abuse* 9 (1997): 103–10; Ralph W. Hingson, Timothy Heeren, and Michael R. Winter, "Age at Drinking Onset and Alcohol Dependence: Age at Onset, Duration, and Severity," *Archives of Pediatrics and Adolescent Medicine* 160, no. 7 (2006): 739, doi:10.1001/archpedi.160.7.739.
42. Caroline Flisher, "Getting Plugged In: An Overview of Internet Addiction," *Journal of Paediatrics and Child Health* 46, no. 10 (2010): 557–59; Kai Yuan et al., "Internet Addiction: Neuroimaging Findings," *Communicative and Integrative Biology* 4, no. 6 (2011): 637–39.
43. S. Choudhury and K. A. McKinney, "Digital Media, the Developing Brain and the Interpretive Plasticity of Neuroplasticity," *Transcultural Psychiatry* 50, no. 2 (2013): 192–215, doi:10.1177/1363461512474623.

44. Flisher, "Getting Plugged In."
45. Yuan et al., "Internet Addiction."
46. Kai Yuan et al., "Cortical Thickness Abnormalities in Late Adolescence with Online Gaming Addiction," ed. Bogdan Draganski, *PLoS ONE* 8, no. 1 (2013): e53055, doi:10.1371/journal.pone.0053055.
47. Yueji Sun et al., "Brain fMRI Study of Crave Induced by Cue Pictures in Online Game Addicts (Male Adolescents)," *Behavioural Brain Research* 233, no. 2 (2012): 563–76, doi:10.1016/j.bbr.2012.05.005.
48. Ibid.
49. Wei-na Ding et al., "Altered Default Network Resting-State Functional Connectivity in Adolescents with Internet Gaming Addiction," ed. Michelle Hampson, *PLoS ONE* 8, no. 3 (2013): e59902, doi:10.1371/journal.pone.0059902.
50. Qi Feng et al., "Voxel-Level Comparison of Arterial Spin-Labeled Perfusion Magnetic Resonance Imaging in Adolescents with Internet Gaming Addiction," *Behavioral and Brain Functions* 9, no. 1 (2013): 33, doi:10.1186/1744-9081-9-33.
51. Ding et al., "Altered Default Network."
52. Dar Meshi, Carmen Morawetz, and Hauke R. Heekeren, "Nucleus Accumbens Response to Gains in Reputation for the Self Relative to Gains for Others Predicts Social Media Use," *Frontiers in Human Neuroscience* 7 (2013), doi:10.3389/fnhum.2013.00439.
53. Suzanne N. Haber and Brian Knutson, "The Reward Circuit: Linking Primate Anatomy and Human Imaging," *Neuropsychopharmacology* 35, no. 1 (2010): 4–26, doi:10.1038/npp.2009.129.
54. Meshi et al., "Nucleus Accumbens."
55. C. W. Korn et al., "Positively Biased Processing of Self-Relevant Social Feedback," *Journal of Neuroscience* 32, no. 47 (2012): 16832–44, doi:10.1523/JNEUROSCI.3016-12.2012.
56. Jennifer H. Pfeifer et al., "Entering Adolescence: Resistance to Peer Influence, Risky Behavior, and Neural Changes in Emotion Reactivity," *Neuron* 69, no. 5 (2011): 1029–36, doi:10.1016/j.neuron.2011.02.019.
57. Ibid.
58. Simone Kühn et al., "Playing Super Mario Induces Structural Brain Plasticity: Gray Matter Changes Resulting from Training with a Commercial Video Game," *Molecular Psychiatry* 19, no. 2 (2014): 265–71, doi:10.1038/mp.2013.120.
59. Simone Kühn et al., "Positive Association of Video Game Playing with Left Frontal Cortical Thickness in Adolescents," ed. Frank Krueger, *PLoS ONE* 9, no. 3 (2014): e91506, doi:10.1371/journal.pone.0091506.
60. S. Kühn and J. Gallinat, "Amount of Lifetime Video Gaming Is Positively Associated with Entorhinal, Hippocampal and Occipital Volume," *Molecular Psychiatry* 19, no. 7 (2014): 842–47, doi:10.1038/mp.2013.100.
61. Amanda Lenhart et al., *Social Media and Mobile Internet Use among Teens and Young Adults* (Washington, DC: Pew Research Center, 2010).
62. David A. Walsh, "The Challenge of the Evolving Media Environment," *Journal of Adolescent Health* 27, no. 2 (2000): 69–72, doi:10.1016/S1054-139X(00)00134-8.
63. Douglas A. Gentile and David A. Walsh, *MediaQuotient: National Survey of Family Media Habits, Knowlege, and Attitudes* (Minneapolis, MN: National Institute on Media and the Family, 1999).
64. Walsh, "Challenge."
65. Kylene Guse et al., "Interventions Using New Digital Media to Improve Adolescent Sexual Health: A Systematic Review," *Journal of Adolescent Health* 51, no. 6 (2012): 535–43, doi:10.1016/j.jadohealth.2012.03.014.

66. Susan R. Tortolero et al., "It's Your Game: Keep It Real: Delaying Sexual Behavior with an Effective Middle School Program," *Journal of Adolescent Health* 46, no. 2 (2010): 169–79, doi:10.1016/j.jadohealth.2009.06.008.

67. Christopher Dede and John Richards, eds., *Digital Teaching Platforms: Customizing Classroom Learning for Each Student* (New York: Teachers College, Columbia University, 2012).

68. *Francis Wyman Technology Blog*, http://fwtech.org/.

69. D. S. Bickham et al., "Characteristics of Screen Media Use Associated with Higher BMI in Young Adolescents," *Pediatrics* 131, no. 5 (2013): 935–41, doi:10.1542/peds.2012-1197.

70. Ibid.

71. Alexander Winkler et al., "Treatment of Internet Addiction: A Meta-Analysis," *Clinical Psychology Review* 33, no. 2 (2013): 317–29, doi:10.1016/j.cpr.2012.12.005.

72. Daniel L. King and Paul H. Delfabbro, "The Cognitive Psychology of Internet Gaming Disorder," *Clinical Psychology Review* 34, no. 4 (2014): 298–308, doi:10.1016/j.cpr.2014.03.006.

73. Daniel L. King and Paul H. Delfabbro, "Internet Gaming Disorder Treatment: A Review of Definitions of Diagnosis and Treatment Outcome: Internet Gaming Disorder Treatment," *Journal of Clinical Psychology* 70, no. 10 (2014): 942–55, doi:10.1002/jclp.22097.

74. Ibid.

75. American Psychiatric Association, *Diagnostic and Statistical Manual of Mental Disorders*, 5th ed. (Arlington, VA: American Psychiatric Association, 2013).

76. Ibid.

77. Daria Kuss, "Internet Gaming Addiction: Current Perspectives," *Psychology Research and Behavior Management* 2013, no. 6 (2013): 125–37, doi:10.2147/PRBM.S39476.

# 4 Neural Correlates of the Multisensory Film Experience

*Luis Rocha Antunes*

Discussions concerning film perception have always been limited by the notion of medium specificity, or that the medium's sensory sources (light and sound) are the only sensory modalities (sight and hearing) at play in our perceptual experience of film. However, what are the perceptual correlates behind our multisensory experiences of film, and how do they support my claim that the perceptual experience of a film can fall into the realm of our perceptual faculties outside the classic five senses? New scientific findings in the field of multisensory studies have been providing abundant support that whereas the film medium is audiovisual—as a recorded visual image with accompanying soundtrack—the spectator's experience of film is multisensory.[1] The *multisensory film experience*, as I define it, is the notion that there is more than just sight and hearing at play when we perceive a film.[2] My account of the multisensory in the context of film perception is in line with Barry Dainton's general account of consciousness, as follows:

> Some experiences are more noticeable than others. In thinking of 'experiences' we tend to think first of what we can see and hear, our thoughts or memories, our more memorable pains and pleasures. We easily overlook the presence of those bodily sensations that form the backdrop of our consciousness: gentle sensations of texture and pressure (e.g. from our clothing), feelings of warmth or coolness, along with feelings in our muscles, organs and joints, and our sense of balance (standing upright feels different from standing on one's head). But these various bodily feelings all have their own distinctive phenomenal character, they all belong to the realm of experience.[3]

This speaks to a redefinition not only of the sensory modalities at play in our perceptual experience of film but also of the notion of embodiment and motor responses from spectators. On one hand, there are minimal motor and embodied responses that go unnoticed, which are a result of the direct perceptual experience of watching a film. Our hands may sweat, our breath may be held, or we may slightly tilt our heads. On the other hand, although we are used to defining experience at the level of the senses through a direct comparison with the motor effects of such experience, we cannot ignore that much of our perceptual experience does not materialize into motor actions—at least visible motor actions. In other words, part of the brain's perceptual processing and integration of the sensory modalities takes place without necessarily motor responses. As Spivey and colleagues have shown, "action is no longer seen as the lonely caboose at the end of a train of sequential modular stages, as once assumed by the traditional information-processing approach in cognitive psychology."[4]

The fact that one individual spectator does not have a strong motor and embodied response to a particular film does not mean that this spectator does not have access to a multisensory experience of film through sight and hearing. Another important aspect is that many motor responses that are traditionally associated with emotional states are not dissociated from sensory perception, because emotions are closely interrelated with our sensory modalities. Although certain scenes in film can be powerful enough to cause visible motor responses, such as the startled response in which we turn our faces away from fast objects tossed toward the screen, these motor responses do not necessarily imply the mimicking of the film characters' motor actions. Our motor actions as spectators do not have to mimic the characters' own motor actions, but they can be aligned in terms of salience. Even if the human brain simulates the motor actions performed by the characters in film, that simulation does not necessarily have to materialize into motor responses and can remain in the realm of neural simulation. This simulation may trigger perceptual imagery, in the sense of neural activity that, although triggered by external sensory information, does not result in motor commands to the periphery of our bodies.

Film perception in its multisensory dimension may seem to be a recent interest in film studies,[5] but as a matter of fact, it goes back to the inception of film theory in the 1910s. In 1916, Harvard psychologist Hugo Münsterberg wrote what can be considered the first scholarly study of film, titled *The Photoplay: A Psychological Study*.[6] In this text, Münsterberg approaches film at the intersection of aesthetics and perceptual experience. Theoretical works that followed Münsterberg's, most notably Arnheim's *Film as Art*,[7] have acknowledged that film aesthetics is not abstract or disembodied, and is not a merely compositional and pictorial element. Rather, it can only be fully understood in perspective with how film style shapes the spectator's perceptual experience of film,[8] and vice versa. In other words, a seminal study such as Münsterberg's shows that film aesthetics is not just about the formal and visual elements displayed by the medium, but it is about how those formal and audiovisual elements combine to shape our perceptual experience of film on the level of the senses, which are closely connected with other layers of perceptual experience, such as emotions, empathy, kinesthetic engagement, memory, perceptual imagery, and others. If the importance attributed to film perception is not new in film studies, the knowledge that can inform us about it certainly needs an update.

Hugo Münsterberg devoted close attention to the impact of the then-new film medium and the role that some of the most fundamental concepts of emotions, attention, and memory play in the shaping of our perceptual experience of film—some of which are still being debated today. However, the historical context of his approach made him place too much emphasis on the mental and psychological levels of perception, as well as a focus on film as a strictly visual art. Nonetheless, the blueprint for our understanding of film perception is already present: "What we need for this study is evidently, first, an insight into the means by which the moving pictures impress us and appeal to us. Not the physical means and technical devices are in question, but the mental means. What psychological factors are involved when we watch the happenings on the screen?"[9]

For a reader today, it may seem obvious for Münsterberg to acknowledge the internal aspects of perception to our experience of film. However, film perception has been studied historically very much in line with the visual, or audiovisual, nature of the medium.[10] In other words, because of the fact that the film medium was earlier seen as a synonym of the screen, film was studied for decades—and to a certain extent still is today—as a visual art form. Of course, this raises aesthetical and methodological questions (one cannot address the other sensory modalities outside a metaphorical framework). This ontology of film is present in the idea that the screen is flat, or two dimensional, and so is our perceptual experience of what we see on the screen.

Here Münsterberg, and later Arnheim, present the contrary argument to this assumption: "The photoplay is therefore poorly characterized if the flatness of the pictorial view is presented as an essential feature. That flatness is an objective part of the technical physical arrangements, but not a feature of that which we really see in the performance of the photoplay."[11] This is one of the fundamental principles behind film perception—there is no necessary direct correspondence between the sensory nature of the medium and the perceptual experience it elicits. This is also the fundamental principle behind my understanding of our perceptual experience of film, or of any other audiovisual medium. Although it is light and sound waves that the medium cues, our perception is multisensory, and thus it overlaps with other senses, modalities and functions of our perception—even senses outside the classic five, such as thermoception, proprioception, nociception, and the vestibular sense. The former conceptualization has been called a sense-to-sense correspondence, where one sensory source corresponds the processing of one sensory modality, say, light to sight or sound to hearing. The sense-to-sense correspondence has recently been dramatically challenged. Many of the aspects behind our multisensory experience of audiovisual media, such as film, rely precisely on this distinction between the medium's sensory sources and our processing of that sensory information. In other words, *the medium is audiovisual, yet our experience is multisensory.* This chapter examines some of the most important research supporting this claim.

We tend to think of perception as access to external stimuli, often forgetting the influence of internal aspects of our bodies and brain. To a certain extent, perception does mean to align us with the sensory world outside our bodies. However, that access is not disembodied; it is not made without the specificity of our bodies, nor without the mental and emotional context of each moment. Internal factors are highly demonstrative of the subjective nature of perception and explain why perception is not merely a mechanical input of sensory information, but rather is mediated by our different states of mind. Münsterberg should also be credited for bringing this aspect to our understanding of film perception: "We see things distant and moving, but we furnish to them more than we receive; we create the depth and the continuity through our mental mechanism."[12] The internal factors of perceptual experience are fundamental to our understanding of why we perceive an audiovisual medium in a multisensory fashion.

Another seminal principle brought by Münsterberg to the understanding of our perceptual experience of film is that, whereas there is a high-order level of *cognition* that allows us to try to exert some control and make sense of what we experience in the film through the use of memory, imagination, and belief-disbelief mechanisms, there is also another fundamental level, a lower level, thought of as *perception*, over which we cannot exert control.

On one hand, Münsterberg's paradigm of film perception is more within the boundaries defined by the notion of sense-to-sense correspondence, but on the other hand, there are the concrete elements of film perception that he proposes, namely, attention, emotions, depth and movement, memory, and imagination, which make his model much more complex. To corroborate Münsterberg's influence on film studies, these elements have all received scholarly attention and are still today central for many scholars. Attention has given rise to an entire theory of film editing.[13] Carl Plantinga and Gregory Smith, among others, have studied emotion in film.[14] Memory has been studied by Laura Marks in the context of transcultural cinema.[15]

All these senses, cognitive modalities, and functions of our perceptual experience of film may fall into sight and hearing, and that is why they have not been problematic for film scholars who believe that our perceptual experience of film is audiovisual.[16] That is why I see as crucial the distinction between multimodality and multisensory. If critics claim that film is a multimodal experience, they are only claiming that these cognitive modalities, such as attention, emotions, memory, imagination, language, are all at play when we view a film. However, that is not really problematic, as these modalities all fall into sight and hearing. The claim that film perception is multimodal does not imply that film perception is multisensory. What is problematic is to understand whether we can perceive senses through film outside sight and hearing, given that the sensory input we receive is mainly audiovisual (and only residually haptic through sound waves that reverberate on surfaces). This is why I explore film perception in the realm of the senses, since I assume that modalities that are not bonded to a specific sensory modality, but can be conveyed through numerous ones (such as sight and hearing), are already well established within the scholarly study of film perception. In other words, there is a strong connection between these cognitive modalities and the senses, and they are exactly what help to explain the ways in which we can perceive one sense by means of another. The only way we have to show that our perceptual experience of an audio-visual medium as film is multisensory is to show that senses outside sight and hearing are physiologically and neurologically elicited. We can further-more make the equation more complex by adding this problematic to the idea that our perception is not only made of the classic five senses but also of sensory modalities that are well established and studied by neuroscience, namely proprioception, thermoception, the vestibular, and thermoception.

The acknowledgment that these modalities take place in our perceptual experience of film also helps to explain the embodied nature of film. For instance, the fact that we may blush, laugh, smile, cry, or hit our partner on the seat next to us serves as evidence of our emotional engagement with the film. This is without dispute for the simple fact that we can justify these responses on the basis of what we see and hear. However, what can be problematic is if some of these emotions and modalities could be working not through sight and hearing, as we may have thought, but through other sensory modalities. This shows that claiming that film is a multimodal expe-rience says little about the problematics involved in film perception, because it does not capture how these modalities are connected to the senses. The McGurk effect (where visual information provided by lip reading changes the way a sound is heard), the ventriloquism effect, and the general modu-lations of sound and sight when a single flash of light is accompanied by multiple beeps causing the light to be experienced as multiple flashes are all important cross-modal cases showing the connection between the senses. These examples, however, do not describe the full range of possible mul-tisensory connections. Moreover, these cross-modal cases may appear to imply that our multisensory experiences are limited to perceptual illusions, when this is not necessarily so.[17]

The historical importance of Münsterberg for the study of film percep-tion is not just that he was the first to address this issue in depth but that he was seminal to the fleshing out of some of the most fundamental aspects of film perception that have attracted film scholars throughout decades. The reason *The Photoplay* caught on in such timely way is that Münsterberg did not limit the notion of film perception to opticality but addressed it from a truly complex perspective. At the same time, he acknowledged that the film medium can help explain part of the equation; however, the spectators' perceptual experiences do not end where the medium ends.

Another paradigmatic contributor to the study of film perception is Rudolf Arnheim, also from Harvard. His book *Film as Art* was first published in the German language in 1932 and a year later in English. Although Arn-heim explains many of the perceptual aspects of film through an audiovisual approach, he did not conceive of the perceptual experience of film to be strictly comprehended by sight and hearing, as the quotations that begin this essay show: "Sensations of smell, equilibrium, or touch are, of course, never conveyed in a film through direct stimuli, but are suggested indirectly through sight."[18] According to Arnheim, the film artist "eliminates entire areas of sensory perception, and thereby brings others into higher relief, ingeniously making them take the place of those that are missing."[19]

Arnheim explored in depth aspects of spatiality, implying that the spectator does not view the film in a disembodied fashion but in an embodied one, in other words, that the space is not just out there, but in here: "Our eyes are not a mechanism functioning independently of the rest of the body. They work in constant cooperation with the other sense organs."[20] Arnheim is historically important because he not only advocated for film as an art form using the tools from fine art, art history and aesthetics, but he claimed that film was an art form relying on its own authenticity and specificity not only as a medium but as a perceptual experience. This means that although he addresses film as a visual art form, Arnheim conceives this art form as a gateway to other sensory realms. He deeply explores film as a medium and apparatus, but he does not limit his conception of perceptual experience to that specificity. The only problematic aspect about Arnheim's work, which is misaligned with my own approach, is that he conceives that "in real life every experience or chain of experiences is enacted for every observer in an uninterrupted spatial and temporal sequence,"[21] which is simply not accurate. We just need to think of eye blinking, selective attention, different states of mind, sleep, and so many other aspects that make our perceptual experience in real life contexts not continuous as he describes it.

Another contribution of Arnheim's *Film as Art* was to lay out a number of stylistic elements of cinematography that are characteristic of films that more prominently address the senses, such as camerawork, lenses, lighting, and color, and how these can shape our perceptual experience of film. He points to the ways in which lighting, for instance, can influence our thermoceptive experience of a scene in a film: "Depending on the lighting, a room may look warm and comfortable, or cold and bare, large or small, clean or dirty."[22] However, he also points out how the scale of shot can be used not only for highlighting a dramatic or emotional moment through the close view of a character's face but to give spectators access to haptic information of objects in the world of the film: "The special delight in getting the sense of the texture of ordinary materials—such as dull iron, shining tin, smooth fur, the woolly hide of an animal, soft skin—in film or photograph is also heightened by the lack of hues."[23] By pointing out these stylistic devices, Arnheim is not only showing that formal elements of film style (such as shot scale) are not enough to understand film aesthetics but also that what could be considered a limitation; that is, the absence of stimuli from other sensory natures, is in fact compensated by the advanced stylistic tools of cinematography. Therefore, film aesthetics is not just formal aspects of cinematography but a certain configuration of our perceptual experience.

## KUBRICK'S *2001*

The intersection between perceptual experience and film aesthetics has been on the mind of not only film theorists but also filmmakers. A paradigmatic example is Stanley Kubrick's *2001: A Space Odyssey* (1968), one of the most influential films of all time[24] and a milestone in further pushing the boundaries between aesthetics and perception.

The film *2001* repositioned and reestablished the film viewing experience on the level of proprioception: it created a cinematic aesthetics based on the physical laws of the outer space, different from those on Earth. There had been films prior to 1969 cueing salient proprioceptive experiences to spectators, but they appeared in isolated scenes, and not on such a fundamental level as in *2001*. The sound design, the use of unusual camera angles, and the motor action of the characters all come together to engage spectators through proprioception, creating sensations of rotation and spinning, and different sorts of gravitational effects that may make one tilt her head to try to make proprioceptive sense of the film. Particularly, *2001*'s sound design is extremely proactive, though often going unnoticed, in shaping the material world of the film, giving information about textures, materials, distances, spatial coordinates, direction of movements, and gravity. The visual image works in partnership with the sound design to create effects of spinning and rotation, which we can only perceive and make sense of because our sense of proprioception is there to help us. The question is, Knowing that spectators are not receiving direct input on their muscles similar to the characters in the film, is it correct to say that this is a proprioceptive experience? Or is it just imagination or even associative memories?

Although perception generally relies not only on the actual external stimuli but also on internal elements such as memory, emotions, multisensory imagery, even language, research shows that there are neural connections between the senses in general, and between proprioception and sight and hearing, as I show later. Some extent of our proprioceptive experience of *2001* is purely perceptual and does not necessarily need to be fully aligned with that of the characters but can be a result of camerawork and sound design. In other words, our proprioceptive experience of a film like *2001* uses sight and hearing as the sensory gateways, but its ultimate level of perception does not end in sight and hearing but in proprioception.

The link between sight and hearing (extrapersonal senses) and proprioception (an interpersonal sense) is a widely accepted idea in neuroscience. A well-known case is that of Ian Waterman, a man who lost his sense of proprioception and relearned successfully through sight how to perform body movements that previously relied on proprioception.[25] His case shows that sight can work in ways to replace proprioception.

Neurologically, studies show that proprioception not only receives input from the receptors located on the joints and muscles but also receives projections from sight and hearing,[26] meaning that there are neural pathways that connect these two sensory modalities, relying on feedback and feedforward processes to optimize percepts. It would seem that the only way for us to think about a proprioceptive experience would be through direct performance of motor action of some sort, and that, as spectators are sitting still, there is no activation of proprioception. Although this is true to some extent, it is also true that the film viewing experience is not one of total stillness.[27] Even what we think of as stillness—say, an upright sitting posture—is not a passive motor position but one that is actively dependent on proprioceptive monitoring. Although spectators are not engaged in locomotive motor actions similar to the characters, they cannot turn their senses off, and they thus still perform many motor actions that often go unnoticed, such as eye saccades or many of Darwin's documented *Expression of the Emotions*,[28] like the raising of the eyebrows in surprise, the baring of the teeth in rage, and the erection of the hair (piloerection) in fear and anger.

I believe we should redefine the idea of motor action in film viewing experiences on three levels: (1) instead of limiting motor action to locomotion, small motor actions should also be considered to be motor actions; (2) there are a number of visceral motor actions that we can not control (respiration, digestion, etc.); and (3) motor action can involve neural processing and the firing of a neural pathway without the execution of a motor command, and emotions as actions tendencies. It can be just a matter of neural representation of space and action, as Fogassi and Gallese suggest: "Parietal areas, together with the frontal areas to which they are connected, constitute cortical networks that process and integrate multisensory information for the purpose of action execution, but also for the purpose of representing the environment in which action takes place."[29]

This is important, for it is known that many of these "small" motor actions have great influence on our proprioception, particularly on our postures. In fact, posture is not a neutral or effortless motor action but rather it is a dynamic and proactive one: "The control of upright posture involves the integration of multiple sensory systems that specify information about the position of body segments relative to each other and to the surrounding environment."[30] Furthermore, "head and body sway induced by an oscillating visual display have been shown to be sensitive to the velocity of the visual stimulus."[31] Other studies have shown the "effect of gaze on postural responses to neck proprioceptive and vestibular stimulation in humans."[32] These findings, which are only a sample of all the research made, show that the audiovisual cues of the film can have a physical, not just imagined, effect on our posture and sense of proprioception. Although one may think that our sitting posture as spectators is static, it is actually a dynamic and subtle motor process.

It is not just that there are neural projections between sight, hearing, and proprioception; in some cases, those projections can modulate our eye movements. In other words, they can influence the targets at which we look.[33] At least since the 1970s, there have been a series of studies on the topic of visual proprioception that address the relationship between sight and proprioception.[34] "It has been shown that the signals from eye-in-orbit and head-on-trunk position as provided by proprioception and efference copies of the motor commands can reorient visually evoked postural responses."[35] For more skeptical readers who believe that, as spectators, they can exert an absolute perceptual control over what they experience in a film, I should point out that many of these findings take place on a low level of perceptual experience, where sight and hearing determine our posture as perceivers. This is corroborated by the research of Ivanenko et al., for instance, when the authors make notice of the shaping of our posture and gaze by high-order cognitive factors: "Cognitive factors such as attention, internal representation or the extent of visual dependence can determine or modulate the influence of gaze on body sway responses."[36]

Hearing has also been well documented as being involved in proprioceptive experiences: "Changes in auditory and visual localization were causally related to changes in apparent arm position."[37] Lakner and Shenker offer an overview of literature exploring the relationship between represented body orientation and the apparent spatial direction. On one hand, there is the idea that some of our perceived movements do not necessarily match an actual body movement; in other words, we may have a certain motor sensation (say, of vertigo and falling off from a tall building) when we are not actually performing that motor action (we are merely watching a camera perspective filming from a tall building). In the words of the authors, "it is possible to create situations in which one perceives oneself to be making movements of directions, amplitudes, or frequencies that differ from those actually being voluntarily executed."[38] On the other hand, actual motor actions are performed from the hearing and seeing of audiovisual stimuli. The question is if those motor actions, in the context of film watching experiences, are not copies of the motor actions of the characters but are subtle movements that we perform, many times unaware, while experiencing films. For instance, in Figure 4.1, we may be tempted to sway our heads to align our gaze with what we perceive as the gravitational orientation of the woman in the whirlpool machine of *2001*

All this evidence that we can have a proprioceptive experience of film through sight and hearing contradicts a fundamental assumption in studies of film perception, namely, the canonical works by Virginia Brooks and Tim Smith, who conceive the perceptual experience of film as strictly audiovisual. Brooks claims that

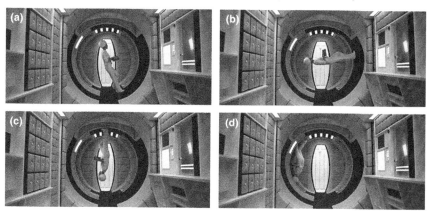

*Figure 4.1*   Proprioception in *2001: A Space Odyssey*

film was first only, and is still primarily, a visual art: that is, it is received by the human organism through the eyes and processed by the visual areas of the brain. It seems odd then that so little interaction has taken place between the study of how this visual processing system works, and how films are perceived and understood.[39]

However, today it is clear that there are many connections and projections between sight and the other senses, and between the senses in general. Although there is a low level of perceptual processing where one can find a clear connection between visual stimuli and visual processing, the whole process of sight is not exclusively visual.[40]

Tim Smith, conversely, claims that "film (cinema) perception refers to the sensory and cognitive processes employed when viewing scenes, events, and narratives presented in edited moving images. . . . Understanding how our perceptual systems deal with the differences between these mediated visual experiences and the real world helps us understand how perception works in both situations."[41] This assumption that film perception is visual and that it is aligned with the audiovisual nature of the film medium is in line with Virginia Brook's notion of film perception as something that exclusively pertains to the realm of sight. However, I believe that by not making a distinction between the medium and the perceptual experience, these authors are perpetuating a false assumption that film perception is audiovisual, when in fact it is multisensory. In other words, it has been inferred that because the medium is audiovisual, so is our perception of that medium. However, I propose that we make this distinction and say instead that the medium is audiovisual, yet our perceptual experience of the medium is multisensory, based on neurophysiological evidence I have shown and will demonstrate in the following.

## THE NEUROLOGY BEHIND THE MULTISENSORY
## PERCEPTION OF FILM

What are the perceptual correlates behind our multisensory experience of film? In other words, what supports the claim that the perceptual experience of a film can fall within the realm of senses outside the classic five? The following are general principles—the actual perceptual content of different viewing contexts and different spectators varies, of course. I focus on the main brain structures and neural processes that are common to the multisensory nature of human perception.

The two and perhaps most important brain structures behind the multisensory experience of film are the hypothalamus and the superior colliculus. The hypothalamus is located within the well-known limbic system, the neural engine room of our emotions, and is simultaneously a key player in the multisensory integration of stimuli[42] and on the processing of emotions through multisensory cues.[43] The role of emotions in shaping our multisensory experience of films is crucial, as emotions can trigger a number of physical responses that makes the spectator aware that her perception of film is embodied and perceptually engaged. At the same time, the hypothalamus and the superior colliculus in multisensory processing show the link between emotions and sensory perception. If we consider that emotions are naturally multisensory, it is not surprising that emotions perceived through visual and auditory stimuli can wire multisensory qualities outside sight and hearing. The most intuitive examples are when we blush because we feel shy or embarrassed for ourselves or for a character on screen (an emotional response on the domain of thermoception).

The superior colliculus offers evidence of neural connection between the senses, as it receives inputs from different senses and determines much of the multisensory integration. The superior colliculus has been brought forth[44] as one of the centers of multisensory integration, and represents a brain structure where the senses connect. It has historical importance, as well. From the findings of Meredith and Stein,[45] the superior colliculus is in the root of their seminal work, the *Merging of the Senses*,[46] which originated the discipline of multisensory studies. The thalamus and the superior colliculus offer physical evidence of where and how the senses connect and the link of emotions in our multisensory perceptual experience of film. There is evidence of the intersection between sight as a gateway to perceptual experience in other domains:

> The locations of the nonvisual receptive fields of SC [superior colliculus] neurons are strongly influenced by the direction of gaze. This ensures that, regardless of the relative eye, head, and body positions, a visual, auditory, or somatosensory cue will activate the same general site in the SC—one that represents the position of the stimulus with respect to the current line of sight.[47]

Meredith and Stein's *The Merging of the Senses* represented a paradigm shift in neuroscience, by calling attention to the fact that

> no part of the nervous system functions in the same way alone as it does in concert with other parts. When a part of the brain is removed in a lesion study, the behavior of the animal afterward is more a reflection of the adjusted capacities of the remaining brain than of the capacities of the part of the brain that was removed. It is unlikely, therefore, that the neural basis of any cognitive function—thought, memory, perception, and language—will be understood by focusing on one region of the brain without considering the relationship of that region to the others.[48]

Meredith and Stein have basically shown the neural evidence that supports my claim that our perceptual experience of an audiovisual medium as film is multisensory. One of the principal underlying ideas to support my claim is based on Meredith and Stein first showing that the auditory cortex is not exclusively a unisensory neural population but, rather, is a center of multisensory integration: "In a more general sense, we surmise that the dynamic interplay of neural populations constitutes a unified temporal framework where the segmented senses unfold and merge, resulting in the seamless multisensory integrated dynamic world we perceive."[49] My claim that film is an audiovisual medium and yet our perceptual experience of it is multisensory can only find support if we assume that our perceptual experience in general is not based on a sense-to-sense correspondence. An example of research showing that there is a connection between the senses in our film watching experiences is Hasson's study "Intersubject Synchronization of Cortical Activity During Natural Vision."[50] This study has shown that watching films causes a network of neural pathways and populations to fire up within the brains of the spectators and that the sensory processing of watching movies is not limited to sight and hearing. This has been followed up and given further evidence in a study by Luo and colleagues, who show that the perceptual experience of film watching is closely aligned with the multisensory experience of natural contexts, if not within the direct sensory sources, at least on a neural level:

> Unlike pairings of transient artificial stimuli used in most previous audiovisual studies, we examined the cross-modal integration effects in presumptively unimodal areas by employing naturalistic audiovisual movies that are ethologically natural and extended in time (30-s film clips). Naturalistic stimuli contain complex structure and rich dynamics in the time domain, and it has been suggested that the relevant neural mechanisms are in part shaped by the statistical structure of natural environments.[51]

There is mounting evidence that our perceptual imagery is multisensory, as well,[52] despite imagery being traditionally looked at from a visual perspective. The idea of perceptual imagery is that the recollection of perceptual experiences can trigger the actual firing up of neural populations that would be associated with that experience. In other words, perceptual imagery shows that some of our perceptual experiences do not need a direct sensory input, or an external stimulus, although, of course, the sensory context can exert a strong influence on that imagery.[53]

The idea of multisensory imagery, or neural networks that fire up to simulate perceptual experiences across the senses, is, I believe, more accurate to describe what I understand by multisensory film experience. I mean this in the sense of a perceptual experience that is not directly cued by the senses beyond sight and hearing but which uses these as entryways to experiences in the realm of the other senses. This multisensory imagery may be internally generated, but it has a material nature on the level of the brain and may imply embodied responses. This is contrary to the commonsense idea of imagination as a disembodied set of processes that takes place in the void. Imagery takes the concept of imagination further by showing the embodied presence of internally generated percepts. In the context of the multisensory experience, it is not just imagery but also concrete processing of sensory information, however indirect, because it is the result of cross-modal interactions where sight and hearing give access to thermoception, proprioceptio, nociception, and the vestibular sense, among others.

## NOTES

I am grateful to Heather Williams, Johan Magnus Elvemo, Lasse Hodne, and Torben Grodal for stimulating conversations about the topic.

1. Not to be confused with synesthesia, as this term has been used by art scholars. Synesthesia is a perceptual condition with a cross-modal nature, but multisensory perception is the general cross-modal way in which we all perceive.
2. Luis Rocha Antunes, "The Vestibular in Film: Orientation and Balance in Gus Van Sant's Cinema of Walking," *Essays in Philosophy* 13, no. 2 (2012): 522–49, doi:10.7710/1526-0569.1436.
3. Barry Dainton, *Stream of Consciousness: Unity and Continuity in Conscious Experience* (London: Routledge, 2006), 2.
4. Michael Spivey, Daniel Richardson, and Rick Dale, "Action Representation as the Bedrock of Social Cognition: A Developmental Neuroscience Perspective," in *Oxford Handbook of Human Action*, ed. Ezequiel Morsella, John A. Bargh, and Peter M. Gollwitzer (Oxford: Oxford University Press, 2008), 242.
5. Laura U. Marks, *The Skin of the Film: Intercultural Cinema, Embodiment, and the Senses* (Durham, NC: Duke University Press, 2000); Thomas Elsaesser, *Film Theory: An Introduction through the Senses* (New York: Routledge, 2010); Vivian Carol Sobchack, *The Address of the Eye: A Phenomenology of Film Experience* (Princeton, NJ: Princeton University Press, 1992); Charles Forceville and Eduardo Urios-Aparisi, eds., *Multimodal Metaphor*, Applications of Cognitive Linguistics 11 (Berlin: Mouton de Gruyter, 2009). Whereas Münsterberg talks about film perception in the sense of actual perceptual sensation, these authors refer to film perception in other senses. Marks

addresses film perception as a result of memories that filmmakers in exile use
to evoke material aspects of their cultures of origin, Elsaesser talks about film
perception as a concept that has given origin to different theories of film, Sobchack writes about the phenomenology or subjectivity of film perception, and
Forceville talks about some multimodal aspects of metaphor. My approach
here is aligned with that of Münsterberg and Arnheim. For instance, Marks
and Sobchack have a holistic idea about perceptual experience; they reject the
idea that segmented sensory modalities take place during our perception of
a film, so they address the multisensory as something that takes place within
the body, generally speaking. Moreover, that sort of diffuse perception across
the body makes them use touch as the sense that metaphorically represents
embodiment in film perception.

6. Hugo Münsterberg, *The Photoplay: A Psychological Study* (New York: D. Appleton, 1916).
7. Rudolf Arnheim, *Film as Art* (Berkeley: University of California Press, 2006).
8. I use perceptual experience of film in a different sense from film experience as meaning of cultural experience, as expressed for instance by Timothy Corrigan, *The Film Experience: An Introduction*, 3rd ed. (Boston: Bedford/ St. Martins, 2012); Miriam Hansen, *Cinema and Experience: Siegfried Kracauer, Walter Benjamin, and Theodor W. Adorno*, Weimar and Now: German Cultural Criticism 44 (Berkeley: University of California Press, 2012).
9. Münsterberg, *The Photoplay*.
10. Michel Chion, *Film, a Sound Art*, English ed. (New York: Columbia University Press, 2009).
11. Münsterberg, *The Photoplay*.
12. Ibid.
13. Tim J. Smith, "The Attentional Theory of Cinematic Continuity," *Projections* 6, no. 1 (2012): 1–27, doi:10.3167/proj.2012.060102.
14. Carl R. Plantinga and Greg M. Smith, eds., *Passionate Views: Film, Cognition, and Emotion* (Baltimore: Johns Hopkins University Press, 1999).
15. Marks, *Skin of the Film*.
16. "Studies investigating the brain areas involved in multi-sensory integration have indicated that the activity in areas traditionally considered to be modality-specific can be modulated by cross-modal signals. Again, the visual cortex has not proved an exception to this rule, having been shown to be affected by tactile and auditory stimulation." Charles Spence and Barry E. Stein, eds., *The Handbook of Multisensory Processes* (Cambridge, MA: MIT Press, 2004), 32.
17. Ibid.
18. Arnheim, *Film as Art*, 34.
19. Ibid., 133.
20. Ibid., 30.
21. Ibid., 20.
22. Ibid., 70.
23. Ibid., 71.
24. Annette Michelson, "Bodies in Space: Film as Carnal Knowledge," *Artforum* (February 1969): 54–63.
25. José Luis Bermúdez, A. J. Marcel, and Naomi Eilan, *The Body and the Self* (Cambridge, MA: MIT Press, 1998), 141.
26. Robert J. Beers, Anne C. Sittig, and Jan J. Denier, "How Humans Combine Simultaneous Proprioceptive and Visual Position Information," *Experimental Brain Research* 111, no. 2 (1996), doi:10.1007/BF00227302; J. Jeka, K.S. Oie, and T. Kiemel, "Multisensory Information for Human Postural Control: Integrating Touch and Vision," *Experimental Brain Research* 134, no. 1

(2000): 107–25. Sherrington established that there is a relationship between proprioception and other senses, namely, sight and hearing. Edward V. Evarts, "Sherrington's Concept of Proprioception," *Trends in Neurosciences* 4 (1981): 44–46, doi:10.1016/0166-2236(81)90016-3. For a review, see James R. Lakner and Barbara Shenker, "Proprioceptive Influences on Auditory and Visual Spatial Localization," *The Journal of Neuroscience* 5, no. 3 (1985): 579–83.

27. Although we are not performing the motor actions of locomotion, we are still processing and perceiving motion, and that is an orientation perceptual task related to motor processing: "Static stimulation in one modality can modulate certain aspects of the perception of dynamic in-formation in another modality." Calvert et al., *Multisensory Processes*, 64.

28. Charles Darwin, *The Expression of the Emotions in Man and Animals* (London: John Murray, 1872).

29. Calvert et al., *Multisensory Processes*, 438.

30. Jeka et al., "Multisensory Information."

31. T. M. Dijkstra et al., "Frequency Dependence of the Action-Perception Cycle for Postural Control in a Moving Visual Environment: Relative Phase Dynamics," *Biological Cybernetics* 71, no. 6 (1994): 489–501.

32. Y. P. Ivanenko, R. Grasso, and F. Lacquaniti, "Effect of Gaze on Postural Responses to Neck Proprioceptive and Vestibular Stimulation in Humans," *Journal of Physiology* 519, Pt. 1 (1999): 301–14.

33. T. Mergner, G. Nasios, and D. Anastasopoulos, "Vestibular Memory-Contingent Saccades Involve Somatosensory Input from the Body Support," *Neuroreport* 9, no. 7 (1998): 1469–73. Of course, this case does not apply directly to *2001*, as I am departing from the audiovisual version of the film, without any sort of haptic input. However, it still shows the connection between sight and proprioception in the sense that sight not only modulates proprioception, but the other way around, as well.

34. D. N. Lane and J. R. Lishman, "Visual Proprioceptive Control of Stance," *Journal of Human Movement Studies* 1, no. 2 (1975): 87–95; G. E. Butterworth and L. Hicks, "Visual Proprioception and Postural Stability in Infancy: A Developmental Study," *Perception* 6 (1977): 255–62.

35. Ivanenko et al., "Effect of Gaze."

36. Ibid., 312.

37. Lakner and Shenker, "Proprioceptive Influences," 582.

38. Ibid.

39. Virginia Brooks, "Film, Perception, and Cognitive Psychology," *Millennium Film Journal* 14, no. 15 (1984): 105.

40. See Calvert et al., *Multisensory Processes*.

41. Tim J. Smith, "Film (Cinema) Perception," in *Encyclopedia of Perception*, ed. E. Bruce Goldstein (Thousand Oaks, CA: Sage, 2010), 458–61.

42. Sascha Tyll, Eike Budinger, and Toemme Noesselt, "Thalamic Influences on Multisensory Integration," *Communicative and Integrative Biology* 4, no. 4 (2001): 378–81.

43. Martin Klasen, Yu-Han Chen, and Klaus Mathiak, "Multisensory Emotions: Perception, Combination and Underlying Neural Processes," *Reviews in the Neurosciences* 23, no. 4 (2012), doi:10.1515/revneuro-2012-0040.

44. Calvert et al., *Multisensory Processes*.

45. M. A. Meredith and B. E. Stein, "Visual, Auditory, and Somatosensory Convergence on Cells in Superior Colliculus Results in Multisensory Integration," *Journal of Neurophysiology* 56, no. 3 (1986): 640–62.

46. Barry E. Stein and M. Alex Meredith, *The Merging of the Senses* (Cambridge, MA: MIT Press, 1993).

47. Calvert et al., *Multisensory Processes*, 248.

48. Stein and Meredith, *Merging*, 365–66.
49. Ibid., 9.
50. Uri Hasson, "Intersubject Synchronization of Cortical Activity during Natural Vision," *Science* 303, no. 5664 (2004): 1634–40, doi:10.1126/science.1089506.
51. Huan Luo, Zuxiang Liu, and David Poeppel, "Auditory Cortex Tracks Both Auditory and Visual Stimulus Dynamics Using Low-Frequency Neuronal Phase Modulation," ed. Robert Zatorre, *PLoS Biology* 8, no. 8 (2010): 8, doi:10.1371/journal.pbio.1000445.
52. Simon Lacey, *Multisensory Imagery* (New York: Springer, 2013).
53. "Perception is not, therefore, a fixed concept, as it is significantly modulated by many contextual factors such as multisensory information, past experiences, internal predictions, associations, ongoing motor behavior, spatial relations, and the nature of the task itself." Calvert et al., *Multisensory Processes*, 135.

# 5 The Reverberatory Narrative
## Toward Story as a Multisensory Network

*Dana Coester*

## STORYVILLE

The bus was crowded and without air conditioning in the middle of July, lurching in fits and starts from LaGuardia to Midtown as I made my crooked journey to Chelsea Market to pick up a beta device for Google's *Project Glass*. I hadn't slept for thirty-six hours, having been on two coasts and four cities in less than a week, and I leaned wearily against the bus window as the city, a mirage of heat-shimmering density, coalesced before my eyes. I began to daydream a different landscape as it might be experienced through augmented reality. Not with Glass. Not yet. I imagined a more distant futurescape of a city lay bare, with all its stories and data and secrets and signage hovering unseen in an invisible digital layer I could access at will.

I smiled at my unintentional reference to New York City's ultimate cliché: there are eight million stories in the naked city. I followed this train of thought to the esoteric 1950s Situationists' project, *The Naked City*,[1] which was part of an artistic and political movement to deconstruct, and reconstruct, urban identity through re-writing and re-contextualizing maps, narratives, networks, and what the authors deemed the "detritus" of a city's life. That the project's imprint was hopelessly ephemeral was part of its appeal, but it suddenly seemed like a half-century-old idea with a promise of resurrection in augmented reality. I made a mental note to revisit *The Naked City* project as a model for an interactive database narrative and assumed its original authors would likely roll over in their graves at the notion. Or delight in it, I wasn't sure which.

I returned my thoughts to the city outside my window. I imagined my view from the simplest perspective of what augmented reality proposes, and saw it transform as all the signage before me fell away. At first I was pleased to see ill-designed billboards disappear, and the layers of mismatched signs evaporate one by one. But as the chaos of advertisements and way-finding cues receded in my reconfigured landscape, I thought, no . . . wait . . . I want to keep the hand-lettered cardboard sign in the window of a shop that tenderly honors an anonymous vet. I want to keep that crudely stenciled graffiti rose with its tangle of thorns on the corner lightpost.

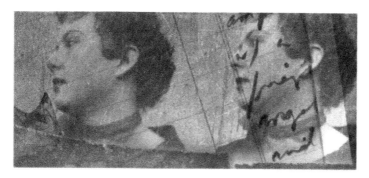

My stories are unravelling. Beads spilling everywhere.

*Figure 5.1*   Opening Photo Illustration Integrating Text and Image, *Pretty* (1998)

I realized, of course, this is precisely the challenge Google faces as it seeks to render unseen data into meaningful, appropriately contextualized experiences for one human at a time. I conducted an inventory of what to keep and what to discard, and wondered: Where in the data of the environment, or, as *The Naked City* project explored, where in that debris and data exhaust of a city's life, do the hidden, the intimate stories live? And then I realized: I was on the last leg of a journey I'd started in 1989.

## PAPER TO GLASS

Over nearly three decades, my interest in fragmented, dispersed, and non-linear narrative has found expression in a series of transmedia works I titled *Pretty*. This evolving series has employed print, film, installation, and digital practices in the assembling and disassembling of lyric essays, poetry, graphic design, photography, and physical artifacts in an experimental documentary of memory, time, and story across media.

This experimental series was naively influenced by a reading of John Anderson's article "The Spreading Activation Theory of Memory."[2] My exposure to this theory was incidental, a reading in a linguistics course. Nonetheless, the theory, which proposed a branching, associative, impressionistic model of memory, set me on a collision path with technology disruption in my field and eventually compelled me to envision new approaches to journalism that performed in digital space in ways that were metaphors for brain space, and which inadvertently anticipated narrative possibilities for journalism in our emerging landscape of augmented reality. This model profoundly altered my trajectory as a young journalist and reframed storytelling in journalism for me as a practice that could operate as nonlinear narrative networks rather than as linear narrative sequences. I began to look to cognitive studies and neuroscience to describe, not brain maps, but *experience networks* that would parallel new forms of digital storytelling and that inevitably brought this work to my current experiments in augmented reality with wearable technology.


**REMEMBRANCE**


Two poets, an art historian, and three photographers were coming to dinner—the evening was intended to be an assembly of different perspectives for Roland Barthes's "The Rhetoric of the Image,"[3] a text we were enthusiastically exploring in a photojournalism seminar. It was 1989, and for visual journalists, it was becoming clear in those early, heady days of the digital revolution that narrative lived equally in analog, digital, and not-yet-cataloged dimensions. We had just begun to abandon darkrooms and had traded the alchemy of light and film for images captured in alterable coded algorithms. Our early whirring Apple machines invoked an entirely new alchemy of creation, and we were beginning to explore the very particles of stories and image, now visible in code. While my colleagues wrung their hands and fretted in what is still an ongoing lament for the loss of traditional journalism practice, for a newly minted journalist with a copy of PageMaker and access to a color Xerox machine, the media world was sweet.

The digital revolution was upon us. The world of typographers, designers, and photographers had changed forever; darkrooms went dark, and professionals lamented the rise of dilettante visual journalists. It was the first wave of amateur-produced content, "citizen media," and few welcomed it with open arms. Professional journalists held their noses and predicted the demise of, well, just about everything. In retrospect, I realize their anxiety stemmed in part from what they perceived to be the loss of a precise, controlled, construct of meaning—a concern at odds with the impressionistic new forms of digital design at the time that favored illegibility over clarity, and ambiguity over certainty. That move toward deconstruction was perfectly expressed through the destruction of typography characterized by the graphic design of digital renegade David Carson. Carson's alternative magazine *RayGun*, which debuted in 1992, represented exactly what professionals feared: this is what happens to content when a dilettante with no formal schooling takes the wheel of newly accessible technology. A surfing icon, Carson influenced communication design in the 1990s with his unique assemblages bridging digital and analog worlds, deftly wielding a Xerox machine and an X-Acto blade to build digital/print assemblages that obscured the point at which print ended and digital began. While my contemporaries predictably dismissed this design chaos as amateur visual noise, to my admiring eye, his experimental, layered and virtually illegible work communicated precisely without a precision of form.

This fed a notion that was just beginning to take shape in my own work—that something broken entirely into fragments could nevertheless impart a compelling and cohesive narrative experience "as is." And while this comfort with chaos and deconstruction may have been alive and well throughout the twentieth-century art world, it was anathema to journalism practice, which favored linearity, an aspiration to objectivity, and controlled narrative formulas designed for an economy of production for print or broadcast media.

At the same time, the Poynter Institute was engaged with its first of many laser "eye-track" studies that revealed how associative the reading path is across and within media. Its key findings seem primitive now—that a reader intuitively constructs meaning from what is essentially a dance of nonlinear reading.[4] It was part of the revolution at hand. And to young, newly digital journalists, it began to free our stories from their century-old constraints.

> The dinner did not happen as planned. A hidden story derailed what may otherwise have been an ordinary winter night and ultimately solidified my inquiry into the potential nature of stories as mere fragments of things:
>
> The poet phoned within hours of dinner and abruptly declined the invitation. In an odd collusion of passions, she revealed she could not attend because the art historian was the victim of a mutual student's stalking. She did not use the term stalking frivolously. It was a fully blown police matter. The poet feared her presence would, under the intermittently clouded light of a mad man's scrutiny, become unreasonably significant. An act of deliberate taunting. A sign of betrayal. Or who knew? She had no wish to feed the insatiable preoccupation that hungered for meaning in every object and every gesture. She described a box the stalker kept where he collected items of misplaced desire. I imagined the inventory: A clothing fiber, strand of hair, lipstick stain, pencil stolen from a desk, a note or two. Each ambiguous at best, yet cherished as evidence of something more.
>
> Years later, when I sifted through a shoebox containing the relics of my husband's and my courtship, I recalled the box the poet described and how we shook our heads sadly at the spectacle of madness. How clearly we saw the boundary the other crossed blindly. Still, it seemed that the box in my lap was a similar harbor of unresolved yearnings. It housed a body of proof accumulated once in its sole intention to attest to our very existence. A jumble of postmarks; a lock of hair; a folded tissue tinged with blood; a tin of aspirin with a note tucked inside; sheaths of negatives where I gazed into his eyes. In horror, for a moment I feared I was as mistaken as that mad man—that I had been

comforted for years by mere props to a delusion. Wasn't all of this—and then I glanced about wildly at what seemed to be the stuff of a marriage: A stranger's tangled debris of cameras on the dining table, a man's large shoes empty by the door—wasn't all of this evidence of our own story?

When for that brief moment I inhabited two separate realms of the very details that bind the stories we imagine to the stories we live, I knew fully the stalker's devotion to his chain of evidence. For the stalker, this flimsy preservation of an imagined story is what tethered him, not to madness, but to reality. Proof of such, damaged pieces of it, to be sure, and tangled in a box, but link by link, the genuine artifacts of having loved. That he had not been loved in return was sadly true enough . . . but it was not the only story to be told.

Our stories are unraveling, I mused. Reassembling them in digital space became a dance of meaning comprised, not of facts and anecdotes and analysis, but one of algorithms, meta tags, contextualized data and layers in nonlinear editing timelines. As a journalist and an art director, my world was already populated with images and content. I experimented daily with

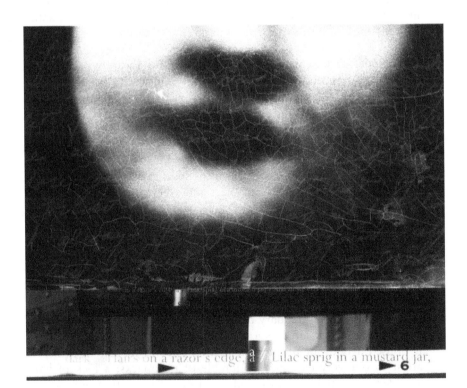

*Figure 5.2*   Overleaf Illustration for Manuscript Merging Film, Documents, and Photographs of Three Women over Three Generations, *Pretty* (1998)

the storytelling properties of the emerging technology and digital tools of the time. I began to contemplate how to use content and artifacts to construct identity and locate stories not only in time and place, but also within platforms, and then eventually within devices themselves. We began to consider that interface was synonymous with story. These confluences nudged me toward a sort of armchair Cubist approach to journalism practice itself: if the Cubists aimed to show objects as the mind, rather than the eye, perceives them, I aimed to impart experience as the mind perceives it, rather than as a journalist reconstructs it. I looked explicitly to Anderson's spreading activation theory of memory for inspiration to this alternative approach and began to experiment.

## STORY AS CONTEXTUALIZED DATA

Anderson's spreading activation theory of memory presented an early model for semantic and contextual relationships that construct meaning—and for my purposes, narrative—by "elaborating" on context through interwoven events in memory and experience, and in which these associations are expressed in terms of weight, or by which "experience establishes a network of nodes connected by links of varying strengths." Anderson also considered a role for images and words as "temporal strings" and which serve as encoded elements of a larger "cognitive unit." For the purposes of envisioning this in a journalism context, I substituted the concept of "the story" in place of the larger "cognitive unit."

Although Anderson's theory proposed a process by which memories are stored and retrieved (and concerned itself primarily with degrees to which this process functions), it intriguingly described a "memory network" that to my journalist's eye provided an impressionistic model for an experience network that could travel across media platforms and by which an experience (or story "at large") might be "retrieved" from discrete, coded elements.

I began experimenting with media inspired by the following process, as described by Anderson, for a viewer's retrieval of a coherent story:

> Memory phenomena can be understood in network structures that encode the to-be-recalled facts and the network structures which surround these fact encodings. . . . When part of a cognitive unit is formed in long-term memory, all of it is encoded. Similarly, when part of a cognitive unit is retrieved from long-term memory, all of it is.

This suggested to me that I might be able to trust fragments of a story to represent the whole, and this became the essential experiment of the documentary and transmedia series *Pretty* as it moved through media, technology, and time.

## FRAGMENTS

To illuminate the implications for journalism practice gleaned through this extended documentary experiment, it is necessary to describe *Pretty* across its platforms (installation, print, film, and digital) and to provide a brief overview of the narrative threads that composed the work.

Its original form was as an installation at the photography gallery *Agnes* in Birmingham, Alabama in 1993. Titled "Undressing Audrey," it was a reading experience in which the viewer had to physically "undress" the book, slipping text from a woman's garments, one button and layer at a time, and moving through the photographic evidence of a hidden love affair from 1924. Once "undressed," the pages of this artist's book were unbound and allowed a series of unique readings by every viewer. In this primitive analog precursor to digital interactivity, the actions of each user shuffled

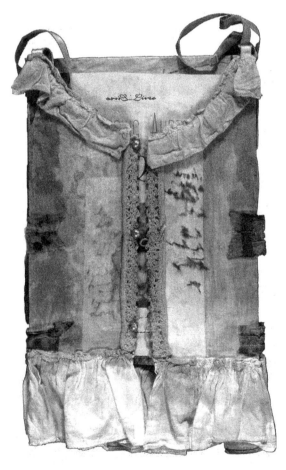

*Figure 5.3*  "Undressing Audrey" (1993)

and reshuffled the content with each reading to cue a unique experience for the next reader.

In its next incarnation in print media, the original poem, "Undressing Audrey," was extended and incorporated into more than 102 illustrations, artifacts, and mixed media assemblages. In a gesture to nonlinearity, the 104 pages of the book remained unbound and placed in a limited edition box to replicate the ability for readers to rearrange content, which remained central to the experience of both the installation artwork the book, and later the film and digital works.

> Our words fell away from us like pages being torn from a book. I gathered the pages up like an archaeologist and read the story backward. Tomorrow we will pause on the stairs of a walkup apartment in 1989 as we once again make the path from kitchen to bed—though it is forever incomplete when we stumble out from under all the desire we'd cooked up at the stove with anchovies and garlic and the breadstuff of hunger and sink into the murmurings of a familiar story, a story being erased as it was told.

Through all of these interpretations, *Pretty* relied on a layered structure that attempted to approximate the original installation experience through a series of overlapping narrative threads that could be sorted and resorted by different contexts and media types, such as time, place, character, artifact, image, audio, and video, among others.

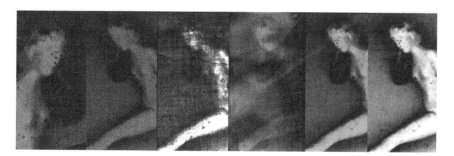

*Figure 5.4* One-Legged Figurine, *Pretty* (1998)

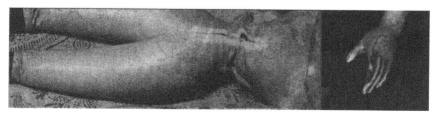

*Figure 5.5* "Torso and Hand," *Pretty* (1998)

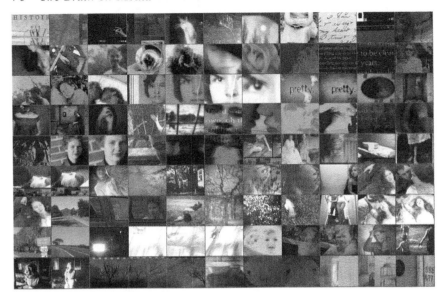

*Figure 5.6*   Selected Multimedia Stills, *Pretty* (2009)

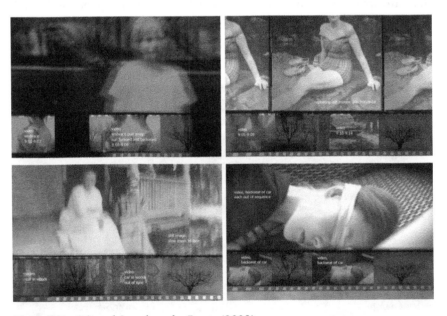

*Figure 5.7*   Selected Storyboards, *Pretty* (2009)

While *Pretty* as a body of work is situated most comfortably in art or literary worlds, it is important to realize that the work was a deliberate challenge to conventions of journalism practice in the 1990s. *Pretty* was intended to be an experimental documentary by a journalist, and not an artwork by an artist.

Documentation, in the form of letters, photographs, video footage, recounted memories, and artifacts, are presented in a series of loosely associated, fragmented vignettes, which are connected by similar "interwoven and web-like structures" as inspired by Anderson's model. Similar to the emerging organization of information in digital content, in which a "weighted list" or

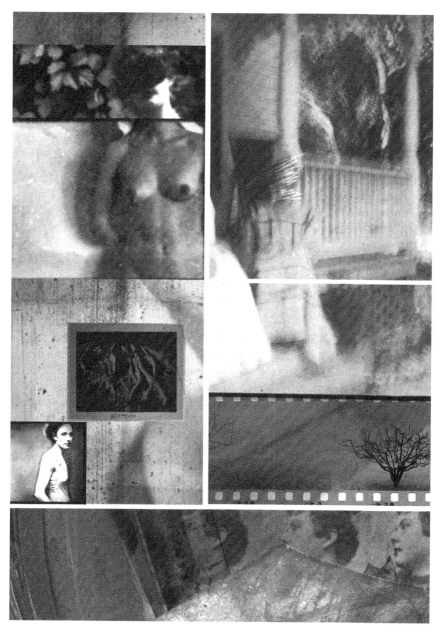

*Figure 5.8*　Page Layout, *Pretty* (1998)

"tag clouds," which emerged as early as the experimental novel *Microserfs*,[5] *Pretty* employed a visual reference for organizing narrative and conformed to the intensely visual approach a designer takes to weighting and ranking meaning, or what graphic designers often refer to as "editing by design."[6]

Although experimental in its multimedia forms, *Pretty* was firmly rooted in the content-driven design traditions that inform classical print media design, in which layouts can be envisioned as streams of competing information presented simultaneously, yet containing strategic visual cues that establish information hierarchy. In this regard, it can be argued that design has always been an associative, "nonlinear" narrative form that makes liberal use of graphically implied webs of context to impart meta-narratives within the meaning-making architecture of a page itself.

## THE TRANSPARENT STORY

This experiment across forms began to suggest that however more deeply we deconstruct content, its nature breaks further down still. I began to muse on content as clusters of like information across an increasingly networked digital space (albeit still in its infancy at that time). Within this emerging spatial metaphor, I began to imagine content as associated networks acquiring density and coalescing under the weight of their own context . . . stories as bodies harboring their own peculiar gravity. I imagined digital content as behaving like matter, pulling in disparate stories, words, images and content along strings of context in a universe of possible narratives.

In *Pretty's* translation from installation to print to film to digital, this called to mind David Boje's *systemicity*, in which he describes a "holographic" narrative form expressed as the "dynamic unfinished, unfinalized, and unmergedness" of content, in which meaning emerges from the "interactivity of complexity properties with storytelling and narrative processes."[7]

Echoing this concept, I frequently described *Pretty* as a process, not a product, and that its intent was not so much to *tell* a story but rather to *accumulate* one. This process reflected parallel literary approaches to hypernarrative that emerged in the 1980s, such as in the experimental narrative database work *Uncle Roger*. In this classic 1986 piece, users were able to access the narrative through keywords, reflecting the contextual relationship established through weighted, semantic content in which narratives operated as networks rather than linear sequences.[8] At the time, I think we may have crudely understood this work to merely allow for alternative endings as a simple variation on a conventional narrative form. However, the creator of *Uncle Roger*, Judy Malloy, compellingly describes her work as much more than that: "I thought of this work as a pool of information into which the reader plunges repeatedly, emerging with a cumulative and individual picture . . . to build up levels of meaning and to show many aspects of the story and characters, rather than as a means of providing alternate plot turns and endings."[9]

It should be noted that Malloy is talking about a literary experiment in 1986 in ways that aptly describe current new practices in journalism narrative, such as the 2010 launch of Storify, an application that allows users to aggregate social media content into a timeline and add additional context curated by users into a dynamically associated story. With the advent of Google's Glass and other wearable technology, we are ushering in an era of immersive, contextualized data driven experiences that bridge the physical, digital, and sensory realms. The devices and applications for creating narratives that span these realms haven't been fully harnessed or even created yet. But there are relevant precedents in these early experimental works by artists, media makers, and technologists that offer alternative paths converging on stories that aren't told but rather are accumulated.

Additionally, an intriguing attribute of Anderson's model illuminated the potential inherent flexibility and stability in the notion of an experiential—or as I was beginning to imagine—a reverberatory story. As described by Anderson, this model "allows activation to reverberate back" and that "contrary to many people's intuitions, these reverberatory possibilities do not change expectations about a stable pattern of activation."

Pre Storify, I began to wonder if these reverberatory possibilities could have implications for harnessing complex, real-time narratives in digital space. In *Pretty*, I'd intended that a loosely choreographed approach accounting for these reverberatory properties—rather than being fragmented, disordered, and chaotic—would impart a transparency of experience. Although this clearly disrupts the conventional structure of an event recounted, it may also suggest a process by which journalists can interact with these properties to choreograph narrative without attempting to re-unite fragments into a whole—allowing this "whole" to emerge across digital, physical, and sensory spaces, its reverberatory, meaning-making properties latent.

An unharnessed example of this possibility is suggested in the chaos of an unfolding event, such as the 2013 Boston marathon bombings. My own experience of this event, as for many of us, was through a tapestry of sources, weaving together direct experience, Twitter feeds, Reddit threads, televised newscasts, citizen media, social media, and other sources. As noted earlier, the application Storify, explicitly, if yet primitively, attempts to harness and amplify these sources as a sense-making, story-making tool, in which the construction of the story is as a network of associations rather than as an event recounted.

This approach in *Pretty* intended to impart a *transparency* of memory, which would disintermediate the act of a memory *recounted* by replacing it with a purer representation of memory *experienced*. This relied on Anderson's faith in the reverberatory properties of memory as well as the premise that memory phenomena can be retrieved as whole networks, and that parts of networks can adequately, and simultaneously, convey the whole.

As one viewer noted in response to a viewing of *Pretty*, "what you sacrifice in clarity you make up for with access to emotional experience."

## PUBLISH THE CITY

Descriptions of how narrative, memory, and consciousness perform in the brain have been refined considerably since the spreading activation theory of memory inspired this meandering experiment nearly twenty-five years ago. One development is the increased understanding of our ability to have unified perceptual experiences when the data that informs these unified perceptions remains highly fragmented in the brain itself. This extends Anderson's and others work to suggest that memory is composed of weighted associations and that the form of a memory itself is not so much an encoded event, but discrete bits of information expressed as relations between and among things.

Neuroscientist Antonio Damasio addresses the seeming paradox, long called the binding problem, in which unified perception can emerge from fragmented data in his description of the making of a memory: "We need to find systems in the brain where signals related to all these different things can converge and code for the simultaneity of the events. Later, converging signals can be reactivated and sent back to the regions they came from, reconstructing a paler version of the original experience."[10]

Although Damasio is speaking narrowly to the behavior of the brain, and I am taking liberties in borrowing this as metaphor, my response as an experimenting journalist is to wonder, might this also be the potential behavior of *story*? Aren't we, as journalists, in our navigation of new platforms, new technology, new forms *"looking for systems where signals related to all these different things can converge and code for the simultaneity of events?"*

Alexis Madrigal, in his piece for *The Atlantic*, asserts the as yet unsolved challenge for intercepting raw data and making sense of it (the meaning-making role that journalists, artists, and others have historically played as part of information ecosystems devoted to rendering our experiences into stories of some sort): "No one publishes a city. They publish a magazine or a book or a news site."[11]

There exists profound potential for new journalism applications that make use of the distribution of content and data across media, between and among threads, and among networks that include neural networks but also social networks and geophysical networks that more closely correlate with direct experience itself. It is reasonable to wonder whether the methods by which journalists have historically structured content in an effort to establish immutable contexts or facsimiles of truth may now counter the potential accessibility, accuracy, and immediacy of experience itself—and that alternative methods may now be available to us as we embark upon ways to "publish the city."

Damasio's, Anderson's, and others' observations about the brain's comfort with stories as merely linked fragments suggest new paths toward data excavation tools that render meaning through increasingly thin interfaces between our brains and our environments. Computer and cognitive scientists notwithstanding, artists, poets, and essayists have long described the fragmented, associative nature of story and have, in their own ways, anticipated the potential of data based narratives in online, digital, and now augmented reality environments. The sense of Boje's "holographic" narrative, Malloy's "pool of information," and Anderson's "interconnected network" independently described the latent meaning-making power of dispersed and fragmented content as a multisensory, or as photo scholar Andrea Noble described, "multisensual" experience, and which may give rise to a new journalism's "alternative ways of knowing."[12]

It was a relatively recent leap for digital journalists to recognize that story was linked to interface at all, the prevailing conceit of "content is king" obscuring an awareness of the invisible spaces between content. This remains a rocky transition in our field; moving journalists to a realization that technology is not merely a tool, and that stories do not live independent of device, user behavior or the very networks data moves through. It is an even greater leap to come to the realization that technology interface is becoming an increasingly thin (and in the case of Glass, transparent) boundary between our senses and our stories. For journalists to marginalize that as a gimmick or "just a tool" is to marginalize the senses, the stories, and the storytellers themselves.

## NOTES

1. Guy Debord, *Psychogeographic Guide of Paris* (Denmark: Permild and Rosengreen, 1955).
2. John R. Anderson, "A Spreading Activation Theory of Memory," *Journal of Verbal Learning and Verbal Behavior* 22, no. 3 (1983): 261–95, doi:10.1016/S0022-5371(83)90201-3.
3. Roland Barthes, "Rhetoric of the Image," in *Image—Music—Text*, 32–51 (New York: Hill and Wang, 1977).
4. Mario R. Garcia, *Eyes on the News* (St. Petersburg, FL: Poynter Institute for Media Studies, 1991).
5. Douglas Coupland, *Microserfs* (New York: Harper Perennial, 2008).
6. Jan V. White, *Editing by Design: Word-and-Picture Communication for Editors and Designers* (New York: R.R. Bowker, 1974).
7. David M. Boje, *Narrative Methods for Organizational and Communication Research* (London: Sage, 2001).
8. N. Katherine Hayles, "Situating Narrative in an Ecology of New Media," *MFS Modern Fiction Studies* 43, no. 3 (1997): 573–76, doi:10.1353/mfs.1997.0059.
9. Judy Malloy, "Hypernarrative in the Age of the Web," National Endowment for the Arts, http://www.well.com/user/jmalloy/neapaper.html.
10. Antonio R. Damasio, *Self Comes to Mind: Constructing the Conscious Brain* (New York: Vintage Books, 2012).
11. Alexis C. Madrigal, "The World Is Not Enough: Google and the Future of Augmented Reality," *The Atlantic*, October 25, 2012, http://www.theatlantic.com/technology/archive/2012/10/the-world-is-not-enough-google-and-the-future-of-augmented-reality/264059/.
12. Alex Hughes and Andrea Noble, eds., *Phototextualities: Intersections of Photography and Narrative*, 1st ed. (Albuquerque: University of New Mexico Press, 2003).

# 6  Embodied Protonarratives Embedded in Systems of Contexts
## A Neurocinematic Approach

*Pia Tikka and Mauri Kaipainen*

## INTRODUCTION: CINEMA AS NARRATIVE WORLD MODEL

Cinematic narratives can be regarded as simulations or models of the world,[1] as even in its most incredible creative visions, cinema generally represents a kind of intersubjectively shared prototype of life. The stories people engage with in narratives typically recycle the experiential knowledge of the everyday social encounters.[2] This is enhanced with one's experiential knowledge of the repetitive patterns of cultural conventions, such as universal stories or film genres. The emergent interaction dynamics of the viewer and the continuously unfolding cinematic narrative form a kind of media ecology, which we argue is to a great extent intersubjectively shared between people. Our conception of media ecology draws from, on one hand, Neisser's cognitive ecology,[3] and, on the other, the McLuhanian concept of media ecology,[4] and is further associated with more recent views of the embodied mind proposed by Varela and collaborators.[5] The inherently temporal nature of narrative experience is characterized by the notion of nowness, as discussed in Varela's neurophenomenological interpretation of philosopher Husserl's experiential structure of temporality and his terms of retention and protention, which usefully describe the dynamical nature of the present moment between the past and the future.[6] In accordance with these theoretical approaches, we have adopted the holistic idea of human being in inseparable continuous interactive coupling with its environment as the fundamental prerequisite for the emergence of narrative cognition.

Cognitive neuroscientists are in an increasing manner applying audiovisual video recordings, interactive games, or movies as stimuli for studying human brain functions in "naturalistic" situations. The attribute "naturalistic," adopted from psychology, refers to experimental situations that aim to bypass the unavoidably artificial and isolated conditions in the neuroimaging laboratories. Such studies typically use complex audiovisual stimuli for creating engaging situations associated more closely to everyday life than is the case with the more traditional stimuli of artificial sounds, abstract test grids, or still images. In the explorative setting of the *free-viewing* paradigm, the test subjects are even not asked to conduct any task but just to view the movie, while their brain behavior is scanned by means of functional magnetic resonance imaging (fMRI). This chapter frames the discussion to a particular approach in naturalistic neuroscience, the *neurocinematics*, coined by Hasson and colleagues.[7] The approach aims at understanding how the established methods of filmmaking and storytelling allow manipulating the intersubjectively shared narrative processes between viewers, even despite their idiosyncratic differences.

According to the *intersubjectivity argument*, human behavior relies to a significant degree on neurobehavioral patterns that relate to the most basic characteristics of being human, such as security, social bonding, or everyday bodily functions and needs. These aspects are likely to have been conditioned by the ontogenetic and phylogenetic evolution of *Homo sapiens* throughout the existence of the species. From the neuroimaging point of view, the significant benefit of movies is that, unlike life itself, same situations can be repeated cross several people allowing the quantification of how similarly they respond to the stimuli. The notion of *intersubjective correlation* refers to the neuroscientifically identified neural phenomenon where the brain activity of viewers is relatively similar and thus in synchrony with each other when viewing the same film sequence.[8]

Until lately, one of the biggest challenges of using naturalistic stimuli with long durations has been the enormous size of brain data collected during any individual experiment.[9] However, due to the rapidly advanced computer capacity together with effective data collection and analysis methods, the challenge of naturalistic neuroscience has gradually shifted from the management of large data sets to the issue of how to match the significant aspects of the stimulus content with the brain data. As we seek to demonstrate in the following, film narrative, an art of conceptualizing storytelling, can guide neurocinematics toward more natural ways of annotating temporal content.

## PROTONARRATIVES AND NEURAL EVENTS

Narratives are essentially temporal sequences of events. Cognitive segmentation of continuous narratives, such as movies, into meaningful sequences, or shorter events, is seemingly an in-built mechanism related to intersubjectively shared sense-making schemata. The event segmentation theory[10] applies the concepts of *event models* and *event schemata* to describe representations of what is happening now and representations of semantic knowledge about events in general, respectively. Zacks and colleagues propose that stimulus-driven event segmentation occurs when the viewers recognize changes in time, space, objects, or character behavior as an onset for a new event.[11] These can be associated with cognitive bottom-up processes. Top-down attention-driven regulation, in turn, allows assuming event continuity based on prior knowledge about ongoing action-goal relations, causes, and intentions, even when there are discontinuities in the stimulus. In line with Zacks and colleagues, in the present discussion we consider *protonarratives*[12] as the smallest events, whose narrative meaningfulness can be identified within the continuous sequence of rich movie stimulus. In our view, the concept of protonarrative is instrumental as a heuristics for the segmentation of film content into shortest meaningful events.

The protonarrative provides a means to identify meaningful events, which support the story coherence and justify character behavior, actions, and decisions. For example, the moment when two people shake hands constitutes a protonarrative that has duration of a few seconds. Protonarratives are closely associated with intersubjectively shared patterns of human behavior and social interactions as they manifest in movies, allowing viewers to recognize and identify with in a largely equal manner. They can therefore be considered as building bricks of the overall narrative, due to their a priori determined significance. They refer to physical and situational engagement with the surrounding world, and they often relate to and gain their semantic significance from spatial and embodied *metaphors*,[13] such as "following a path" or "falling like a stone." In this sense, they form the basis for a narrative "language." As an example of how protonarratives can relate to broader contexts, the protonarrative of rejection (a person turning away from another person in a negative manner) or the protonarrative of eating (lifting a spoon from a soup bowl to one's mouth) is sufficient to be recognized in an eyeblink and on a relatively low level of abstraction. However, independent protonarratives only become interrelated and provide explanatory contexts for each other when organized by montage (editing) and thereby contributing to narrative coherence and continuity.

Based on the recent neuroscientific findings,[14] we assume that the short temporal receptive windows (TRW) in the brain determine the neural duration of protonarratives. The TRW of a cortical microcircuit is defined as "the length of time before a response during which sensory information may affect that response."[15] While in the earlier sensory areas, TRW can be described in milliseconds, the higher cognitive regions, such as posterior lateral sulcus (LS), temporal parietal junction (TPJ), and frontal eye field (FEF), responded to information accumulated over longer durations ($\approx$36 s) than, for instance, superior temporal sulcus (STS) and precuneus ($\approx$12 s).[16] Consider, for instance, the immediate response to seeing the event of a snake moving on the ground as a shortest possible protonarrative. Altogether, these studies allow the overall hypothesis that the more complex the contextual embedding of a protonarrative, the longer the duration of the TRW of neural processing. We go further assuming that while the protonarrative "snake moving" carries highly prioritized ecological validity related to staying alive, the richer the content and the longer the context-bearing temporal durations, the higher is the situational and social validity of the event-level narrative stimulus. At the same time, however, the cost of this is that interpretation of the brain activity against the narrative becomes more demanding. Based on the accumulated evidence, two human brain functions appear to contribute to the understanding of narrative, namely, *mirroring* and *mentalizing*.[17] These complementary aspects of neural dynamics are discussed in the following sections.

## MIRRORING AS EMBODIMENT OF PROTONARRATIVES

Neural *mirroring* refers to the brain phenomenon of same neural networks activating when a person performs an action and when she just views same action performed by another person.[18] This amounts to simulating other people's behavior based on brain activity deeply anchored to corresponding own motor activity, a phenomenon of a deeply embodied nature. The phenomenon of neural mirroring has been considered as the foundation of social interaction.[19] Furthermore, as the neural mechanism behind the human ability to imitate the others, it may also be the embodied basis of learning[20] and of language.[21] From the point of view of cinema, mirroring can be seen as the basis of the viewer's ability to identify with the goal-directed actions of the screen characters even beyond visual observation. For example, merely hearing words is enough to activate motor areas that they are associated with.[22]

Neurocinematics studies have shown that viewing other people in action, we tend to look particularly at their faces, hands, and body movements in an intersubjctively synchronized manner.[23] Intersubjectively shared brain processes of action observation not only appear to form the neural foundations of understanding other people, but can be assumed to support the identification of protonarratives as events structures on the neural level of embodied simulation. Obviously, mirroring is then one of the very universally shared neural prerequisites of cinematic art, at the same time anchoring to each viewer's own embodied experience. We also suggest that the phenomenon of mirroring also contributes to the experience of *nowness* constituted by protonarratives. Relying on Merleau-Ponty's conceptualization of nowness as an anchoring to the environment,[24] protonarrative nowness does not occur in context-void vacuum. This, together with the technical possibility of viewing entire films in experimental neuroimaging settings, demands for methods to account for long-span context dependency in term of retention and anticipatory protention.

## MENTALIZING AS CONTEXTUALIZATION OF PROTONARRATIVES

The cognitive function of *mentalizing*[25] relies on the idea that human mind is fundamentally context dependent, continuously reflecting the ongoing events and changes in the environment against the previous experiences in order to predict what happens next. In the neurocinematic discourse, mentalizing refers to cognitive construction of narrative, for example, elaborated inferences about screen character's intentions and motivations. Mentalizing harnesses the momentarily present experiential information and accumulated contextual information of the (story) world for constructing consequent anticipations for future narrative events.

While mirroring, with its roots in evolution, refers to automated neural reactions, mentalizing is usually interpreted against contextual situatedness. Mentalizing allows inferences about narrative events even in their absence from the screen. These aspects can be studied by focusing on basic bodily actions, such as grasping an object, in different context. Becchio and colleagues noticed that socially intended movements elicited stronger activation both in the brain areas associated to mirroring and mentalizing compared to non-social movements. Even in the absence of context information, "social information conveyed by action kinematics modulates intention processing, leading to a transition from mirroring to mentalizing."[26]

The cultural tradition of storytelling assumes that the listeners or the viewers are aware that the story they live by is fiction. Indeed, following Frijda and Tan, one of the necessary preconditions of narrative media ecology is the *interest* to listen or view people interacting with one another in a situation that one *both* knows *and* recognizes as enacted "as if," or "pretended."[27] Whitehead and others showed that pretend-play of, for instance, showing videos with someone playing banjo with a tennis racket, activated additional areas "previously associated with theory of mind tasks and listening to narrative" (including medial prefrontal cortex, posterior STS and temporal poles), while videos of playing tennis with a tennis racket involved mirror system regions.[28] Gazzaniga has proposed that there is a interpreter in the brain that fills up gaps and missing information for the favor of constructing coherent narratives. This is the case even by the expense of truth, thus resulting stories that make sense but are false.[29] For instance, in the psychiatric practice traumatized people are known to invent coherent false stories about past painful experiences.

In itself, the role of context as the condition of behavior has been recognized along the history of psychology. In a limited sense, context was already a part of Pavlov's experiments and behaviorist conditioning. More relevantly, at least since the 1980s, context effects have been studied by means of priming tasks, in which the priming stimuli is presented before the presentation of the actual stimuli. Priming that immediately precedes the measurement thus sets a context condition for the actual stimulus. However, these experiments have typically used artificial stimuli, such as short sounds or still images, open to the criticism concerning the ecological validity.

The effects of context are well known in the art of cinema. As Pavlov's contemporary the Russian film director Lev Kuleshov demonstrated, the viewer's response to faces is not fixed but varies depending on various contextual factors. The same neutral face of a man (Ivan Nozhukin) together with either a bowl of soup, a child, or a woman in coffin resulted in three different interpretations of the man's emotions and situation.[30] Contextual factors determine emotional attributions[31] and whether the faces of people are assumed a priori to be hostile or friendly.[32] Well known to storytellers and filmmakers, the better the context is framed by the cinematographic methods (plot, camera, sound design, editing, etc.), the better the attention of the viewers is controlled. In the circumstances of such guidance, even the viewers' brain responses to the same event are similar to each other.[33] In terms of temporal durations, observations of mentalizing may well match with broader scales of cinema narratives beyond the immediate nowness, in which chains of individual events take place and are interpreted against their contexts.

Free viewing of films in an fMRI scanner has allowed studying the context dependency of human brain functions in increasingly broader and therewith more ecologically valid conditions. As an example, Lahnakoski and colleagues found differences in intersubject correlation between two groups that viewed the same film clip but with different narrative priming. When the viewers were primed to assume the role of a crime detective, or alternatively that of a set decorator, their brain activation was different correspondingly.[34] This result suggests that the mental perspective from which the viewer observes the social interaction of other people matters and can be detected in the brain.

Several studies seem to confirm that the more complex the stimulus content and higher contextualization level, the more global the brain's involvement. For example, Xu and colleagues showed that this was the case with reading of words, sentences, and full narratives in fMRI, respectively. In addition, they saw the increase in right hemisphere activation correlate with the contextual complexity and seemingly related to the story resolution, while left hemisphere was more involved in the onset of the narrative meaning-making process.[35] Beyond language, the same relation seems to hold also with cinematic stimuli. As mentioned earlier, the studies of TRWs in the brain imply a correlation of a spatial hierarchy and a scale of frequency bands in brain signals, the highest frequencies occurring mainly in the posterior and lowest in the most anterior parts of the brain.[36]

In particular, complex processes of emotion regulation are strongly affected by the context. An fMRI study by Raz and colleagues[37] tracked the psychophysiological measures and brain behavior in fMRI while the viewers watched two emotionally engaging movie scenes about the mother-child separation shadowed by death. They showed that the internal dynamic coordination within the core limbic system (automatic emotional responses) correlated similarly with the subjective sadness ratings across both movie conditions. However, they also observed significant differences in the areas involved in cognitive control over emotional reactions (cognitive motor system) and in monitoring own and others' emotional states in social contexts (medial prefrontal cortex) across the conditions.[38] These differences in the functional connectivity patterns are explained by the contextual differences of the narrative situatedness dealing with more normal life situatedness versus inevitable death at the Nazi concentration camp. According to the researchers, the findings indicate, respectively, "a dichotomy between regulated empathy toward determined-loss and vicarious empathy toward a real-time occurrence."[39]

To understand other people's emotional behavior, both the rapid identification of emotional expressions (mirror system) and the interpretation based on identification (mentalizing) are assumed to interact.[40] Mentalizing of the other person's intentions may become more accurate the more time one has for observing them. For example, the duration of direct gaze activates also emotional evaluation related brain regions (medial prefrontal cortex, orbitofrontal and paracingulate regions).[41] Film's emotional engagement relies heavily on the first ten minutes of the character introduction, during which the viewer learns about and starts to share the main character's personal desires, goals, and personal motivations. As during these first minutes the main character turns from a "stranger" to a "friend," the results by Meyer and colleagues could be extrapolated for the film experience. The researchers showed strong synchronization in the brain's functional connectivity in the medial prefrontal cortex and affective pain regions when people observed social maltreatment of friends, while observing strangers' social suffering seemingly involved more processes related to mentalizing.[42]

Interestingly, Singer and colleagues revealed gender differences in an fMRI study, where they compared people's brain responses in situations where the test people observed distinct persons characterized as "fair" or "unfair" to receive pain. A group of male subjects showed activation in the reward-related areas, when the unfair screen persons experienced pain.[43] Considering the number of films with the good guy chasing and finally revenging the bad guy, Singer and colleagues might have revealed, perhaps unintentionally, the neural foundation of a specific type of genre movies. In the case of revenge, for example, the long-lasting effect of context dependency is likely to be maintained due to the strong emotional priming during the first ten minutes of the film, say, in the case a violent act is committed against innocent people.

## FILM ANNOTATION AS A PREREQUISITE OF NEUROCINEMATIC RESEARCH

The common means of neurocinematics to map observed brain activity to content is to annotate prominent features of the stimuli at each moment in time. Typically the features referred to are such that are immediately present, for instance, faces, hands, objects, or perhaps a seductive gaze. These annotations can then be matched against the time series of brain scanner data recorded from viewers while viewing the film. However, even if successfully annotating the content of momentary events, the present neu-rocinematic annotation paradigms fall short of explaining neural process-ing of narrative comprehension against broader situational contexts beyond immediate nowness. It is unavoidable that the analysis of brain activity by means of match with mere moment-specific annotations will focus rather on the momentary audiovisual information observed in isolated stimuli than fully context-aware narrative cognition. In terms of neuroanatomy, it may be quite broadly hypothesized on the basis of findings related to intersub-ject correlation during free viewing of movies[44] that moment-specific stimuli rather contribute to the identification of activity in posterior than anterior regions.

If it is the desire to understand narrative cognition and emotion in response to the cinematic nowness as it is experienced against its full con-textual situatedness, it is compelling to take into account the entire *retentive* context accumulated since the opening scene, altogether comprising the *nar-rative ontology*, the full description of all so far induced narrative elements that can *protentively* be significant. In terms of a spatial metaphor, this can be described as a very highly dimensional *narrative ontospace*, leaning on the spatial conceptualization of Kaipainen and colleagues.[45]

## NARRATIVE PERSPECTIVE MODEL

With regard to nowness, however, there are no grounds to assume that all of the contextual factors conceivable as dimensions of the narrative onto-space would contribute to the experience simultaneously and equally. Nei-ther would such assumption yield much explanatory power. It is more likely that the experience of nowness is determined by a lower dimensional set of narrative dimensions of focus, termed *narrative perspective*. It is quite safe to suggest that there are various constraints to human memory capacity and attention, limiting the number of context factors effective at one time. These limits may or may not relate to something like Miller's classical notion of plus minus seven,[46] but in no case would it cover tens or hundreds of simul-taneously effective context dimensions. Which ones are effective at a given point of time (nowness window) may be influenced by a number of factors, including (1) the narrative guidance the cinematic storytelling induces in a relatively intersubjective manner, (2) the interplay of different memory lay-ers from short-term or working memory to the memory spanning the entire duration of the film, as well as even broader knowledge-related layers of context contributing to, for example, the sense of genre or film history, and these colored by (3) previous individual experience. All mentioned above are among the prerequisites of holding contextual elements of different time spans as actively retentive and protentive triggers. The narrative perspec-tive, in terms of a spatial metaphor, is a continuously changing point of view to the landscape determined by a number of narratively meaningful dimensions, something like the view through a train window speeding through a landscape.

We infer that detailed content annotation alone will not suffice for a full analysis of the experience corresponding to narrative at a particular point of nowness. Quite obviously, this may apply to a range of experiences in life situations beyond cinema. As we see it, to progress toward more encompassing ecological validity and more naturalistic neuroscience, it is compelling to assume some kind of a dynamical model that simulates the way cinematic storytelling regulates the attention and memory associated to the retentive contexts constituted by previously introduced events. It should account to whatever is known about attention and memory and the way how it relates to anticipation of future events, protention, respectively. We refer to the implied hypothetical model as the *narrative perspective* model, specifying the dimensions of the view through a nowness window moment by moment. The narrative perspective model should be conceived of as an algorithmic model putting out multidimensional arrays of narrative dimensions, calculating the influence of each moment by moment.

## CONCLUSIONS

The medium of film, interpreted as a model of the experienced world, imposes challenges to neurosciences, because experiences of nowness as they occur when viewing films are dependent on a vast system of contexts. One may generalize this even further to experiencing events in the world.

A range of observations from brain studies contribute to the understanding of the experience of cinematic nowness by means of brain activity in distributed networks. Some, such as the findings revealing neural mirroring or action observation networks, enrich the understanding of meaningful windows of nowness in terms of protonarratives. Others, such as the findings related to the processing of different time scales, are among the bases of seeing nowness within the system of overlapping and embedded temporal contexts.

Despite the goal of "naturalism" common to today's neuroscientific experiments, the methodological repertoire to account for context dependence of the nowness experience is still rather limited. The temporal extent to which present stimuli are dependent on contextual priming is typically not considered to reach much longer than the immediately preceding events. To proceed toward scales of backward looking retention that determine meaningful narrative tensions, it is compelling to reconsider and further elaborate the current approaches to stimulus annotation.

In this chapter, we suggested that the notion of dynamically evolving narrative perspectives may serve this purpose and lead the way toward extended priming studies, in which the primer is not a point-like factor but rather a system of concepts. It may provide explanations for what constitutes the narrative drive apparently behind intersubjective synchronization in response to cinematic narration, as established by the paradigm of neurocinematics. We believe that the suggested narrative perspective model will also provide keys to explain the variation of experience from one individual to another, and even an individual's varying experiences depending on the context.

To simulate how the viewer's brain handles high-dimensional narrative contexts, we propose the narrative perspective model as a means to simulate relative effects of various factors regulating the selection and prioritization of contexts as interpretation keys to the nowness of a protonarrative. These include memory decay and refresh in the course of the narrative flow, attentional mechanisms, even genre-specific, cultural and political settings, and so on. Implying a broad multidisciplinary challenge, a spectrum of interdisciplinary collaboration between at least psychology and sociology besides neurosciences and film studies is required. Understanding the artillery of cinematic narration that has proven its power to regulate these factors provides crucial insights to the construction of such a model.

## NOTES

We thank Dr. Janne Kauttonen for his valuable insights. The research group aivoAALTO and Aalto Starting Grant at the Aalto University, as well as the Foundation for Baltic and East European Studies, provided the frameworks and resources that made this work possible.

1. Pia Tikka, *Enactive Cinema: Simultatorium Eisensteinense* (Saarbrücken: Lambert Academic Publishing, 2010).
2. Raymond A. Mar and Keith Oatley, "The Function of Fiction Is the Abstraction and Simulation of Social Experience," *Perspectives on Psychological Science* 3, no. 3 (2008): 173–92, doi:10.1111/j.1745-6924.2008.00073.x.
3. Ulric Neisser, *Cognition and Reality: Principles and Implications of Cognitive Psychology* (San Francisco: W. H. Freeman, 1976).
4. Marshall McLuhan, *Understanding Media: The Extensions of Man* (New York: McGraw-Hill, 1964).
5. Francisco J. Varela, Evan T. Thompson, and Eleanor Rosch, *The Embodied Mind: Cognitive Science and Human Experience* (Cambridge, MA: MIT Press, 1991).
6. Francisco J. Varela, "The Specious Present: A Neurophenomenology of Time Consciousness," in *Naturalizing Phenomenology: Issues in Contemporary Phenomenology and Cognitive Science*, ed. Jean Petitot, 266–314 (Stanford, CA: Stanford University Press, 1999).
7. Uri Hasson et al., "Neurocinematics: The Neuroscience of Film," *Projections* 2, no. 1 (2008): 1–26, doi:10.3167/proj.2008.020102.
8. Andreas Bartels and Semir Zeki, "The Chronoarchitecture of the Human Brain: Natural Viewing Conditions Reveal a Time-Based Anatomy of the Brain," *NeuroImage* 22, no. 1 (2004): 419–33, doi:10.1016/j.neuroimage.2004.01.007; Uri Hasson et al., "Enhanced Intersubject Correlations during Movie Viewing Correlate with Successful Episodic Encoding," *Neuron* 57, no. 3 (2008): 452–62, doi:10.1016/j.neuron.2007.12.009; Iiro P. Jääskeläinen et al., "Inter-Subject

Synchronization of Prefrontal Cortex Hemodynamic Activity during Natural Viewing," *The Open Neuroimaging Journal* 2 (2008): 14–19, doi:10.2174/1 874440000802010014; Juha M. Lahnakoski et al., "Stimulus-Related Independent Component and Voxel-Wise Analysis of Human Brain Activity during Free Viewing of a Feature Film," ed. Mark Alexander Williams, *PLoS ONE* 7, no. 4 (2012): e35215, doi:10.1371/journal.pone.0035215; L. Nummenmaa et al., "Emotions Promote Social Interaction by Synchronizing Brain Activity across Individuals," *Proceedings of the National Academy of Sciences* 109, no. 24 (2012): 9599–604, doi:10.1073/pnas.1206095109.

9. Nikos K. Logothetis, "What We Can Do and What We Cannot Do with fMRI," *Nature* 453, no. 7197 (2008): 869–78, doi:10.1038/nature06976.

10. Jeffrey M. Zacks et al., "Event Perception: A Mind-Brain Perspective," *Psychological Bulletin* 133, no. 2 (2007): 273–93, doi:10.1037/0033-2909.133.2.273.

11. Ibid.; Jeffrey M. Zacks et al., "The Brain's Cutting-Room Floor: Segmentation of Narrative Cinema," *Frontiers in Human Neuroscience* 4 (2010), doi:10.3389/fnhum.2010.00168.

12. The notion of protonarrative has been previously used in philosophical discourse by Philip Lewin. See http://www.focusing.org/apm_papers/Lewin.html. The concept of *narrateme* coined by Vladimir Propp describes a limited number (thirty-one) of smallest possible narrative units that carry the fairytale forward and can be found repeating cross cultures and ages. Vladimir Propp, *Morphology of the Folktale*, 2nd ed. Publications of the American Folklore Society 9 (Austin: University of Texas Press, 1968).

13. George Lakoff and Mark Johnson, *Philosophy in the Flesh: The Embodied Mind and Its Challenge to Western Thought* (New York: Basic Books, 1999).

14. Uri Hasson et al., "A Hierarchy of Temporal Receptive Windows in Human Cortex," *Journal of Neuroscience* 28, no. 10 (2008): 2539–50, doi:10.1523/JNEUROSCI.5487-07.2008; Jukka-Pekka Kauppi et al., "Inter-Subject Correlation of Brain Hemodynamic Responses during Watching a Movie: Localization in Space and Frequency," *Frontiers in Neuroinformatics* 4 (2010): 5, doi:10.3389/fninf.2010.00005; Y. Lerner et al., "Topographic Mapping of a Hierarchy of Temporal Receptive Windows Using a Narrated Story," *Journal of Neuroscience* 31, no. 8 (2011): 2906–15, doi:10.1523/JNEUROSCI.3684-10.2011.

15. Lerner et al., "Topographic Mapping."

16. Hasson et al., "Hierarchy."

17. For a review, see Frank Van Overwalle and Kris Baetens, "Understanding Others' Actions and Goals by Mirror and Mentalizing Systems: A Meta-Analysis," *NeuroImage* 48, no. 3 (2009): 564–84, doi:10.1016/j.neuroimage.2009.06.009.

18. R. Hari et al., "Activation of Human Primary Motor Cortex during Action Observation: A Neuromagnetic Study," *Proceedings of the National Academy of Sciences of the United States of America* 95, no. 25 (1998): 15061–65; Pascal Molenberghs, Ross Cunnington, and Jason B. Mattingley, "Brain Regions with Mirror Properties: A Meta-Analysis of 125 Human fMRI Studies," *Neuroscience and Biobehavioral Reviews* 36, no. 1 (2012): 341–49, doi:10.1016/j.neubiorev.2011.07.004; Giacomo Rizzolatti and Maddalena Fabbri-Destro, "The Mirror System and Its Role in Social Cognition," *Current Opinion in Neurobiology* 18, no. 2 (2008): 179–84, doi:10.1016/j.conb.2008.08.001; Giacomo Rizzolatti et al., "Premotor Cortex and the Recognition of Motor Actions," *Cognitive Brain Research* 3, no. 2 (1996): 131–41, doi:10.1016/0926-6410(95)00038-0.

19. Vittorio Gallese, "Before and Below 'Theory of Mind': Embodied Simulation and the Neural Correlates of Social Cognition," *Philosophical Transactions of the Royal Society of London, Series B, Biological Sciences* 362,

no. 1480 (2007): 659–69, doi:10.1098/rstb.2006.2002; R. Hari and M. V. Kujala, "Brain Basis of Human Social Interaction: From Concepts to Brain Imaging," *Physiological Reviews* 89, no. 2 (2009): 453–79, doi:10.1152/physrev.00041.2007; Marco Iacoboni, "Imitation, Empathy, and Mirror Neurons," *Annual Review of Psychology* 60, no. 1 (2009): 653–70, doi:10.1146/annurev.psych.60.110707.163604.

20. B. Calvo-Merino, "Action Observation and Acquired Motor Skills: An fMRI Study with Expert Dancers," *Cerebral Cortex* 15, no. 8 (2004): 1243–49, doi:10.1093/cercor/bhi007; C. M. Heyes and C. L. Foster, "Motor Learning by Observation: Evidence from a Serial Reaction Time Task," *Quarterly Journal of Experimental Psychology Section A* 55, no. 2 (2002): 593–607, doi:10.1080/02724980143000389.

21. Michael A. Arbib, "From Grasp to Language: Embodied Concepts and the Challenge of Abstraction," *Journal of Physiology-Paris* 102, no. 1–3 (2008): 4–20, doi:10.1016/j.jphysparis.2008.03.001.

22. Lisa Aziz-Zadeh and Antonio Damasio, "Embodied Semantics for Actions: Findings from Functional Brain Imaging," *Journal of Physiology-Paris* 102, no. 1–3 (2008): 35–39, doi:10.1016/j.jphysparis.2008.03.012; Olaf Hauk, Ingrid Johnsrude, and Friedemann Pulvermüller, "Somatotopic Representation of Action Words in Human Motor and Premotor Cortex," *Neuron* 41, no. 2 (2004): 301–7.

23. U. Hasson et al., "A Hierarchy of Temporal Receptive Windows in Human Cortex," *Journal of Neuroscience* 28, no. 10 (2008): 2539–50, doi:10.1523/JNEUROSCI.5487-07.2008; Iiro P. Jääskeläinen et al., "Inter-Subject Synchronization of Prefrontal Cortex Hemodynamic Activity during Natural Viewing," *The Open Neuroimaging Journal* 2 (2008): 14–19, doi:10.2174/1874440000802010014; Juha M. Lahnakoski et al., "Stimulus-Related Independent Component and Voxel-Wise Analysis of Human Brain Activity during Free Viewing of a Feature Film," ed. Mark Alexander Williams, *PLoS ONE* 7, no. 4 (2012): e35215, doi:10.1371/journal.pone.0035215; L. Nummenmaa et al., "Emotions Promote Social Interaction by Synchronizing Brain Activity across Individuals," *Proceedings of the National Academy of Sciences of the United States of America* 109, no. 24 (2012): 9599–604, doi:10.1073/pnas.1206095109.

24. Maurice Merleau-Ponty and Donald A. Landes, *Phenomenology of Perception*, trans. Donald A. Landes (New York: Routledge, 2013).

25. P. C. Fletcher et al., "Other Minds in the Brain: A Functional Imaging Study of 'Theory of Mind' in Story Comprehension," *Cognition* 57, no. 2 (1995): 109–28; Chris D. Frith and Uta Frith, "Mechanisms of Social Cognition," *Annual Review of Psychology* 63, no. 1 (2012): 287–313, doi:10.1146/annurev-psych-120710-100449.

26. Cristina Becchio et al., "Social Grasping: From Mirroring to Mentalizing," *NeuroImage* 61, no. 1 (2012): 240–48, doi:10.1016/j.neuroimage.2012.03.013.

27. Nico H. Frijda, *The Emotions* (Cambridge: Cambridge University Press, 1986); Ed S. Tan, *Emotion and the Structure of Narrative Film: Film as an Emotion Machine* (New York: Routledge, 2011).

28. Charles Whitehead et al., "Neural Correlates of Observing Pretend Play in Which One Object Is Represented as Another," *Social Cognitive and Affective Neuroscience* 4, no. 4 (2009): 369–78, doi:10.1093/scan/nsp021.

29. M. S. Gazzaniga, "Cerebral Specialization and Interhemispheric Communication: Does the Corpus Callosum Enable the Human Condition?," *Brain* 123, no. 7 (2000): 1293–326, doi:10.1093/brain/123.7.1293.

30. L. V. Kuleshov, *Kuleshov on Film: Writings* (Berkeley: University of California Press, 1974), 18, 192.

31. D. Mobbs, "The Kuleshov Effect: The Influence of Contextual Framing on Emotional Attributions," *Social Cognitive and Affective Neuroscience* 1, no. 2 (2006): 95–106, doi:10.1093/scan/nsl014.
32. Harald G. Wallbott, "In and Out of Context: Influences of Facial Expression and Context Information on Emotion Attributions," *British Journal of Social Psychology* 27, no. 4 (1988): 357–69, doi:10.1111/j.2044-8309.1988. tb00837.x.
33. Hasson et al., "Neurocinematics."
34. Juha M. Lahnakoski et al., "Synchronous Brain Activity across Individuals Underlies Shared Psychological Perspectives," *NeuroImage* 100 (2014): 316–24, doi:10.1016/j.neuroimage.2014.06.022.
35. Jiang Xu et al., "Language in Context: Emergent Features of Word, Sentence, and Narrative Comprehension," *NeuroImage* 25, no. 3 (2005): 1002–15, doi:10.1016/j.neuroimage.2004.12.013.
36. Hasson et al., "Hierarchy"; Kauppi et al., "Inter-Subject Correlation"; Lerner et al., "Topographic Mapping."
37. Gal Raz et al., "Portraying Emotions at Their Unfolding: A Multilayered Approach for Probing Dynamics of Neural Networks," *NeuroImage* 60, no. 2 (2012): 1448–61, doi:10.1016/j.neuroimage.2011.12.084.
38. Ibid.; Gal Raz et al., "Cry for Her or Cry with Her: Context-Dependent Dissociation of Two Modes of Cinematic Empathy Reflected in Network Cohesion Dynamics," *Social Cognitive and Affective Neuroscience* 9, no. 1 (2014): 30–38, doi:10.1093/scan/nst052.
39. Raz et al., "Cry for Her."
40. Robert P. Spunt and Matthew D. Lieberman, "An Integrative Model of the Neural Systems Supporting the Comprehension of Observed Emotional Behavior," *NeuroImage* 59, no. 3 (2012): 3050–59, doi:10.1016/j. neuroimage.2011.10.005.
41. Bojana Kuzmanovic et al., "Duration Matters: Dissociating Neural Correlates of Detection and Evaluation of Social Gaze," *NeuroImage* 46, no. 4 (2009): 1154–63, doi:10.1016/j.neuroimage.2009.03.037.
42. Meghan L. Meyer et al., "Empathy for the Social Suffering of Friends and Strangers Recruits Distinct Patterns of Brain Activation," *Social Cognitive and Affective Neuroscience* 8, no. 4 (2013): 446–54, doi:10.1093/scan/nss019.
43. Tania Singer et al., "Empathic Neural Responses Are Modulated by the Perceived Fairness of Others," *Nature* 439, no. 7075 (2006): 466–69, doi:10.1038/nature04271.
44. Uri Hasson, "Intersubject Synchronization of Cortical Activity During Natural Vision," *Science* 303, no. 5664 (2004): 1634–40, doi:10.1126/ science.1089506.
45. Mauri Kaipainen and Antti Hautamäki, "Epistemic Pluralism and Multi-Perspective Knowledge Organization: Explorative Conceptualization of Topical Content Domains," *Knowledge Organization* 38, no. 6 (2011): 503–14; Mauri Kaipainen et al., "Soft Ontologies, Spatial Representations and Multi-Perspective Explorability," *Expert Systems* 25, no. 5 (2008): 474–83, doi:10.1111/j.1468-0394.2008.00470.x.
46. George A. Miller, "The Magical Number Seven, plus or Minus Two: Some Limits on Our Capacity for Processing Information," *Psychological Review* 63, no. 2 (1956): 81–97, doi:10.1037/h0043158.

# 7 Seeing In, and Out, to the Extended Mind through an EEG Analysis of Page and Screen Reading

*Robert C. MacDougall*

In the *Mechanical Bride*, Marshall McLuhan sought to understand the "public mind" by closely reading American advertising. Thereafter, with *The Gutenberg Galaxy, Understanding Media, Verbi-Voco-Visual Explorations,* "The Brain and Media," and posthumously, with his son Eric, *The Laws of Media*, McLuhan's attention turned squarely to questions about the human mind, brain, cognition, and consciousness.[1] In his Centre for Culture and Technology at the University of Toronto, a map of the bicameral human brain hung on the wall near his desk. McLuhan was fascinated with neurology, emerging brain research, including the study of hemisphericity, and specifically, the localization of brain function that was beginning to be revealed. Indeed, McLuhan remained convinced until his death in 1980 that communication media play a constitutive, formative role as extensions of the human cognitive and perceptual apparatus, in all its manifestations.

McLuhan's writings can be seen as forming part of an early, paradigm-shifting theory of mind that was also being articulated in various ways by mathematician Norbert Weiner, perceptual psychologist J.J. Gibson, and anthropologist Gregory Bateson, among others. McLuhan's entire corpus might even distill down to this one essential point: to understand human cognition and consciousness, we have to embrace the notion of extensions—extension of the body, brain, and mind through a wide variety of material and symbolic means. On this view, having a brain is certainly a necessary condition, but it is by no means a sufficient condition for having a mind. Indeed, this might even suggest that a brain alone cannot produce mental activity in the absence of an external environment. Of course, this is a notion that is impossible to test because we cannot separate a brain from its environment (e.g., the body and external world surrounding it). Nonetheless, this basic intuition of a disembodied, decontextualized brain persists today as the core legacy of Descartes's cogito.

However, although there has been a groundswell of support for the "extended mind" thesis over the last couple of decades,[2] stout opposition to the general position continues. A newly emboldened reductionist outlook has gained traction in large enough swaths of the neuroscientific community to substantially redirect both research funding and public opinion concerning the relationship between brain function—specifically function registered at the neuronal level—and states of mind (i.e., the particularities of conscious experience). This heightened attention surrounds the application of newer measurement tools and methods of analysis, including MRI, fMRI, and MEG, and a resurgence and reapplication of some older tools, such as EEG and PET.

Emblematic of the more conventional mind/brain identity thesis, Stanislas Dehaene writes, "In reality, a direct one-to-one relation exists between each of our thoughts and the discharge patterns of given groups of neurons in our brains—states of mind *are* states of brain matter."[3] This perspective of course has deep intellectual roots. While the essential idea behind mind/brain identity was first given formal treatment by Rene Descartes in his *Discourse on Method* in 1637, intermediate tracings can be found in Locke's *mental tokens* and Kant's *vorstellungen* (or mental representations). While there is no easy way to determine even general proportions, published research reports available to the public indicate that a significant majority of the neurophysiological research conducted of late is being marshaled in service of the brain/mind identity thesis and the representational theory of mind (RTM) undergirding it. This chapter details one research initiative that constitutes a formal critique of both constructs. Before describing the research let us first consider the nature of tools as both perceptual enhancers and inhibitors.

Dubbed "the law of the instrument" by Abraham Kaplan in 1964, we find a core tenet of media ecology. The essential idea is that tool use can be deterministic. If sometimes determining, however, our tools (conceptual and material) have consequences that play out in thought and action. One powerful way ideas and apparatuses can be consequential is the manner in which they function like lenses that can focus and sharpen our vision. Indeed, anyone who has paid even the slightest attention to the nature of optics knows that enhanced focus and sharper vision typically results in a narrowed view. Let us proceed carefully then. For now, more than ever, with all of this powerful technology at our disposal, we may find that the *devil* is in the extended, out-of-brain, and even out-of-body details.

The next section of this chapter offers a brief review of media-related electroencephalographic (EEG) research spanning more than forty years. Keeping the pertinent history and our contemporary techno-cultural context in mind, an original empirical investigation employing an EEG measurement apparatus is then described that sought, in part, to retest an early media-related EEG project. The experiment was designed to detect changes in cognitive activity during, and between, screen and page reading conditions in a small sample of college students ($N = 12$) ranging from eighteen to twenty-two years of age. Directly challenging Dehaene and many others who subscribe to the *brain-mind identity* thesis, we can now reliably extend McLuhan's efforts to articulate why, to better understand human cognition, we need to move away from that Cartesian story and embrace an extended, "brain-body-world" explanation of human thought, cognition, and consciousness.

EEG, PET, MEG, MRI, fMRI, and several other neurophysiological measurement tools no longer sit at the periphery of media research. Today, in fact, they are moving to the center of inquiries considering the relationship between communication media and the *brains* interacting with them. If some investigators, including Richard Restack and Stanislas Dehaene,[4] do seem to be engaged in a reductionist story of mind-brain identity, not all new research employing the scientific tools and methodologies now at our disposal is necessarily reductive.

The meta-analytic study of EEG research described here also suggests why a reductionist approach is not the most productive way to proceed as we build new knowledge about the relationship between media, minds, and brains in the world today. Media researchers can adopt a robust ecological perspective in the analysis of human-technological systems by taking to task McLuhan's suggestion that we shape our tools, and they, in turn shape us. Framed and prefigured by some of these new tools, recent investigations of media use have revealed an unprecedented focus on the units and sub-units of the biological brain. Instead of a reductive story, however, it seems more likely that brains, media, and the resultant minds (of various kinds) have always blended and bled into each other. No doubt, taking this idea of the extended mind seriously prompts a return to a quasi-metaphysical position[5] whereby physical minds or body-brains are additionally constituted in the process of integrating with both external physical artifacts (including paper notepads, icons, smart phones, etc.) and non-physical artifacts (including a cultural extension such as clock time or a bio-cultural extension such as language).

## THE MEASUREMENT OF NEUROPHYSIOLOGICAL ACTIVITY USING EEG

Ostensibly, EEG measures levels of attention, consciousness, awareness, and memory function, and this suggests that it is possible to capture a physiological index of psychological processes. What follows are the traditional parameters of EEG measurement, with brief descriptions of the most commonly accepted cognitive, perceptual, and/or phenomenological states associated with each:

> *Delta* (0–3 Hz) is associated with deep sleep.
> *Theta* (4–7 Hz) is associated with the transition from wakefulness to sleep (might experience dreamlike/hypnagogic imagery).
> *Alpha* activity (8–13 Hz) is primarily associated with withdrawal of visual attention and information processing, along with an internal focus.
> *Beta* (14–18 Hz and high beta, 18–30 Hz) is associated with "paying attention" to novel, interesting or important aspects of our visual world. Paying attention also seems to mean using motor control to focus and direct the eyes toward a source of stimulation.

*Gamma* (30–40 Hz) is associated with higher order thinking, binding of perceptual properties of objects (e.g., integrating color, shape, form, and size), and associative thinking.

These parameters are generally accepted by the scientific community to reliably measure particular "psychological" events at the physiological level. A reductive and decidedly materialist framing is evident here. Such a framing suggests also that there is a general consensus around the notion of a distributed or modular network that gives rise to human cognitive processes. That is to say, in given conditions like reading from page or screen, there is measurable activity in left-hemispheric regions of the neocortex, the frontal and posterior cortices, hippocampus, and cerebellum.

The argument being put forward in this chapter, however, is that the distribution of cognitive labor currently being described through such framings, and indeed, in the lion's share of extant neuroscience literature on "brain mapping," does not go far enough. Before we can begin to understand why such a localized or tight framing must be inadequate, however, it may be instructive to review several earlier EEG-based media research projects.

## SOME PREVIOUS NEURO-ANOTOMICAL MEDIA RESEARCH

From John J. Burns and Daniel R. Anderson,[6] we get a well-rounded history of EEG research and experimentation centered upon comparisons of page-based and screen-based media use. The first study reviewed is Herbert Krugman's 1971 project measuring brainwaves of subjects using media.[7] This is the research study sometimes highlighted by Marshall McLuhan as demonstrating empirical support for his own implicit neuro-media philosophy.

Krugman's work is notable as a pioneering effort but can be critiqued for providing only one "case study" of media effects. Only a single research participant was hooked up to Krugman's EEG apparatus to gather data for this study. While a significant difference in alpha and beta output between the page and screen conditions was recorded (showing the predicted increase in alpha waves during the screen condition), these findings are not generalizable according to any standard.

We can critique Krugman's work for being either methodologically flawed or perhaps merely indicative of an idiosyncratic brain. There was an appreciable lull in media-related EEG research for nearly a decade following Krugman's study. However, a group of new studies appeared at the end of the decade, beginning with Gregg Featherman et al.[8] Their project was conducted at Hampshire College and made possible through an NSF grant.

[Featherman et al.] hypothesized that, when compared with reading, television viewing would result in reduced levels of cortical activation

in the occipital region. Decreased cortical activation was operational-
ized as increased alpha along with decreased beta and theta activity. In
an effort to minimize the environmental differences between the two
activities Featherman et al. (1979) displayed reading material on a television screen. They found a significant decrease in both theta and beta
activity during television when compared to reading. However, while
television did produce a higher level of alpha than reading, this difference was not significant.[9]

The following year, Weinstein, Appel, and Weinstein continued in a similar
vein.[10] Both of these studies represent enhancements upon Krugman's project
for different reasons. Weinstein and company gathered thirty research participants, so their ability to claim generalizability was significantly enhanced.
However, for some undisclosed reason, their study involved only women.
More to our core methodological point, however, Featherman et al. did
their best to fix the content across both page and screen conditions. For this
reason, the research described immediately after this review is based as well
upon Featherman et al.

Media-related EEG investigations continued into the next decade with
James L. Walker and Michael S. Radlick,[11] but the findings from those
studies did not do much to shake the emerging picture. Only very modest
evidence for differences along the EEG spectrum was percolating to the
surface in the academy, and elsewhere. It seemed as though McLuhan's
*light-on/light-through* distinction was losing distinction. A collection
of methodological peculiarities might account for some of the lacklus-
ter findings, but something else seems to have been amiss when we look
closely at the way earlier EEG researchers were thinking about the media
employed in these experimental contexts. Almost two decades passed
before the glimmerings of a conceptual problem in all of this previous
research became apparent. It was an oversight that often triggered a
cascading collection of procedural missteps. The contours of the brain
became the default limits of mind. Researchers also seem to conflate the
medium and the message—or, the formal properties, and the content
afforded by pages and screens.

## A NEW CONCEPTUALIZATION (AND SOME OLD
METHODOLOGICAL PROBLEMS)

Robert Kubey and Mihaly Csikszentmihalyi suggest that it is the frequency
of the formal features (the camera cuts, pans, zooms, etc) that triggers the
"orienting response" most directly affecting brain wave activity, not the
visual complexity of content.[12] The investigators highlight one of the perennial difficulties associated with such research when it comes to ferreting out
a distinction between form (technological format or medium) and content
in our symbolic environments. For some observers, camera cuts, pans, and

zooms might be considered a kind of content or at least begin to blur the line between format and content—or medium and message.

However, such an assessment ignores the simple fact that camera cuts, pans, and zooms are impossible in other media formats like radio or print, or even still photography. It seems reasonable, then, to suggest that these examples are emergent manifestations (or something perceptual psychologist J. J. Gibson called *affordances*)[13] of the formal or structural features of the medium of television and, it could be argued, conventional and digital film technologies as well.

It is notable that all of the studies mentioned earlier found paltry EEG-based differences between television viewing and reading, so a nagging worry remains. Did the experimenters accidentally (or even purposively) select TV shows or video content that contained few if any of the aforementioned features? If this is the case, then we should be ready to qualify scenarios where the over-control of experimental variables becomes systematic in such research contexts. That is to say, locating television content containing minimal cuts, pans, and zooms, and so on, is at once a hard-to-find television viewing condition today (as it was already becoming rare in the 1970s) and, because of this, a fairly uncommon expectation in viewers as well.

Another moral here is that media researchers need to be especially careful about over-constraining and over-determining the actual contexts that are built out and enacted by real-world media users. In situ media use is what we should always strive to access as researchers, and with as little disruption as possible. Of course, this is precisely why sitting a research participant down in a lab and hooking electrodes up to their scalp immediately problematizes our efforts to cull meaningful data. But there are some steps we can take to help increase the likelihood of obtaining an accurate picture of what's happening both in and outside of biological brains.

There is no question that the observation frame and selection biases present in contemporary media-based EEG research may help account for the small differences measured in many of the output tables being published and disseminated. It seems also to be the case, however, as with the effort described below to *retest* different aspects of the Krugman-inspired studies, that some research teams scrutinizing alpha and beta waves (where the differences between television watching and reading are minor) did not look as closely at theta patterns, or the very fast hi-beta and gamma waves where the drop-off during television watching can become quite large.

## The Current Study

With all of these caveats in place regarding "natural" or "real-world" media consumption contexts, our primary interest was to see if some of these subtle differences could be detected between page and screen reading while holding the "content" variable as constant as possible across conditions. Reading from screens tends to elicit different postures and perceptual patterns than watching screens, so special attention was given to these reading conditions. In other words, total equivalance here would be both undesirable and impossible. Our efforts to achieve these near-equivalencies was therefore a highly nuanced enterprise, as we had to be careful not to obliterate those features most common and central to real-world uses of these media systems and formats.

For example, in our more "static" screen versus page reading research model, every effort was made to fix the content by aligning as closely as possible the text on the page and the "text" presented to research participants on various screens. We accomplished this via verbatim word matching, font/ font size, contrast, brightness, and so on. However, there were some cases where it was impossible and, indeed, probably detrimental to our aims to occlude all of the peripheral information (and stimuli of various sorts) at the margins of the screens. Again, we saw this as providing an accurate picture of the way this new population of users access media content through screens both online and offline.

## The Custom EEG Apparatus

We used the anterior, frontal location (Fz in the 10–20 International Electrode System) because this location is part of the anterior, attention system in the brain. We used the right occipital-parietal location (O2-P4) because it is part of the posterior attention system that provides a reliable baseline reading during the "at rest, eyes closed" condition to help ensure that the system was functioning properly. The EEG from both locations was recorded with bipolar electrode placements.

The EEG was amplified with two V75–02 bio-amplifiers manufactured by Coulbourn Instruments. These units transmitted their data to a National Instruments Interface that performed an analog to digital (A-D) conversion of the EEG signal. The A-D conversion used 512 EEG data samples in each 500 milliseconds of the data recording trial. The digitized values of the EEG were collected and evaluated with custom designed software that analyzed the power spectrum of the EEG in two hertz frequency bins, from two to thirty-two hertz.[14] The real-time, analog EEG signal was recorded on a Lenovo laptop computer using WindaQ Pro+ software.[15]

The dependent variable for the study consisted of the power spectrum measurements of the EEG in each of the two hertz frequency bins of interest. These data also were collected every half second and downloaded to an Excel spreadsheet at the end of the recording trial. Power spectrum averages were calculated for each EEG location and stimulation condition using a Hewlett-Packard d325 desktop computer. The real-time EEG records were scanned on the laptop, and any EEG epochs containing recording artifacts were eliminated from the data stream.

Each subject received a computer/screen reading and a text/page reading of chapter 11 of Mary Shelley's *Frankenstein*. Each of the reading sessions was repeated at the anterior and posterior electrode locations while we recorded the EEG. In addition, we tested each subject with a low and high demand visual attention battery in the form of a ready-made instrument developed by Clifford Nass and associates at Stanford University that was accessed via the *New York Times* website.[16] The two forms of the attention test were repeated at each EEG site while the EEG was recorded.

We went into the lab giving all legitimacy to McLuhan's "light-on" (page) versus "light-through" (screen) probe. However, given that the vast majority of laptops and tablet computers are a combination of back-lit (the Kindle and other e-ink devices are not) and in-lit matrices, we were also updating McLuhan to account for the increased use of what really are "light-in" technologies purchased for reading and watching in a fast-growing segment of the population. The liquid crystal display (LCD) matrix is emerging as the industry standard and cultural default, assuming the current trend to replace the contents of student's backpacks, school libraries, and college bookstores with iPads, tablets, and e-readers continues.

McLuhan's original, if mostly tacit, neuro-media philosophy is rooted in something we might call the "pixilation hypothesis." According to this infamous probe, the tiny rectangles of light—or *pixels*—projected onto the surface of a conventional cathode ray tube (CRT)/television screen demand more participation from the viewer than, say, traditional film because the blurry images appearing on the phosphor-coated screen require additional decoding and completion to allow meaningful pattern recognition. Again, whereas Krugman employed the extant screen-based media of his day (CRT/light-through), we used LCDs almost exclusively. The latter are a hybrid form of light-in/light-through technology given the nature of their active matrix and often backlit screens. Even though LCD displays produce a legitimate kind of pixilation, it is still a higher resolution image than most conventional CRT systems (even without an HD matrix and accompanying signal). This is one material difference between the outputs of a scanning-electron-beam-fired CRT and a liquid crystal display. This means that McLuhan's pixilation hypothesis may no longer apply in today's media milieu.

While we found no significant differences in alpha and beta output in the aggregate data between the two reading conditions, some interesting patterns were detected within-subjects that warranted further scrutiny. Three of the twelve participants exhibited noticeable differences along the EEG spectrum between the screen and page conditions. This finding ran directly counter to both McLuhan's original probe and Krugman's results. We elected to pay closer attention to this minority. The analog waveforms illustrated in Figure 7.1 clearly show an inversion of the difference Krugman originally detected between screen and page reading within select subjects.

The upper waveform in both images registers the anterior lead which in these cases provided the baseline/control reading. The lower waveform shows the output recorded at the very active occipital-parietal, posterior location, which is the main visual processing area of the brain. In the first image, the tell-tale low-frequency alpha waveform with its broad chasms reveals an unexpected reversal of the predicted alpha-beta pattern. This

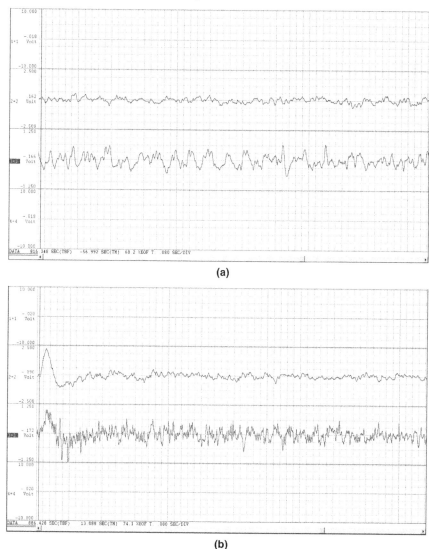

*Figure 7.1* EEG of Page and Screen Reading: (a) Page, (b) Screen

kind of pattern has been associated with screen and page reading in some EEG research completed by others at the time of this writing.

This particular participant was an outlier. While the biological ages of all participants ranged between eighteen and twenty-two years, subsequent interviews suggest subtle yet potentially significant experiential differences in the research pool. A series of brief qualitative questions were posed between the reading conditions, with more probing follow-up questions asked upon completion of the EEG battery. Answers and explanations provided throughout suggest that the paperback reading experience was less exciting or less engaging in some way. The book experience prompted some participants' attention to wander, and even made some of them feel tired. Such reporting typically emerged after just 90–120 seconds of reading from the page.

During the follow-up interviews, we also sought details about the morning's breakfast, regular food and drug habits, and general media usage. Participants were explicitly advised to avoid any appreciable amounts of sugar or caffeine prior to the lab visit, but sugar, caffeine, nicotine, marijuana, alcohol, and a variety of attention-deficit, anti-anxiety, and anti-depression drugs were mentioned by a majority of the twelve.[17]

All of this and other related information was taken into consideration in an effort to ensure the highest quality data. For example, some anomalous micro-volt readings were correlated with reports of recent intake of stimulants and removed during the data-cleaning phase. Spikes and flatlines produced when a participant coughed, moved their head erratically, pulled out a lead accidentally, or disrupted the normal signal flow in some way were eliminated as well. As stated earlier, there was some concern about the potential for over-cleaning the data. The combinations of chemical and technological media reported by our co-investigators—using a variety of somewhat unconventional drug-media salads—seems to be an increasingly common synergy. Naturally, then, our cleaned datasets might not be particularly faithful representations of the way these drug-media mixes could be triggering new modes of awareness and attention. Put another way, the latest drug-media practices are likely contributing to some very different kinds of brains, and minds, roaming the world today.[18]

In addition to the substance queries, then, we asked a series of open-ended questions, including requests to describe "how you felt" after the different reading conditions. To reiterate, participants also answered a series of questions about their experiences with pages, screens, and other media as children. As might be expected, not everyone in this small collection of what is sometimes dubbed "digital natives"[19] grew up with regular interaction with books or physical pages of different sorts. Before we even had a look at the EEG outputs, it was apparent that the screen was a more familiar media form for seven of the twelve given their descriptions of media use as children and in the way they showed an immediate sense of comfort with the laptop or iPad in front of them during those reading conditions. A few, by contrast, seemed uncomfortable with the old paperback copy of *Frankenstein* lent to them.

## EVIDENCE OF MEDIA GENERATIONS

There was simply no group-level consistency in the way these young people were orienting to and interacting with the media systems placed before them. According to Prenski's digital native hypothesis, this should have been a well-aligned collection of media users, yet some of the diametrically opposed EEG readouts suggested something else all together. Of course, a broad array of media habits takes place among members of the same biological generation. The core idea behind the digital native construct is that anyone born after, say, 1980 will process the world very differently due to their regular immersion in digital tools of various sorts. Prenski in fact described both digital natives and digital immigrants. The latter, born sometime prior to 1980, do not exhibit the same kind of perfunctory familiarly with digital tools according to the author.[20]

But while Prenski's construct has come under fire in the intervening years, he still generally subscribes to the proposition that new media structures are causal with respect to the way media users process information, and even the emergence of new brain structures. It is the notion of a media generation that seems to have more credence here, however.[21] A media generation is not bound to any particular biological generation and appears to align and separate persons much more reliably in terms of media use and the information and symbolic processing habits and patterns that use entails. So, for example, a person born in the year 2000 who was "brought up" on the oral rendering of story books (instead of their digital counterparts) would not be a digital native accustomed to the non-linear logics of television, film, and hypertextual displays. They would instead be most steeped in the linear, sequential logic of the written word. The media generation idea allows us to make more subtle and accurate generalizations about media users today.

Indeed, even within the collection of participants in their late teens and early twenties who participated in our small study, there were notable differences between self-reports regarding past experiences with, and current use of, books. If all were adept screen users, and while all initially claimed to be regular readers of books, it was obvious that some were more comfortable handling the paperback than others. Three grasped the book in palpably awkward ways (variably crouched, almost crumpled over the splayed pages, as if striving to look more intently at the words, to focus, concentrate, or perhaps stay awake). After follow-up questions, some of these college students even admitted to not spending much time reading physical books at all, including course texts. Four admitted to having never read a single book from "cover to cover" since they were very young children.

In addition to redoubling our awareness of a patterned set of self-reports posted by young people on social networks, noted in the popular press, and gathered in formal research of this sort, the trend is newsworthy because it reveals a fairly specific phenomenological feel to reading from pages, as opposed to screens. This may be why so many iPad advertisements and commercials depict users in comfortable positions—typically supine characters reading in bed, on the beach, or curled up on sofas. An effort is apparent in the promotional material to conjure some of the aesthetics and experiential benefits often associated with conventional book reading. But even while the messaging suggests idealized contexts of use, do these postures and physical contortions mask deeper differences between screen and page reading? Or, to borrow a line from Gregory Bateson, is there a *difference that makes a difference?*

To reiterate, we noted different experiences in the qualitative data compared across this cohort of college students who are often dubbed "computer kids" or "digital natives" (born into a world of highly active screens, mice, joysticks and remote controls of various kinds). However, reported differences in upbringing with and through new media suggest that we are not talking about a homogenous collection of user experiences at all. The alpha/beta inversion described earlier bolsters these qualitative details and points to a media-specific, not age-specific set of experiences.

Again, if the lack of significant differences in EEG output between the screen and page conditions in the aggregate raises serious questions about McLuhan's original light-in versus light-on distinction, there was some evidence for a difference in alpha and beta waveforms within-subject. This prompts a revisiting of Gumpert and Cathcart's notion of a media generation,[22] a direct extension of McLuhan's core observation that the media environment an individual is born in, raised through, and essentially inhabits, will introduce certain representational biases to the organization/encoding/reception and decoding/interpretation patterns of the media user-qua-inhabitant. Strangely, we might even be talking about a brand of the RTM here. In this case, however, it is an "extended" version of that story, where components of mind are embedded in certain media and artifacts surrounding biological brains. If the current project tacitly critiques the traditional RTM by heavily qualifying it, the debate between proponents of representational and non-representation minds is a profound one that deserves much more attention than this chapter can allow.

What's clear is that questions of *media habitation* should become central questions that guide our efforts to ferret out the subtle differences in media experience among users. Gumpert and Cathcart hypothesized meaningful differences between the various "media generations" that have been postulated, albeit in less-formal ways, by media theorists dating all the way back to Plato. Certainly the works of McLuhan are elaborations of this same idea.[23] Gumpert and Cathcart contend, as with spoken language, people orient in particular ways to the world through the media cultivating them. According to the authors,

1. there are sets of codes and conventions integral to each medium
2. such codes and conventions constitute part of our media consciousness
3. the information processing made possible through these various grammars influence our perceptions and values
4. the order of acquisition of media literacy will produce a particular world perspective which relates and separates persons accordingly[24]

For example, some eighteen- to twenty-two-year-olds were raised into a relatively full awareness of, and ready orientation to, the active nature of the visual display attending such an environment. These individuals most often come to expect a continuous, if non-linear, and what often amounts to a non-logic-based kind of content issuing from the screens in front of and around them. That is to say, while one certainly can locate static rows of typographic language appearing on television and computer screens, this is not the default content of such devices anymore. Evidence for a beta spike during the screen condition with some participants seems to bolster a "media generation" explanation. They know what they can expect from screens and, indeed, many reported wanting—or expressed a felt need to look for—something else to happen/appear in the back-lit (or in-lit) window before them.

So the possibility, based upon unique media histories, that different research participants were bringing different modes of perception and kinds of consciousness to our EEG laboratory along with them further complicated our efforts to interpret the data.

## SOME IMPLICATIONS OF THE RESEARCH

All of this carries practical significance for teaching, both formal and informal learning, the general acquisition of information, and knowledge production. With the dissemination of small, powerful devices with extended battery life, reading practices continue to shift from a focus on pages to screens, as our more general information-gathering behaviors progressively involve fewer words and more images, both moving and still. Primary and secondary schools, and colleges and universities, are ideal environments to investigate these pressing questions, with a broad array of learning styles and pedagogical traditions still represented.

It seems tenable that a combination of user habituation, the formal features of modern screen technology, and the active natures of our immediate experiential milieus have introduced a confounding set of variables that the theory and practice of EEG research (or any other neuro-method alone) is simply ill-equipped to detect, let alone measure, effectively. One worry is that MRI, fMRI, EEG, and other neuro-recording methods can prompt investigators to keep tightening their focus and reduce these phenomena to their neurophysiological manifestations. The question is, should we primarily be looking so far down and in, simply because we can now do so with such high intensities of resolution?

While many contemporary theorists and practitioners, including Stanislas Dehaene, Daniel Dennett, and Paul and Patricia Churchland, seem more or less settled on brain/mind identity, a host of problems tend to arise in brain-centered media studies that warrants continued questions about the relationship between brains and minds. One issue is that we are dealing with an incredibly complex, distributed network of neuronal connections that seem almost designed to elude efforts at encapsulation or localization. But this is not to require any kind of nefarious cosmic designer, as much as suggest the reality of a subtle dynamic of feedback systems, off-loading and outsourcing between neurons in brains as well as between brains and media of various kinds external to them.

Did the theta spike detected in some of the data streams during this study signal a physical, chemically induced, or some externally derived condition in the participant that was already in effect before the EEG readings commenced? Or were these expectancy effects generated by the medium itself? Perceptual physiologist Don Berlyne's work surrounding something he called "collative stimulus properties" should be taken into consideration here.[25] According to Berlyne, these properties concern the nature and function of novelty in the perceptual field. He claims that specific stimulus characteristics, for example, color, shape, form, or complexity (described as "collative" stimulus properties), are capable of eliciting interest or orienting on the part of the observer. This may happen because the stimuli elicit arousal of the nervous system automatically, or at least in some pre-conscious manner.

Unless we pay close attention to the way people use and orient to media of various kinds, it is highly unlikely that such emergent, synergistic effects can be explained nor reliably predicted given the variety of medium-user combinations occurring today. Indeed, these entities and components are not easy to delineate because they always work as a system, in conjunction with and through the other. For example, it is possible that user recognition (at or below the level of conscious awareness) of the properties, capacities, and general affordances of a laptop used as a reading device prompts some page-oriented readers to be distracted, or possibly even lulled by the experience of merely anticipating additional stimulation. By the same token, and depending on their media histories, habitual screen readers may be stimulated and become more focused by the same condition. This could, in any case, be what was indicated by the theta spike detected in some participants' EEG data.

The argument here is that there is no obvious nor consistent matching between particular brains and particular EEG outputs (or MRI, or fMRI outputs for that matter). More to the point, no direct one-to-one relation necessarily exists between our thoughts-qua-states of mind and the discharge patterns of different groups of neurons in our brains. In sum, and in line with research and theorizing accomplished to date under the broad "extended mind" umbrella, the present project suggests that states of mind are always woefully underdetermined by states of brain matter. We need the world in the equation, just as we always have, to understand the mind's complexity. Otherwise we might begin thinking, as my research colleague did once jest, that we're seeing "a dead fish doing math." To be sure, all kinds of things can be read into and out of an EEG output (or an fMRI animation).

## A FUTURE FOR NEURO-MEDIA RESEARCH

New research of this sort will have to take more of the world into consideration. It was suggested at the beginning of this chapter that arguments postulating the brain-bound distribution of cognitive labor do not go far enough to explain brains or minds and will not be very helpful in enhancing our understanding of how in situ media users perceive and experience the world around them. Counterintuitively, perhaps, many of the latest brain-centered approaches toward understanding intention, states of mind, human consciousness, and cognition in general remain constrained by an outmoded allegiance to the notion that *brain=mind* or, perhaps, even that mind-qua-consciousness is a nagging fiction altogether. A quick survey of the questions asked and conclusions drawn in virtually all of the highest profile and most well funded research initiatives involving EEG, fMRI, and other tools suggest that an unmistakable media logic is at work. To be sure, untangling the subtle and varied technological biases bound up in the instrument-specific methods and methodologies of modern neuro-anotomical research undoubtedly deserves a separate chapter.

It will have to suffice for now to point out that any research enterprise designed around particular investigative tools like EEG, CAT, PET, MRI, and fMRI are especially susceptible to being prefigured and framed by the affordances of these technological innovations. Of course, the caveat is not to suggest an abandonment of such enterprises, only that they proceed under special scrutiny, including a high degree of self-awareness and reflexivity.[26] There is ample evidence suggesting that such methods call forth very particular units of analysis (neurons or clusters of neurons), and a "natural" level of analysis (that methodologically amounts to the disembodied, decontextualized human brain). The systematic reduction we are seeing of late appears to be one part technological determinism and one part procedural logic deriving from scientific method, with a healthy dose of anthropocentrism thrown in.

Research tools and methods, including their laboratory contexts, have always impacted the way investigators see the world, and these latest tools-in-use have the effect of procedurally framing cognitive processes along the contours of the physical brain like never before. Letting our tools do too much of the talking becomes an especially worrisome development given the way educational policy is becoming increasingly dependent upon "brain-based" and various other species of neuro-research. This is not to mention the manner in which the theorists most impressed by the new brain sciences are proposing quite narrow answers to wider questions of subjective experience and consciousness.

With these new practices we find old modes of thinking coming back with a vengeance. A serious concern is that this re-appropriation of outmoded theory has a cascade effect that ultimately aids in the reification of arbitrary methodological constraints and over-simplifies definitions of thinking and learning. It also helps conjure dubious theoretical constructs like multiple intelligences[27] and learning styles[28] and certainly constrains what potentially constitutes mind and cognitive activity.

Contrary to many professional opinions based in large measure upon this onslaught of brain-centered research, minds are not brains; they are thinking systems often distributed across a wide range of substrates, material and otherwise. Unfortunately, this kind of experimental and technological bias is especially prominent as a kind of echo or afterimage that gets peddled in popular media representations of a theory being generated, and perhaps the research that takes place to accomplish some larger work. Indeed, so much of this depends on how we read our new tools and devices and requires that we think carefully about the kinds of information they provide, including the levels of explanation and analysis they imply. Otherwise, this new science of the mind will have the tendency to systematically over-simplify the study of the brain (and mind) to the point that it begins to look very much like that questionable effort of searching for one's lost keys under the single street lamp.

A different story has been emerging that suggests that encapsulating the important action within skin and skull gives short shrift to the way thinking, and even perception occurs. Some representatives of the cognitive scientific community are looking at these tools in a different way. They are tracking multiple variables, processes and effects both in and outside of the skull and proceeding carefully, and self-reflexively, in their efforts to understand not merely brains but also the functional minds all that gray stuff helps instantiate.

A much broader and more nuanced story is manifesting. It is our biological system writ-large as an environment-based organism coupled to and constituted by various kinds of technology and media that prompt different modes of being-in-the-world. These structures help create different kinds of minds, and which eventually manifest in different kinds of brains, and even functionally different human organisms. As McLuhan put it, "man is an extension of nature that remakes the nature that makes the man."[29] Contemporary work in these areas should therefore extend the systems-theoretic approaches of Gibson and McLuhan, and cognitive philosophers like Andy Clark and David Chalmers. It's becoming increasingly clear, as Clark suggests, that we are natural-born cyborgs.[30] Given that modern humans are often different variations on the bio-mechanical-electro-digital-symbolic hybrid, we cannot productively study neurons, brains, or minds without systematically getting outside of our heads.

Future investigations involving brain measurement apparatuses of any kind (including EEG, CAT, MRI, and fMRI) should consider ways of first grouping research participants according to their habitual "media-couplings" and then make note of the different cognitive and perceptual affordances and capacities those new environments seem to represent for particular users before attempting to make sense of the outputs of those apparatuses. J.J. Gibson, an early proponent of the "extended mind" camp, bolsters McLuhan's core thesis regarding communication media as prostheses or extensions of the humans who use them.[31] Gibson suggested that "the words 'animal' and 'environment' make an inseparable pair. Each term implies the other. No animal could exist without an environment surrounding it.

Equally, though not so obvious, an environment implies an animal (an organism with particular capacities and capabilities) to be surrounded."[32]

## NOTES

This chapter is based on "Reading Into, and Out of, McLuhan's Neuro-philosophy: Preliminary Observations from an EEG Investigation Comparing Screen and Page Reading," a paper presented at McLuhan's Philosophy of Media conference in Brussels, 2012, and included in the conference proceedings. I would like to thank Dr. Bruce Steinberg, who guided and assisted with the original research featured in this chapter.

1. Marshall McLuhan, *The Gutenberg Galaxy* (Toronto: University of Toronto Press, 1962); McLuhan, *Understanding Media: The Extensions of Man*, ed. W. Terrence Gordon (Corte Madera, CA: Gingko Press, 1994); Marshall McLuhan, *Verbi-Voco-Visual Explorations* (New York: Something Else Press, 1967); Marshall McLuhan, "The Brain and the Media: The 'Western' Hemisphere," *Journal of Communication*, 28, no. 4 (1978): 54–60; Marshall McLuhan and Eric McLuhan, *Laws of Media: The New Science* (Toronto: University of Toronto Press, 1988).
2. Cf. also "extended cognition," "embodied cognition," "enactive cognition," "existential cognition," etc. Anthony Chemero and Michael Silberstein, "Defending Extended Cognition," http://philsci-archive.pitt.edu/archive/0000 3204/; Andy Clark, *Being There: Putting Brain, Body, and World Back Together Again* (Cambridge, MA: MIT Press, 1996); Andy Clark, "Linguistic Anchors in the Sea of Thought," *Pragmatics and Cognition* 4, no. 1 (1996): 93–103; Andy Clark, *Natural Born Cyborgs* (Oxford: Oxford University Press, 2003); Andy Clark, "Beyond the Flesh: Some Lessons from a Mole Cricket," *Artificial Life* 11, no. 1–2 (2005): 233–44; Antonio Damasio, *Descartes' Error: Emotion, Reason and the Human Brain* (New York: Putnam Books, 1994); Antonio Damasio, *The Feeling of What Happens: Body and Emotion in the Making of Consciousness* (New York: Harcourt-Brace, 1999); Antonio Damasio and Hanna Damasio, "Minding the Body," *Daedalus* 135, no. 3 (2006): 15–22; Ron McClamrock, *Existential Cognition: Computational Minds in the World* (Chicago: Chicago University Press, 1995); Jessica Lindblom and Tom Ziemke, "Interacting Socially through Embodied Action," in *Enacting Intersubjectivity: A Cognitive and Social Perspective on the Study of Interactions*, ed. Francesca Morganti, Antonella Carassa, and Giuseppe Riva, 49–63 (Amsterdam: IOS Press, 2008); Robert Logan, *The Extended Mind: The Emergence of Language, the Human Mind and Culture* (Toronto: University of Toronto Press, 2008); N. Katherine Hayles, *How We Think: Digital Media and Contemporary Technogenesis* (Chicago: University of Chicago Press, 2012).
3. Stanislas Dehaene, *The Reading Brain: The New Science of How We Read* (New York: Penguin Books, 2009), 257.
4. Richard Restak, *The New Brain: How the Modern Age Is Rewiring Your Mind* (New York: Rodale, 2004); Dehaene, *Reading Brain*.
5. For example, McClamrock describes a non-reductive, though non-dualist position in line with a functional understanding of the human cognitive apparatus that is variously described in the philosophical literature as a form of extended, embedded, or *existential cognition*. McClamrock, *Existential Cognition*.

6. John J. Burns and Daniel R. Anderson, "Cognition and Watching Television," in *The Neuropsychology of Everyday Life: Issues in Development and Rehabilitation*, ed. David E. Tupper and Keith D. Cicerone, 93–108 (Norwell, MA: Springer, 1990).
7. Herbert E. Krugman, "Brainwave Measures of Media Involvement," *Journal of Advertising Research* 11 (1971): 3–9.
8. Gregg Featherman et al., *Electroencephalographic and Electrooculographic Correlates of Television Viewing: Final Technical Report*, National Science Foundation Student-Oriented Studies (Grant SP178–03698) (Amherst, MA: Hampshire College, 1979).
9. Burns and Anderson, "Cognition," 100.
10. Valentine Appel, Sidney Weinstein, and Curt Weinstein, "Brain Activity and Recall of TV," *Journal of Advertising Research* 19, no. 4 (1979): 7–15.
11. James L. Walker, "Changes in EEG Rhythms during Television Viewing: Preliminary Comparisons with Reading and other Tasks," *Perceptual and Motor Skills* 51, no. 1 (1980): 255–61; Michael S. Radlick, *The Processing Demands of Television: Neurophysiological Correlates of Television Viewing* (Troy, NY: Rensselaer Polytechnic Institute, 1980).
12. Robert Kubey and Mihaly Csikszentmihalyi, "Television Addiction Is No Mere Metaphor," *Scientific American*, February 2002, http://www.sciam.com/2002/0202issue/0202kubey.html.
13. James J. Gibson, *The Ecological Approach to Visual Perception* (Boston: Houghton Mifflin, 1979).
14. LabView 8.5 software, National Instruments.
15. DataQ Instruments.
16. "Test Your Focus," *New York Times*, http://www.nytimes.com/interactive/2010/06/07/technology/20100607-distraction-filtering-demo.html.
17. Indeed, this all seemed hard to avoid for most of the research participants. This is not to mention talk of standard regimens that included "morning doses" of Facebook, Twitter, Instagram, and other digital social media.
18. Cf. Robert C. MacDougall, ed., *Drugs and Media* (New York: Continuum, 2012).
19. Marc Prensky, "Digital Natives, Digital Immigrants," *On the Horizon* 9, no. 5 (2001): 1–6.
20. Ibid.
21. Gary Gumpert and Robert Cathcart, "Media Grammars, Generations and Media Gaps," *Critical Studies in Mass Communication* 2, no. 1 (1985): 23–35.
22. Ibid.
23. McLuhan, *Gutenberg Galaxy*; McLuhan, *Understanding Media*; McLuhan and McLuhan, *Laws of Media*.
24. Gumpert and Cathcart, "Media Grammars," 24.
25. Don Berlyne, *Conflict, Arousal and Curiosity* (New York: McGraw-Hill, 1960).
26. Cf. Bruno Latour, *Science in Action: How to Follow Scientists and Engineers through Society* (Cambridge, MA: Harvard University Press, 1987); Latour, *Aramis or the Love of Technology*, trans. Catherine Porter (Cambridge, MA: Harvard University Press, 1996); Latour, *Reassembling the Social: An Introduction to Actor-Network-Theory* (Oxford: Oxford University Press, 2005).
27. Howard Gardner, *Frames of Mind: The Theory of Multiple Intelligences* (New York: Basic Books, 2011).
28. David A. Kolb and Ronald E. Fry, "Toward an Applied Theory of Experiential Learning," in *Theories of Group Process*, ed. Cary L. Cooper, 33–58 (London: John Wiley, 1975).

29. Marshall McLuhan and Barrington Nevitt, *Take Today: The Executive as Dropout* (New York: Harcourt, Brace, Jovanovich, 1972), 66.
30. Clark, *Natural Born Cyborgs*.
31. Gibson, *Ecological Approach*.
32. Ibid., 8.

# 8    On the Origins of Propaganda
## Bio-Cultural and Evolutionary Perspectives on Social Cohesion

*Bob Schapiro and Stanley H. Ambrose*

## INTRODUCTION: MEMES AT WORK

The ability to form social groups based on shared ideas and beliefs is uniquely human. Other species, such as wolves or lions, form groups based on genetic kinship, reproduction, shared territories and immediate survival, but never, as far as we can tell, around an idea. Our closest cousins, chimpanzees and other primates, live in groups called troops, also based, in part on genetic kinship. They display many behaviors that, among humans, might commonly be associated with the formation of dominance hierarchies and "in-groups" or coalitions, which may play several roles:

> The formation of coalitions may result in the maintenance or the increase of the dominance of an individual, in the expulsion of certain lower ranked individuals from a group, in taking over a group, in the defense of the home range against other groups, in getting access to estrus females, and in the protection of an infant or adult female. The degree of cognition involved in coalitions is unclear.[1]

Modern propaganda often leads to the same results as primate coalitions: Raising the status of a group leader, expelling people from the group, uniting members in defending the group's homeland, and so on. The degree of cognition of the properties of coalitions among humans is, of course, significantly higher.

We shall develop the thesis that our modern human propensities for cooperation and coalition formation have deep evolutionary biological roots, and that some aspects of our biology, including the effects of some hormones on our brains and our behavior, influence our susceptibility to the modes of communication often labeled as propaganda. We shall draw on the behaviors and biology shared with our primate relatives for evidence for the foundations for human coalition formation in cooperation and competition, and for propaganda.[2]

One is tempted to abandon the word *propaganda* as hopelessly vague, yet it remains very popular in the American vocabulary. The well-regarded textbook *Propaganda and Persuasion* details no fewer than fifteen different definitions.[3] Clearly propaganda represents a concept that people wish to communicate. Furthermore, the United States and other countries have laws against certain types of propaganda. Without a solid definition, these laws can become the basis for indiscriminate censorship, or even censorship that no one intends.

We will propose a concise definition of propaganda that is applicable across human cultures and trace its roots in our biological heritage. This will, at times, take us back and forth between biology and culture, before we see how the two unite in defining propaganda. In the end it turns out that what we discover is not really a new definition, but one that is consistent with the seemingly diverse uses of the word *propaganda* throughout most of history.

We begin by identifying aspects that are consistent in most uses of this word: we often use the term *propaganda* to refer to what they say, as opposed to what we believe. You can take your pick of who they are: Big corporations, foreign governments, the mainstream media, liberals or conservatives, ethnic groups, social classes, and so on.[4] This leads to the second consistent aspect: propaganda concerns groups. We rarely use the word to refer to interpersonal communication, although similar strategies may be used between individuals.

The roots of propaganda may be embedded deeply in our ancestry, with the beginnings of syntactic language, or perhaps even earlier, when our primate ancestors began to live in social groups with dominance hierarchies and defended territories. Moreover, it likely began with inter-individual one-on-one communication rather than one-to-many communication. For example, an assertive individual in a chimpanzee troop, lion pride, or elephant seal herd uses physical and vocal threats against other individuals to rise in the dominance hierarchy; lower ranked individuals sort themselves in a similar interactive fashion down the line, sometimes forming coalitions of a few individuals.[5] When the pecking order stabilizes it seems likely that the troop members have accepted their position or rank within the social order.[6] Stability can be maintained by occasional threats and warnings by dominant members, which can settle hierarchical disputes without physical injury. We consider this kind of communication to be a pre-adaptation for more complex sub-group and group level goal-oriented communication that can be considered propaganda.[7]

Indoctrinability is a closely related concept. It is defined by Polly Wiessner as the universally human "predisposition to be inculcated with values or loyalties that run contrary to immediate individual interest."[8] She proposed that this predisposition began with the development of formal kinship systems, and the extension of kinship terms to unrelated individuals. Calling someone brother, sister, or father may be a strategy for building individual alliances, and the foundation for uniting group members for intergroup competition, as with soldiers who call themselves brothers-in-arms.

Among humans, propaganda is about the socially cohesive ideas and behaviors that may hold one group together and tear another group apart. These are different sides of the same coin. Very often we are talking about exactly the same ideas: the speeches that seem routine at an American Fourth of July parade would be foreign propaganda in much of the world. Any human social group that fails to actively propagate its memes—its ideas and behaviors—is as doomed as one that fails to propagate its genes. The people of ancient Carthage likely had a vibrant propaganda when they followed Hannibal across the Alps, but Carthage's belief system does not survive today; or rather, the genes and memes of Carthage are so scattered that they are no longer recognizable as the traits of a group. Our propaganda, then, is important to our survival.

## OUR BIOLOGY

Among most primate species, cooperation occurs *within* groups, but conflict predominates *between* groups. The great evolutionary advantage of human beings is our ability to cooperate over extended social landscapes with other social groups, and to communicate complex ideas with spoken language. In our long evolution on the African savanna, an individual early hominid was ill-equipped to survive alone. We are weaker and less agile than chimpanzees, slower than cheetahs (and almost anything else larger than a chicken) and we have nothing like the big teeth and claws of lions, tigers or even wolves. Not only are we physically outclassed by our predators and competitors, we are sometimes outclassed by our prey; as individuals our early Stone Age ancestors were probably unable to hunt larger prey, such as buffalo, elk, or wooly mammoth. But humans hunting in groups were likely able to dominate their environment.

Thus group cohesion is at the center of the human experience. Furthermore, we often form non-kinship groups, not just the troops common among other primates. This begins with an extremely high level of trust. Paul J. Zak, who studies the role of the neurologically active hormone oxytocin in trust, cooperation, and reciprocity, notes that our ability to walk down a city street is remarkable, considering that many other hunting species would worry that every stranger they encounter might attack. Instead we are able to see most strangers as members of a group to which we also belong.[9] Biologist Martin Nowak is more illustrative in calling human beings nature's "super-cooperators":

> In this respect, our close relatives don't even come close. Take four hundred chimpanzees and put them in economy class on a seven-hour flight. They would, in all likelihood, stumble off the plane at their destination with bitten ears, missing fur and bleeding limbs. Yet millions of us tolerate being crammed together this way so we can roam the planet.[10]

We expect cooperative behavior at an early age. Wiessner describes indoctrination of six-month-old infants with the ethos of gift giving and of young men with the standards, practices, and values of their society during extended initiation ceremonies.[11] You may recall your first day of kindergarten, when you were required to sit quietly with a roomful of strangers, accepting them as your new group. Most of us were able to master this skill as five-year-olds, at least for a short while. In terms of biology, this is really a momentous achievement: virtually no other primates can do this, no matter how they are raised, yet all healthy humans can be raised this way.

Furthermore, as five-year-olds, we understood that our new group was "Miss Brown's class" and that we were there to learn things. Some of what we learn includes socially cohesive beliefs such as American citizenship, reinforced by daily pledging allegiance to the flag. Many people don't send their children to public school precisely because they see it as a threat to the beliefs and cohesion of a group. Teaching evolution, for example, can be a threat to the cohesion of a fundamentalist group that believes that the world is only about six thousand years old. One group may consider evolution to simply be a scientific fact; another group may label it propaganda.

On the flip side, most of us have, at times, been part of some arbitrary task-oriented group that dissolved once the task was complete. These groups seemingly have no propaganda, no shared cohesive beliefs of much consequence. Yet when experimental psychologists manipulate these temporary groups in opposition to each other, they can exhibit many of the negative behaviors of long-standing groups. Ironically, classroom teachers have seen the same thing when they form a random group to help students understand the detrimental effects of labeling a group as the "other."[12] Why should we care so much about the Blue Team versus the Red Team? Why are sports fans so passionate that we have soccer riots? On a more positive note, can a school pep rally do more than just fill the stands at a football game?

We have seen that communication and cooperation are intertwined; each gives an enormous boost to the usefulness of the other. So, too, are biology and culture intertwined in studying these fields, yet it is important to recognize when we are seeing one and not the other. A smile is a good illustration of a natural human biological behavior. It's in our genes. A healthy human baby can be raised in any culture and it will naturally understand what a smile is about. In fact, people from many different cultures show roughly the same frequency of deciphering whether or not a smile is sincere.[13] Shaking your head yes or no, however, is a cultural behavior. It may seem like "second-nature" to us, but in India many people do a head bobble that is entirely different. Cultural behaviors, such as shaking your head, depend on biology to a certain extent—such as our ability to understand symbols and gestures—but they are specific to certain cultures. Culture may also mediate biological behaviors; people in different cultures smile at different things.

The ways in which modern human beings form social groups reflect unique biologically based social abilities. There is mounting evidence that

Neanderthals—a branch of humanity that survived until roughly forty thousand years ago—did not match our social abilities for cooperation.[14] During the last ice age, Neanderthals apparently continued to live in small, closed territories with limited intergroup interactions, often involving interpersonal violence and cannibalism. Conversely, African moderns (anatomically modern humans) apparently adopted a very different social and territorial organization strategy to reduce risk during this era of harsh and unpredictable climates: they apparently began to forge strong networks of cooperation with distant social groups, reinforced by reciprocal gift giving. African moderns thus behaved more like human tribes, Neanderthals more like primate troops. These differences in social and territorial organization and information sharing may have contributed to the eventual replacement of Neanderthals by African modern humans during the last ice age.

Were Neanderthals deficient in, or relatively insensitive to, pro-social variants of hormones such as oxytocin, serotonin, and vasopressin, and did they have an excess of anti-social ones, such as testosterone? We are far from a definitive answer. Although the genetic basis for variation in behavior in relationship to variation in these hormones in a wide range of animal species—including humans—is becoming well understood,[15] the DNA of Neanderthals has not yet been analyzed this way. However one remarkable feature of Neanderthal skulls may reflect their hormonal status. Among humans, facial masculinity or robusticity—a strong jaw and prominent brow, among other features—is correlated with testosterone levels.[16] Chimpanzees and gorillas also show this relationship, as well as the fossilized skulls of our early hominid ancestors. The robust faces of Neanderthals suggest that they also had extremely high levels of testosterone.[17] This hormone can have anti-social effects, at least in males, as will be discussed later.

Neanderthals likely referred to competing groups in ways that many people today would consider to be propaganda. Conversely, like the hunter-gatherers of the Kalahari Desert of southern Africa studied by Polly Wiessner, early modern humans may have promoted an ethos of sharing, cooperation, and trust with members of other social groups within their region by using inclusive kinship terms and reciprocal gift-giving.[18]

While the success of modern humans is the result of many factors, at this point we can see that the evolution of greater cooperation and trust is quite important. "Propaganda" can't be all bad if it propagates socially cohesive beliefs. Yet some people have a vague sense that propaganda is inherently negative. Let's jump right into the heart of that debate.

## AXIS SALLY

While there are differing definitions of propaganda, we should also note that there are areas of general consensus. Most analysts would agree that the World War II radio hosts called "Axis Sally," "Berlin Betty," and other names were broadcasting propaganda; after all, they worked for the German Ministry of Propaganda. Let's imagine a scene from an old World War II movie. The American soldiers are sitting in a foxhole, listening to music played by Axis Sally. The sergeant says, "Turn off that damned propaganda," but the GIs assure him that they're just listening to the music, they don't believe any of "those lies." The problem is that the enemy broadcasters are not lying—and that's why they're dangerous.

Between songs, Axis Sally is *not* arguing that national socialism is a superior socio-economic system to American capitalism. She is not even saying that the Germans are winning the war, a claim that would seem rather hollow by the time American troops were well established in France. Instead she is reminding soldiers that while they're in Europe, their poor gray-haired mother is working the farm all by herself, or that their father's small business is suffering because he has to make all the deliveries "and he's not as young as he used to be." And what's more, "your wife can't be happy, being alone so long." For a number of soldiers, these statements ring true. If Axis Sally can create tension between their roles as soldiers and their roles as sons, boyfriends, and husbands, then her propaganda is effective. Normally these things are not in conflict, but if Axis Sally can create turmoil in the soldier's mind, she's doing her job.

We can be more precise by examining what Axis Sally is not doing. When she reminds soldiers that their families miss them, she is not lying, she is not persuading them of something they did not believe before, she is not giving them "bad" information—in fact, she's not giving them any new information at all, she is merely reminding them of a reality that may be distant from their thoughts. In psychological terms, Axis Sally's job is to create cognitive dissonance, the disconcerting feeling you sometimes have when you hold two opposing ideas in your mind at the same time. Human beings can experience cognitive dissonance over group identity in ways no other animal can experience, because only humans can have the mental capacities for being in several different idea-based groups at one time.

While other animals may have the specialized role of fighting on behalf of the group, the group itself is never half a world away. That is one reason why propaganda tends to be noticeable among soldiers; if we are not fighting for the immediate needs of a small kin-related group, ideas are needed for group cohesion. Thus we are fighting for democracy, we are fighting for Mother Russia, we are fighting to bring religion to the heathens, we are fighting for the glory that is Rome, we are fighting for the Emperor. When soldiers begin to question what they are fighting for, their army is in trouble.

It is difficult to get people to question their core beliefs. That's why Axis Sally is taking an easier route: she is taking the beliefs we already have and putting them in cognitively dissonant opposition.

Armies have many ways of creating group cohesion: parades, medals, flags, and many shared experiences of hardship and exultation. These are what sociologist Émile Durkheim described as "a rhythm of collective life" that enhances idea-based groups, observing that "man has a natural faculty for idealizing, that is, for substituting for the world of reality a different world to which he is transported by thought."[19] Most of us are aware of times when we willingly seek cohesive propaganda. We know what to expect when we go to the school pep rally or the Fourth of July parade, what ideas will be communicated. If we already agree, then this propaganda does not persuade us, but it motivates us. To use psychological terms once again, these events help create cognitive consonance, reinforcing the beliefs we already have and making us feel good about the group.

Up to this point, then, we can define propaganda as communication that affects group cohesion, creating either cognitive dissonance or cognitive consonance. In military circles this is often called "the information war," but as we can see, both sides may be using the same information. Clearly there is an additional element at work. The late Neal Postman and his New York University colleague Terence Moran find that element in the context of answers to the following questions that create one's personal belief system:[20]

1. Who am I? (A son or daughter, a wife or husband, a citizen, a farmer, a lawyer, an inventor.)
2. Where do I come from? (What group am I in? Where does the group come from?)
3. What is my status? (My rank; my place within the group.)
4. What is my quest? (What am I supposed to do?)

Your family is almost always your first group—you know your place at a young age. Yet for human beings, other group identifications develop very quickly. It is fairly easy to see how your religion and nationality can answer multiple "belief system" questions, although we sometimes fail to appreciate how other group identifications answer multiple questions as well. For example, readers of a certain age will recall John Denver's song, "Thank God I'm a Country Boy," in which a host of wholesome practices and beliefs are inferred simply by declaring one's self a country boy.

If you ask someone the open-ended question "Please tell me about yourself," he or she may say "I'm from Texas" (a regional identity); "I'm Catholic" (religion); "I'm a vice-president at IBM" (occupation); or "I'm the mother of three boys" (family). Of course, one person can be all of these things. Our belief systems often provide more than one answer to the same question. Yet at any given moment we generally don't consider ourselves to be some agglomeration of our various beliefs and identities. A "system" is singular—we know who we are. Most of us would like to believe that we choose our own primary group at any given moment, but if you think about it, that is often not the case. Imagine yourself at work. The phone rings. If it is someone you supervise, then you are the boss. If it is your boss, then obviously you are the employee. So far you are just in your work group, but it can quickly become more complex. If your daughter calls, you are a parent; you are suddenly in your family identity. If your spouse calls, you are in a different family identity. If the call is from the mechanic who still hasn't fixed your car, you might be quite demanding. But if it is from someone to whom you are trying to sell your car, you are in no position to make demands. Your position in the social hierarchy can be different each time you answer the phone. Sometimes you are consciously aware of this, sometimes not. Psychologist Kenneth Gergen points out that this change in our media environment occurred in an eyeblink of human history and that we did not evolve to handle such sudden changes.[21]

Earlier we discussed how certain animals display a pre-adaptation for propaganda when they utilize threat displays or submissive posturing instead of actual violence. But for animals, it is only about hierarchy. They don't have multiple belief-based groups. So we must add to our definition of propaganda to complete it: *Propaganda is communication that utilizes your personal belief system to affect group cohesion, creating either cognitive dissonance or cognitive consonance.*

Neal Postman said that the authority of a definition rests entirely on its usefulness, not its correctness.[22] We believe that the preceding definition is useful when applied to examples that most Americans consider propaganda, and it is also consistent with the biological roots of human coalition formation. Propaganda may be positive or negative, true or false, but it is generally more effective when it has some truth for you. It concerns your personal belief system. In the "Axis Sally" example, the propaganda has little effect on those who do not feel any conflict between their obligations overseas and at home.

What about the issue of intent? When a high school teacher says, "It doesn't matter whether you vote for a Democrat or a Republican, the important thing is that you vote," the teacher may not intend the statement as propaganda. There is, however, a message: "Trust and believe in the system. Participate in it." Sometimes that is non-controversial, but when groups on the left or right are loudly declaring "our system is broken," then the previously innocuous statement about voting can become propaganda. French theorist Jacques Ellul would consider that to be sociological propaganda.

In his influential book *Propaganda*, Ellul admits that his definition of sociological propaganda is "vast." [23] We think it is often too vast to survive Postman's test of usefulness outside of a scholarly context, and Ellul might agree. Think of a young mother teaching basic moral values to her toddler. She may use facts, logic, a story—and propaganda. That last one may jump out at you; we generally don't think of young mothers as propagandists with their own children. By the same token, we don't consider her to be teaching literary analysis when she asks her child the meaning of a fairy tale, although in a strict sense, she is. But it is not always useful to look at things in such a pedantic way. This example may, in fact, cross the blurry boundary between propaganda and indoctrination as defined by Wiessner.[24] Propaganda is a type of communication, just as facts are, and can be modified with the same commonly used words. There are simple facts and complicated facts, as well as nasty facts and pleasant facts. And although a "fact" is supposed to be true, few people have difficulty understanding the oxymoron "false facts." Various types of propaganda can be described in much the same way, without inventing a specialized language.

Once again: Propaganda is communication that utilizes your personal belief system to affect group cohesion, creating either cognitive dissonance or cognitive consonance. Is this definition consistent with our biology and our history? The modern use of the word *propaganda* is generally traced back to 1622, when Pope Gregory XV established the Sacred Congregation for the Propagation of the Faith (Propaganda Fide). This group propagated ideas that directly utilized people's belief systems. These ideas generally increased the cohesion of Catholics and disrupted the cohesion of people who were not Catholic. If the propaganda was effective, it caused cognitive consonance or cognitive dissonance, depending on which group you were in.

Human beings and other social animals have a biologically based propensity in the ways they form groups. To what degree does our biology work with culture in the way we actually form groups today? This is one small facet of the much larger issue of nature versus nurture in human behavior that includes the extent to which we are born with a blank slate versus genetically "wired" for culture,[25] good natured,[26] born to be good,[27] angelic,[28] and moral,[29] or Machiavellian,[30] or cooperative in competition with others, as Darwin proposed in *The Descent of Man*.[31]

## ALTRUISTIC PUNISHMENT

Propaganda has a great deal to do with the evolution of our pro-social behaviors. A good example may be "altruistic punishment." This is when we punish someone who violates the norms of the group, even when it is against our individual interests to do so. While these norms are often cultural in origin, altruistic punishment appears to be a species-wide behavior in modern humans.[32] To illustrate, picture a highway where two lanes must merge at a popular exit. Traffic in these two exit lanes is backed up a quarter-mile, while cars on the main highway whiz by. A selfish driver decides to cut in near the exit itself and succeeds in getting into the left lane of the two exit lanes. Drivers on the right see this. They now cooperate in blocking the malefactor from merging onto the exit ramp, even though it costs each of them precious time in their commute and may even risk denting their car. In narrow economic terms, they would each come out ahead if they just continued to obey the traffic sign that says "Alternate Merge," but they want to punish the transgression. Some drivers engage in altruistic punishment reflexively while others are thinking ahead, believing that they themselves will benefit in the future if selfish driving is deterred. Either way, the behavior benefits the group.

What does this have to do with modern propaganda? Plenty: many popular World War I propaganda posters said simply, "Remember Belgium." Everyone knew the context: Germany had violated international law by ignoring the neutrality of Belgium. The mere fact that Germany had violated the norms of the group was enough to motivate people. Nothing on the posters said that protecting Belgium would benefit us directly; in fact, the posters usually called for people to make sacrifices. Similarly, today we have an active debate about military strikes against nations that use chemical weapons, with many people saying that we must punish such nations for violating international law, even if that is not in our immediate self-interest. Both today's debate and the World War I debate are examples of our tendency toward altruistic punishment. Of course both international law and traffic laws arise mostly from culture. Yet our biological evolution has much to do with the way we choose to enforce group norms.

## TWO SIMULTANEOUS EVOLUTIONS

Human beings, like other animals, evolved over time as we both competed and cooperated with other individuals. But unlike other animals, human beings also competed and cooperated as members of groups organized, in part, around fairly complex cultures. Recent discoveries indicate that the influence of such culture may go back much earlier than previously thought.

As we have stated, social cohesion and propaganda are two sides of the same coin, a coin that may have gained special currency once human beings developed settled agriculture. The Agricultural Revolution—or Neolithic Revolution—occurred eight thousand to twelve thousand years ago, when human beings moved from being hunter-gatherers to producing and storing a reliable surplus of food. When people settled down, farmed the land, and stored food, their population densities began to increase by orders of magnitude; competition for resources may have intensified. With the "the rise of civilization," we got really serious about forming larger, non-kinship-based groups. But a reliable surplus of food is merely an economic condition. The biological and language communication equipment necessary for modern social cohesion—and propaganda—was already in place. The question is not whether these faculties came together suddenly for this purpose but whether propaganda was useful far earlier in our evolution.

There is increasing evidence that our ancestors may have developed cooperative social networks more than seventy thousand years ago or even earlier, when we were certainly hunter-gatherers, not farmers. This may have been a nascent social security system, similar to that of Kalahari Desert hunter-gatherer communities in southern Africa studied by anthropologist

Polly Wiessner. She explains the logic of this system in her paper titled "Taking the Risk Out of Risky Transactions" as follows:[33]

> For the better part of our history as foragers, the well-being of any individual rested heavily in the hands of others. With no grain in the larder, no meat stored on the hoof, and no money in the bank, humans had little option other than to build savings in the form of social ties that could be drawn on to cover unforeseen losses caused by environmental or social hazards. . . . In other words, risk, the probability of loss, was pooled within social networks.

One notable feature of the Kalahari peoples studied by Wiessner is that every stranger that speaks their language is considered a priori a potential partner to be added to their widespread social networks of trusted, reciprocating cooperators. Similar strategies are adopted by Australian desert Aborigines, foragers in the American Great Basin, and the Turkana herders of the harsh lowlands of the Kenya Rift Valley. Looking further into the past, during the last ice age, when large areas of the world were colder, drier, and more unpredictable, Late Paleolithic modern human hunter-gatherers seem to have developed similar large-scale social networks, uniting local groups into regional networks that could be considered tribal in geographic scale. Conversely, Neanderthals seem to have refuged in more predictable humid forested enclaves where they could defend their local group territorial boundaries. In terms of territorial defensiveness, archaic Neanderthals behaved more like primate troops than human tribes.

We can now examine the extent to which there is biological basis for this new strategy of intergroup reciprocity. Was our modern human capacity for cooperation and trust facilitated by the increased prevalence of pro-social variants of the genes for hormones that influence social behaviors? If so, then when and how did we make this biological transition?

## THE BIG BOOST

To paraphrase Virginia Woolf, on or about 71,800 BCE, human behavior began a period of rapid change. That is the approximate time of the fiery Toba supereruption, the largest explosive volcanic event of the last 23 million years. Ash and dust from this Sumatran volcano have been found in the sediments beneath the Yellow Sea on the east, and Lake Malawi and South Africa on the west.[34] A layer of sulfuric acid-infused ice that lies more than two and a half kilometers below the surface of the Greenland ice sheet suggests that Toba may have caused an icy six-year volcanic winter followed by two millennia of the coldest temperatures of the last ice age. After a brief respite from this instant ice age, extreme cold returned between seventy and sixty thousand years ago. The anomalously low genetic diversity of the human species today indicates a rapid decline of global human populations during this era.[35] If we'd had the foresight to create an endangered species list, we'd have nearly been on it.

Not to spoil the ending, we survived—but not unchanged. Patterns of genetic diversification show population growth and range expansion beginning sixty thousand years ago, during the middle of the last ice age, as modern humans expanded within, and then out of, Africa. Humans already likely had modern capacities to communicate and cooperate. The volcanic winter and its ensuing mini ice age may have boosted what has been called the troop-to-tribe transition by creating environmental conditions that further favored extended social networks and the "super-cooperators" who functioned well within them.

Anthropologists rarely, if ever, use the term *troop* for even the earliest tool-using human ancestors. Territoriality and the absence of intergroup pro-social interaction are key features of troop-level organization. Most primate species have extremely limited and usually antagonistic and defensive inter-troop territorial boundary relationships. Conversely, the Kalahari San and other "band" level societies in arid, risky environments are integrated into larger regional intergroup cooperative networks that extend over long distances.[36] Regional integration makes such hunter-gatherer "band" societies more like tribes, as traditionally defined in anthropology. Yellen and Harpending take the implications of regional networks even further, arguing that agriculturalists living in endogamous villages with defended territories and limited intergroup interactions have a band level of organization.[37] We agree with Watts that the role of propaganda in the origins of social cohesion is closely tied to the evolution of within- and between-group competition and cooperation in our primate relatives and ancestors.[38] The scale of dissemination of propaganda likely increased with the troop-to-tribe transition, and with subsequent increases in scale and complexity of social formations such as chiefdoms, states, and empires.[39]

During this prolonged era of extremely harsh and variable climates, greater cooperation may have been essential for survival. Perhaps those individuals with the genetic predisposition for greater cooperation, mediated by their pro-social variants of genes related to the functions of oxytocin,[40] serotonin,[41] and vasopressin,[42] had greater survivorship, while those with the anti-social variants, and those with high levels of testosterone may have largely, but not completely, died out.[43] Our modern ancestors may have emerged from this bottleneck with the biologically enhanced toolkit to facilitate survival through trust, reciprocity, and cooperation. Neanderthals, as noted earlier, retain the kind of robust skull features that are associated with high levels of testosterone[44] and thus may have been less predisposed toward trust, cooperation, and reciprocity.

We should pause to define our terms. Henceforth, for clarity, we will refer to serotonin, vasopressin, and oxytocin as "pro-social" hormones. This is an oversimplification because each hormone is part of a complex system that has both pro- and anti-social genetic variants, and other neurotransmitters and endorphins can also influence sociality.[45] People who take Prozac and other such medications may know that modulating serotonin in the brain can elevate mood and lead to pro-social behaviors. Similarly, testosterone is a steroid hormone that, in certain degrees, can lead to aggressive or anti-social behavior, similar to what has been popularly called 'roid rage.

Oxytocin is related to an increase in trust reciprocity, and empathy, the ability to perceive another's affective state ("I feel your pain"). Neuroeconomist Paul Zak designed an economic game—"The Trust Game"—in which two strangers, who never learn each other's identities and who communicate only by computer, are given a certain amount of cash. The optimal result is that they can increase each other's money by 200 percent, but this only happens when they display optimal trust and reciprocity. Zak administered oxytocin to some subjects with an inhaler to determine if trust and reciprocity increased. In repeated experiments, Zak found that greater trust and reciprocity was associated with a 47 percent increase in oxytocin from baseline. This is an indication that this hormone has a direct influence on pro-social behavior and displays of empathy. In experiments of similar design with testosterone, Zak and colleagues found an increase in distrust and anger among male subjects in response to unfair transactions, whereas females responded by matching degrees of unfairness. Put simply, men get mad, women get even.[46]

If oxytocin plays a role in our susceptibility to propaganda, is there evidence that levels of this hormone can be manipulated by vocal communication? Several studies have indeed shown that social support and expression of empathy increase oxytocin and reduce cortisol (a stress-induced hormone) levels.[47] Indeed, empathetic text messages do not have this effect.[48] Like physical grooming[49] empathetic speech and perhaps flattery may increase oxytocin and other pro-social hormones.[50] The charming car salesman may manipulate your trust hormone levels with a few strategic compliments before making the pitch for a model with accessories that you cannot afford, but will increase his sales commission.

To see this in an evolutionary context, first remember that primates include, among others, monkeys, the great apes, and human beings. A primate troop is a group whose world essentially ends at the boundary of their home range. Their interactions with other troops are nearly always antagonistic.[51] The exception is when a breeding-age individual may cross over into another troop. This is a one-way trip. They do not go home again.[52]

The troop-to-tribe transition[53] emphasizes the aspect of the definition of tribes involving the formation of macro-regional networks of local groups with positive reciprocal relationships. They can be permanent agricultural villages but they can also be mobile herders or hunter-gatherers. Their economy is not a determining factor in their social evolution.

These regional networks are organized around ideas; the earliest ones likely shared only the simple idea that, as stated, "social ties . . . could be drawn on to cover unforeseen losses caused by environmental or social hazards." It is good to have someone to cover your back when bad things happen.[54]

After the Toba supereruption, we begin to see evidence of modern humans taking an increasingly pro-social direction.[55] If you have more social ties, you are a member of more groups. To be clear, we are not suggesting that the volcanic winter and instant ice age caused any genetic mutations. However, if the environment changed abruptly, then those humans that may have squeezed through a population bottleneck may have had preexisting genetic traits that became much more advantageous in the risky ice age environment, and spread rapidly when populations rebounded.

This hypothesis is further supported by evidence of what happened to Neanderthals. After the Toba eruption, their population declined just as modern humans did.[56] Much later, around forty-five thousand years ago, modern humans, who had now expanded out of Africa, began to encounter Neanderthals, and Neanderthals became extinct around five thousand years later.[57] In a one-on-one match, Neanderthals were bigger and stronger than our modern human ancestors. However, if Neanderthal troops could not form intergroup coalitions, then they could not compete with modern human tribes. As we noted earlier, anatomical and archeological evidence indicates a hormonal difference: Neanderthals may have had higher levels of anti-social hormones than our ancestors, whereas modern humans had already gone the other direction, utilizing more pro-social hormones. In short, modern humans were more effective cooperators, perhaps because our ancestors had the biological equipment to facilitate the troop-to-tribe transition, whereas Neanderthals lacked this ability.

Thus conformity of individuals and groups to the social order of hierarchies has deep roots in primate social evolution.[58] Simple "leader" propaganda is common in modern times, whether the leader is Der Fuhrer, Mao Zedong, or George Orwell's "Big Brother" from the novel *1984*. "Leader" propaganda is generally not about obedience but often to make us feel that the leader understands our group and thus has empathy for us.

To illustrate empathy in propaganda, successful presidential candidates strive to show us not that they are exceptional, but that they are in the same groups as we are. Their propaganda message is often not directly about themselves but about us: how we work hard, live straight, tighten our belts, and do the right thing. The implication is that because they understand us so well, they are one of us. When they do talk about themselves, they try to demonstrate empathy, not just toughness. Bill Clinton's "I feel your pain" defines that; George W. Bush also campaigned on empathy and "compassionate conservatism." Some Tea Party candidates may campaign on "I share your anger" ("I'm mad as hell . . ."), which is also a strategic empathic appeal to group solidarity.

## PROPAGANDA AND TRUTH

We must confront the fact that many people use *propaganda* as a synonym for *lies*. We agree with Jacques Ellul that *truth* is not the relevant term; Ellul preferred "accuracy of facts." A belief that is true for you may not be true for me, but we still may agree on the accuracy of the facts. Ellul felt that "the idea that propaganda consists of lies" could make it "seem harmless, and even a little ridiculous," to those who are confident they can distinguish truth from lies.[59]

Propaganda began to acquire its modern malodor in the middle of the nineteenth century, for reasons that are understandable. Let's use as our benchmark the America of 1840, before the telegraph became widespread. At that time, the rhythms of daily life did not put you or your children in touch with the belief systems of other groups. You went to the local church and your children read only the books approved by the local school board. Then came urbanization and, more importantly, the mass media: the cheap newspapers of the penny press, paperbacks, nickelodeons, silent films, radio, Technicolor extravaganzas, and television. Suddenly your children encountered other belief systems just by getting up early on Sunday and turning on the TV, even if they were just looking for the cartoons. Today people who don't like what they believe to be propaganda often use the term interchangeably with "the media," citing both as untrustworthy.

Crowded, multi-ethnic cities and mass media force us to encounter other people's beliefs all the time. As noted, beliefs that we don't share can seem false to us, hence the uneasy perception that they are "propaganda." In reality, we are encountering more of the propaganda that causes cognitive dissonance. We are probably also encountering more propaganda that reinforces what we already believe, but we tend not to notice that.

The popular perception of propaganda changed markedly in the aftermath of World War I. Just as it was becoming obvious that the war did not "make the world safe for democracy," several prominent people responsible for "war information" began to boast about the job they had done, explicitly using the word *propaganda* in a number of ways, many of them contradictory. Most notable was a book called *How We Advertised America*, written in 1920 by George Creel, who had headed the U.S. wartime Committee on Public Information (CPI).[60] Creel was from the school that maintains that what they say is propaganda, what we say is not, referring to

> . . . the barrage of lies that kept the people of the Central Powers (Germany and its allies) in darkness and delusion; we sought the friendship and support of the neutral nations by continuous presentation of facts. We did not call it propaganda, for that word, in German hands, had come to be associated with deceit and corruption.[61]

In Creel's day, the work of the CPI was indeed quickly labeled as propaganda by a number of social critics, although they differed on exactly what that meant. Walter Lippmann, in his book *Public Opinion*, asked, "But what is propaganda, if not the effort to alter the picture to which men respond, to substitute one social pattern for another?"[62] Lippmann's definition here is in sync with what this chapter would consider intentional propaganda. But Lippmann keeps expanding his definition, as when he notes how French generals over-reported German casualties and under-reported their own: "We have learned to call this propaganda. A group of men who can prevent independent access to the event, arrange the news of it to suit their purpose."

Much of what Lippmann is describing is actually censorship. It would be best to recognize that and treat it as such. He is also discussing the use of misinformation, which can be a technique of propaganda, but it isn't always propaganda. This is where a definition can become so broad that it subverts itself. For example, the U.S. military defines "misinformation" as a type of propaganda, which we found, in our time in Afghanistan, to be confusing to our own public affairs officers.[63] Consider misinformation in its own right. It was common in World War II, when the navy would let it be known that a troop ship was leaving port at midnight, when in fact it was leaving hours earlier. By itself, that is not propaganda. It does not affect group cohesion, hierarchy, or belief systems.

The only lies that are inherently propaganda are those that utilize our belief systems. Consider this passage by Edward Bernays,[64] who sought to speak favorably of propaganda:

> . . . [Ralph Waldo] Emerson uses propagandist as an adjective not at all suggestive of the stealthy spread of some pernicious creed or notion. He describes the British as "still aggressive and propagandist, enlarging their dominion of their arts and liberty"—a passage that associates propaganda not with alien subversion but the most enlightened rule.

Emerson was writing in 1856, just one year before more than one hundred thousand people died in the 1857 Great Rebellion in India. Certainly those people did not consider British rule "the most enlightened." One can see why the propaganda debates of the 1920s gave many people the impression that propaganda is about lies, but it is more useful to discuss whether propaganda is effective or ineffective. Advertising agencies are well aware of this.

## ADVERTISING, PROPAGANDA, AND BIOLOGY

The strategy of most modern advertising is to create trust between strangers. Although an ad that says a store has the lowest price on a standard item may induce you to make a purchase, an ad convincing you that a particular store almost always has the lowest prices (or best service, most reliable delivery, etc.) has a far greater payoff. The only logical way to convince you of what is "almost always" true is consistency over time, but advertising is designed to work right now. Ads must create instant credibility or, in other words, trust between members of a group. That brings us back to the communication and cooperation that were necessary for the earliest humans to acquire much of anything. The content of someone's message was always a distant second to trust; if you gesture "come here," nothing will happen if I don't trust you. Precisely how someone wanted us to help stampede a wooly mammoth or kill an antelope mattered far less than whether we could trust that person.

We'd like to believe that our important decisions are motivated by logic: "just give me the facts." But if you turn on the television, you will find a preponderance of commercials that contain little or no information. These ads appeal to our group identifications to create trust. As one of the authors of this chapter drives a Volvo, we were interested in a particular television ad: you see a man picking up his wife in a howling rainstorm. The storm continues as they drive their Volvo down a twisting road by the sea, with waves battering the rocks. They encounter a large sea turtle in the middle of the road. In a quick montage, the man returns the turtle to the ocean, despite getting soaked in the process.

Although there is a bit of narration, there is no mention whatsoever of specific luxury features, styling, acceleration, gas mileage, or price. The message is in the montage. This commercial will only persuade you to buy a Volvo if you identify with the man who is driving it, if he is the person you want to be. And why shouldn't you? He is handsome. He is neither too young nor too old. He has a beautiful, successful wife and a good-looking car. He is responsible. He is wearing a shirt and tie, yet he is not reluctant to get his hands dirty. He is athletic. He cares. This man drives a Volvo.

Many commercials feature beautiful people. This one illustrates that Volvo owners are people who really care. If that is how you see yourself, this ad is for you. It creates cognitive consonance. Speaking for a moment in the first person, is this man . . . me? I wish. This man is an idealized version of how I'd like to see myself. The idealized individual, the person you want to be, is crucial for advertising and for many forms of propaganda. Furthermore, it is an essential part of human nature that began evolving even before our ancestors were human. Anthropologist Robert Trivers describes much of this in his book *The Folly of Fools: The Logic of Deceit and Self-Deception in Human Life.*[65] He discusses the way in which an animal will puff up its fur during a confrontation to deceive its opponent into thinking it is bigger than it really is. Adopting a powerful pose can increase testosterone and decrease cortisol.[66] This may facilitate our ability to deceive ourselves into thinking we are smarter, stronger and more likely to prevail than we really are. Self-confidence gives us a boost and, within certain limits, increases our chances of actual success.

## PROPAGANDA, DIRECT-RESPONSE ADVERTISING, AND RELIGION

Some definitions of propaganda say that it must motivate us to take action. This is not always true, but propaganda that gets you to take a desired action is certainly successful. Direct-response advertising, sometimes called an infomercial, is a perfect example, not only because it requires action but also because the products themselves are about a person's status within the group. The infomercial persuades you that the tooth whitener will not only whiten your teeth, you'll find yourself smiling more. You'll win more friends. You'll look more confident and, more importantly, you'll feel more confident. Other people will notice. You'll get the girl or get the guy, receive the promotion, and be respected and envied by the group.

Any product that is marketed as a status symbol links us to our long evolutionary heritage. Status—or "pecking order"—is vitally important to many species. The postures and vocalizations that convey status are, as we have said, pre-adaptations for propaganda. In an animal world, status is determined among members of the group. The high-status individuals may get to eat when the low-status animals go hungry or, at least, go last.

Human beings can have different kinds of status. Even in hunter-gatherer societies with little food, individuals may undertake a dangerous fast to please the gods. In doing so, they achieve a higher religious status. Once again, our biology and culture intertwine. All human groups have the neurological equipment for multiple idea-based notions of status and hierarchy. This takes the group inside our own heads, in ways that direct-response advertisers understand.

Direct-response products are often sold through "empowerment." Even a car polish is portrayed as raising your status. This motivates people off the sofa and to a phone or website with a credit card in hand, to buy something they weren't even thinking about before. Indeed, there is new evidence linking pro-social hormones to a willingness to part with more money directly after viewing a television commercial. In one study, people who received oxytocin gave 56 percent more money after viewing public service advertisements.[67]

There are three notes that such an infomercial must hit and they are very similar to religion. Religion—at least a certain type of religion—says three things:

1. You are a sinner. You know that. Late at night, deep in your heart, you know it. You are probably going to hell, if your life is not already sheer hell.
2. It's not your fault. Blame it on the devil. Temptation is everywhere, no wonder you sin. Eve ate the apple. People in our society don't stand a chance. Whatever can fill your soul has been lacking . . . until now.
3. Now the Savior has come. Accept the Savior and your life will be transformed.

An infomercial strikes the same chord, with almost the same three notes:

1. You don't measure up. You know it. You are not as attractive, smart, or well liked as other people (the group). You could stand to lose a few pounds. Your car is an embarrassment. Don't get me started on your breath. You're always one step behind other people, now aren't you?

2. It's not your fault. Blame it on the media. Temptation is everywhere, no wonder you're fat. People in our society don't have time to go to the gym, file every receipt, and change their oil every three thousand miles. Who has the money to paint their house every three years, shine their car, and seal every crack by their windows and gutters? Whatever can deal with your problem quickly and easily either has not been invented or was available only to the rich . . . until now.

3. Now the Product has arrived. Accept the Product and your life will be transformed.

The product will give you cognitive consonance. To become happy, to become your best self, you propagandize yourself.

## PROPAGANDA, WAR, AND FEAR

We function differently in a state of fear; many of us have experienced the fight-or-flight (or freeze) response of immediate fear and the physical stress of long-term fear. Neuroscientists, most notably Joseph LeDoux of New York University, are detailing the ways in which fear affects the brain.[68] The relationship between fear and receptivity to certain types of propaganda has long been under scrutiny. We tend to recognize propaganda after a war has ended, in part because the sense of fear dissipates.

Today the U.S. military defines propaganda exclusively in negative ways, as what they say, as reflected in a recent official glossary:[69]

Propaganda—Any form of adversary communication, especially of a biased or misleading nature, designed to influence the opinions, emotions, attitudes, or behavior of any group in order to benefit the sponsor, either directly or indirectly.[70]

If you examine this definition, it is obvious that you can toss out the first subordinate clause, "especially of a biased or misleading nature." Imagine a law or regulation that said you cannot cross an intersection when the light is red, especially if you do so in a careless manner. Would that mean it is okay to run a red light if you do so in a careful manner? Of course not. The rest of the clause is circular; it considers propaganda to be biased and misleading, but the implied definition of those terms is that they are propaganda. The second clause, "designed to influence opinions, emotions, attitudes, or behavior," is too broad to mean anything; a simple statement like "the zoo will close at noon today" may influence my behavior—I won't go to the zoo. What we are left with, in the military definition, is simply that propaganda is "any form of adversary communication."[71] Unfortunately, this allows U.S. adversaries to decide what is and is not propaganda.

## CONCLUSION

Propaganda, as communication regarding group cohesion and beliefs, is inherently value neutral. American democracy is founded on the decision of "one people to dissolve the political bands which have connected them with another," as it says in the first sentence of the Declaration of Independence. Yet propaganda can also be used for terrible ends. Any time someone tries to re-define who you are, whether it is a country, a corporation, or a commercial, you should think long and hard. The first step is recognizing when this re-definition is occurring.

If one were to draw a Venn diagram, there would be a great deal of overlap between the circle labeled propaganda and the circles representing "beliefs," "education," "religion," "social psychology," "identity," "behavioral norms," and just plain "upbringing." But none of the other circles would precisely be propaganda. The unique word persists because the unique concept endures. Continued exploration of the bio-cultural and evolutionary origins of propaganda will, we hope, lead to greater clarity.

Our definition: *propaganda is communication that utilizes your personal belief system to affect group cohesion, creating either cognitive dissonance or cognitive consonance.* This definition is, we believe, concise, consistent, and rooted in our history, culture, and biological heritage. As long as we have groups based around ideas and beliefs, we will have propaganda.

## NOTES

1. Charlotte K. Hemelrijk and Jutta Steinhauser, "Cooperation, Coalition, and Alliances," in *Handbook of Paleoanthropology*, vol. 3, ed. Winfried Henke, Ian Tattersall, and Thorolf Hardt, 1321–46 (Berlin: Springer, 2007).
2. Alan H. Harcourt and Frans B.M. de Waal, "Coalitions and Alliances: A History of Ethological Research," in *Coalitions and Alliances in Humans and Other Animals*, ed. Alan H. Harcourt and Frans B.M. de Waal, 1–19 (New York: Oxford University Press, 1992); Christopher Boehm, "Segmentary 'Warfare' and the Management of Conflict: Comparison of East African Chimpanzees and Patrilineal-Patrilocal Humans," in *Coalitions and Alliances in Humans and Other Animals*, ed. Alan H. Harcourt and Frans B.M. de Waal, 37–173 (New York: Oxford University Press, 1992); Margaret C. Crofoot and Richard W. Wrangham, "Intergroup aggression in primates and humans: the case for a unified theory," in *Mind the Gap Tracing the Origins of Human Universal*, ed. Peter M. Kappelar and Joan B. Silk, 171–95 (Berlin: Springer, 2010); David P. Watts, "Dominance, Power, and Politics in Nonhuman and Human Primates," in *Mind the Gap: Tracing the Origins of Human Universal*, ed. Peter M. Kappelar and Joan B. Silk, 109–38 (Berlin: Springer, 2010).
3. Garth S. Jowett and Victoria O'Donnell, *Propaganda and Persuasion*, 6th ed. (Los Angeles: Sage, 2014).
4. Jacob M. Rabbie, "The Effect of Intragroup Cooperation and Intergroup Competition on In-Group and Out-Group Hostility," in *Coalitions and Alliances in Humans and Other Animals*, ed. Alan H. Harcourt and Franz B.M.

de Waal, 175–205 (New York: Oxford University Press, 1992); Boehm, "Segmentary 'Warfare,' " 37–173.

5. Harcourt and de Waal, "Coalitions and Alliances," 1–19.
6. Watts, "Dominance, Power, and Politics in Nonhuman and Human Primates," 109–38.
7. Ibid.
8. Polly Wiessner, "Indoctrinability and the Evolution of Socially Defined Kinship," in *Indoctrinability, Ideology and Warfare*, ed. Irenäus Eibl-Eibelsfeldt and Frank K. Salter, 133–50 (New York: Berghan Books, 1998).
9. Paul J. Zak's comments come from our conversations specifically for this chapter. Zak is the founding director of Claremont University's Center for Neuroeconomics Studies and the author of *The Moral Molecule: The Source of Love and Prosperity* (2013).
10. Martin A. Nowak and Roger Highfield, *Super Cooperators: Evolution, Altruism and Human Behaviour or Why We Need Each Other to Succeed* (Edinburgh: Cannongate, 2011), xvi.
11. Wiessner, "Indoctrinability," 140–41.
12. L. F. Pendry, D. M. Driscoll, and S. C. Field, "Diversity Training: Putting Theory into Practice," *Journal of Occupational and Organizational Psychology* 80, no. 1 (2007): 27–50.
13. Paul Ekman, *Darwin and Facial Expression: A Century of Research in Review* (New York: Academic Press, 1973).
14. Stanley H. Ambrose, "Coevolution of Composite-Tool Technology, Constructive Memory, and Language," *Current Anthropology* 51, no. S1 (2010): S135–47.
15. Zoe R. Donaldson and Larry D. Young, "Oxytocin, Vasopressin and the Neurogenetics of Sociality," *Science* 332 (2008): 900–904.
16. Nicholas Pound, Ian Penton-Voak, and Alison K. Surridge, "Testosterone Responses to Competition in Men Are Related to Facial Masculinity," *Proceedings of the Royal Society, Series B* 276, no. 1654 (2009): 153–59; Ian S. Penton-Voak and Jennie Y. Chen, "High Salivary Testosterone Is Linked to Masculine Male Facial Appearance in Humans," *Evolution and Human Behavior* 25, no. 4 (2004): 229–41.
17. Jessamy Doman, Andrew Hill, and R. Bribiescas, "A New Osteological Approach to Inferring Hominin Social Behavior: Seeking Facial Indicators of Testosterone Level," in Paleoanthropology Society Meetings Abstracts, Honolulu, HI, April 2–3, 2013, *PaleoAnthropology* (2013): A10.
18. Polly Wiessner, "Taking the Risk Out of Risky Transactions: A Forager's Dilemma," in *Risky Transactions: Trust, Kinship, and Ethnicity*, ed. Frank K. Salter, 21–43 (Oxford: Berghan Books, 2002).
19. Émile Durkheim, *The Elementary Forms of the Religious Life*, trans. Joseph Ward Swain (London: George Allen and Unwin, 1915), 316, 338.
20. The late Dr. Neal Postman and his colleague Dr. Terence Moran maintained a fluid discourse on the nature of propaganda in the Media Ecology department at New York University. The specific version included here was presented in a lecture by Dr. Moran in 2010 and was later confirmed with him in discussions specifically for this chapter.
21. Kenneth Gergen, *The Saturated Self: Dilemmas of Identity in Contemporary Life* (New York: Basic Books, 1991).
22. Neil Postman, *Conscientious Objections: Stirring up Trouble about Language, Technology, and Education* (New York: Vintage Books, 1992).
23. Jacques Ellul, *Propaganda: The Formation of Men's Attitudes* (New York: Knopf, 1965).

24. Wiessner, "Indoctrinability," 133–50.
25. Mark Pagel, *Wired for Culture: Origins of the Human Social Mind* (New York: W. W. Norton, 2012).
26. Frans B. de Waal, *Good Natured: The Origins of Right and Wrong in Primates and Other Animals* (Cambridge, MA: Harvard University Press, 1996).
27. Dacher Keltner, *Born to Be Good: The Science of a Meaningful Life* (New York: W. W. Norton, 2009).
28. Steven Pinker, *The Blank Slate: The Modern Denial of Human Nature* (New York: Penguin, 2003); Pinker, *The Better Angels of Our Nature: The Decline of Violence in History and Its Causes* (New York: Penguin, 2011).
29. Paul J. Zak, *The Moral Molecule: The Source of Love and Prosperity* (New York: Dutton, 2013).
30. Richard W. Byrne and Andrew Whiten, *Machiavellian Intelligence: Social Expertise and the Evolution of Intellect in Monkeys, Apes, and Humans* (Oxford: Oxford Science, 1989).
31. Charles Darwin, *The Descent of Man, and Selection in Relation to Sex* (London: John Murray, 1871).
32. Amots Zahavi and Avishag Zahavi, *The Handicap Principle: A Missing Piece of Darwin's Puzzle* (New York: Oxford University Press, 1997); Dominique J.-F. de Quervain, Urs Fischbacher, Valerie Treyer, Melanie Schellhamer, Ulrich Schnyder, Alfred Buck, and Ernst Fehr, "The Neural Basis of Altruistic Punishment," *Science* 305 (2004): 1254–58; Rebekka A. Klein, "The Neurobiology of Altruistic Punishment: A Moral Assessment of Its Social Utility," in *Philosophy of Behavioral Biology*, ed. Kathryn S. Plaisance and Thomas A. C. Reydon, 297–313 (Dordrecht: Springer, 2012).
33. Wiessner, "Taking the Risk Out of Risky Transactions," 21.
34. Martin A. J. Williams, Stanley H. Ambrose, Sander van der Kaars, Carsten Ruehlmann, Umesh Chattopadhyaya, Jagganath Pal, and Parth Chauhan, "Environmental Impact of the Toba Mega-Eruption Inferred from Paleosol Carbonate Stable Isotopes in Central India," *Palaeogeography, Palaeoclimatology, Palaeoecology* 284 (2009): 295–314; Eugene I. Smith, Amber Ciravallo, Panagiotis Karkanas, Curtis W. Marean, Erich Fisher, Naomi Cleghorn, Christine Lane, and Minghua Ren, "Cryptotephra Possibly from the 74 Ka Eruption of Toba Discovered at Pinnacle Point, South Africa: Implications for Resolving the Dating Controversy for Middle Stone Age Sites in Southern Africa," *PaleoAnthropology* (2014): A24; C. S. Lane, Ben T. Chorn, and Thomas C. Johnson, "Ash from the Toba Supereruption in Lake Malawi Shows No Volcanic Winter in East Africa at 75 ka," *Proceedings of the National Academy of Sciences* 110, no. 20 (2013): 8025–29.
35. Stanley H. Ambrose, "Late Pleistocene Human Population Bottlenecks, Volcanic Winter, and Differentiation of Modern Humans," *Journal of Human Evolution* 34 (1998): 623–51.
36. Polly Wiessner, "Risk, Reciprocity and Social Influences on !Kung San Economics," in *Politics and History in Band Societies*, ed. Eleanor Leacock and Richard B. Lee, 61–84 (Cambridge: Cambridge University Press, 1982); Polly Wiessner, "The Pathways of the Past: !Kung San Hxaro Exchange and History," in *Überlebenstrategien in Afrika*, ed. M. Bollig and F. Klees, 110–24 (Cologne: Heinrich-Barth-Institut, 1994); Richard B. Lee, "!Kung Spatial Organization: An Ecological and Historical Perspective," *Human Ecology* 1, no. 2 (1972): 125–47.
37. John Yellen and Henry Harpending, "Hunter-Gatherer Populations and Archaeological Inference," *World Archaeology* 4, no. 2 (1972): 244–53.
38. Watts, "Dominance, Power, and Politics," 109–38.

39. Robert Carneiro, "On the Relationship between Size of Population and Complexity of Social Organization," *Southwestern Journal of Anthropology* 23 (1967): 234–43.

40. Paul J. Zak, "The Neurobiology of Trust," *Scientific American* 298, no. 6 (2008): 88–95; Aleksandr Kogan, Laura R. Saslow, Emily A. Impett, Christopher Oveis, Dacher Keltner, and Sarina Rodrigues Saturn, "Thin-Slicing Study of the Oxytocin Receptor (OXTR) Gene and the Evaluation and Expression of the Prosocial Disposition," *Proceedings of the National Academy of Sciences* 108, no. 48 (2011): 19189–92.

41. Joan Y. Chiao and Katherine D. Blizinsky, "Culture–Gene Coevolution of Individualism–Collectivism and the Serotonin Transporter Gene," *Proceedings of the Royal Society, Series B* 277, no. 1681 (2010): 529–37; Sue Howell, Greg Westergaard, Beth Hoos, Tara J. Chavanne, Susan E. Shoaf, Allison Cleveland, Philip J. Snoy, Stephen J. Suomi, and J. Dee Higley, "Serotonergic Influences on Life-History Outcomes in Free-Ranging Male Rhesus Macaques," *American Journal of Primatology* 69, no. 8 (2007): 851–65; Jens R. Wendland, Klaus-Peter Lesch, Timothy K. Newman, Angelika Timme, and Hélène Gachot-Neveu, "Bernard Thierry and Stephen J. Suomi, Differential Functional Variability of Serotonin Transporter and Monoamine Oxidase A Genes in Macaque Species Displaying Contrasting Levels of Aggression-Related Behavior," *Behavior Genetics* 36, no. 2 (2006): 163–72.

42. Heather K. Caldwell, Heon-Jin Lee, Abbe H. Macbeth, and W. Scott Young III, "Vasopressin: Behavioral Roles of an 'Original' Neuropeptide," *Progress in Neurobiology* 84, no. 1 (2008): 1–24; R.R. Thompson, K. George, J.C. Walton, S.P. Orr, and J. Benson, "Sex-Specific Influences of Vasopressin on Human Social Communication," *Proceedings of the National Academy of Sciences* 103, no. 20 (2006): 7889–94.

43. Paul J. Zak, K. Borja, W.T. Matzner, and R. Kurzban, "The Neuroeconomics of Distrust: Sex Differences in Behavior and Physiology," *American Economic Review Papers and Proceedings* 95, no. 2 (2005): 360–64; Peter A. Bos, David Terburg, and Jack van Honk, "Testosterone Decreases Trust in Socially Naïve Humans," *Proceedings of the National Academy of Sciences* 107, no. 22 (2010): 9991–95.

44. Doman et al., "New Osteological," A9.

45. Robin I.M. Dunbar, "The Social Role of Touch in Humans and Primates: Behavioural Function and Neurobiological Mechanisms," *Neuroscience and Biobehavioral Reviews* 34, no. 2 (2010): 260–68; Wendland, "Differential Functional Variability," 163–72.

46. Zak et al., "Neuroeconomics of Distrust," 360–64.

47. Markus Heinrichs, Thomas Baumgartner, Clemens Kirschbaum, and Ulrike Ehlert, "Social Support and Oxytocin Interact to Suppress Cortisol and Subjective Responses to Psychosocial Stress," *Biological Psychiatry* 54, no. 12 (2003): 1389–98; Leslie J. Seltzer, Toni E. Ziegler, and Seth D. Pollak, "Social Vocalizations Can Release Oxytocin in Humans," *Proceedings of the Royal Society, Series B* 277, no. 1694 (2010): 2661–66; Frances S. Chen, Robert Kumsta, Bernadette von Dawans, Mikhail Monakhov, Richard P. Ebstein, and Markus Heinrichs, "Common Oxytocin Receptor Gene (OXTR) Polymorphism and Social Support Interact to Reduce Stress in Humans," *Proceedings of the National Academy of Sciences* 108, no. 50 (2011): 19937–42.

48. Leslie J. Seltzer, Ashley R. Prososki, Toni E. Ziegler, and Seth D. Pollak, "Instant Messages vs. Speech: Hormones and Why We Still Need to Hear Each Other," *Evolution and Human Behavior* 33, no. 1 (2012): 42–45.

49. Dunbar, "The Social," 163–72.

50. Ambrose, "Coevolution," S135–47.

51. Margaret C. Crofoot and Richard W. Wrangham, "Intergroup Aggression in Primates and Humans: The Case for a Unified Theory," in Kappelar and Silk, *Mind the Gap*, 171–95.

52. Bonobos (aka the pygmy chimpanzee, *Pan paniscus*) are the only significant exception to this pattern. When bonobo troops meet, females typically engage in non-threatening "truly friendly and affinitive" interactions, whereas males are more reserved. Genichi Idani, "Relations between Unit-Groups of Bonobos at Wamba, Zaire: Encounters and Temporary Fusions," *African Study Monographs* 11, no. 3 (1990): 153–86. Bonobos are close relatives of chimpanzees yet are much more socially tolerant, not showing significant increases in testosterone in competitive situations. Victoria Wobber, Brian Hare, Jean Maboto, Susan Lipson, Richard Wrangham, and Peter T. Ellison, "Differential Changes in Steroid Hormones before Competition in Bonobos and Chimpanzees," *Proceedings of the National Academy of Sciences* 107, no. 28 (2010): 12457–62.

53. Ambrose, "Late Pleistocene," 623–51; Ambrose, "Coevolution," S135–47.

54. Wiessner, "Taking the Risk," 21–43.

55. Ambrose, "Late Pleistocene," 623–51; Ambrose, "Coevolution," S135–47.

56. Love Dalén, Ludovic Orlando, Beth Shapiro, Mikael Brandström-Durling, Rolf Quam, M. Thomas P. Gilbert, J. Carlos Díez Fernández-Lomana, Eske Willerslev, Juan Luis Arsuaga, and Anders Götherström, "Partial Genetic Turnover in Neandertals: Continuity in the East and Population Replacement in the West," *Molecular Biology and Evolution* 29, no. 8 (2012): 1893–97.

57. Jean-Jacques Hublin, Sahra Talamo, Michèle Julien, Francine David, Nelly Connet, Pierre Bodu, Bernard Vandermeersch, and Michael P. Richards, "Radiocarbon Dates from the Grotte du Renne and Saint-Césaire Support a Neandertal Origin for the Châtelperronian," *Proceedings of the National Academy of Sciences* 109, no. 46 (2012): 18743–48; R. Pinhasi, M. Nioradze, N. Tushabramishvili, D. Lordkipanidze, D. Pleurdeau, M.-H. Moncel, D.S. Adler, C. Stringer, and T. F. G. Higham, "New Chronology for the Middle Palaeolithic of the Southern Caucasus Suggests Early Demise of Neanderthals in this Region," *Journal of Human Evolution* 63 (2012): 770–80.

58. Watts, "Dominance, Power, and Politics," 109–38.

59. Ellul, *Propaganda*.

60. George Creel, *How We Advertised America: The First Telling of the Amazing Story of the Committee on Public Information That Carried the Gospel of Americanism to Every Corner of the Globe* (New York: Harper, 1920).

61. Ibid.

62. Walter Lippmann, *Public Opinion* (New York: Free Press Paperbacks, 1997), 27.

63. One of the authors of this chapter, Bob Schapiro, observed public affairs operations in Kabul in 2009. An unclassified definition of misinformation can be found in Joint Chiefs of Staff, "Psychological Operations," *Joint Publication U.S. Department of Defense* (January 7, 2010), B-9.

64. Edward L. Bernays, *Propaganda* (Brooklyn, NY: Ig, 1928), 10.

65. Robert Trivers, *The Folly of Fools: The Logic of Deceit and Self-Deception in Human Life* (New York: Basic Books, 2011).

66. Dana R. Carney, Amy J.C. Cuddy, and Andy J. Yap, "Power Posing Brief Nonverbal Displays Affect Neuroendocrine Levels and Risk Tolerance," *Psychological Science* 21, no. 10 (2010): 1363–68.

67. Pei-Ying Lin, Naomi Sparks Grewal, Christophe Morin, Walter D. Johnson, and Paul J. Zak, "Oxytocin Increases the Influence of Public Service Advertisements," *PLoS One* 8, no. 2 (2013): e56934.

68. Joseph E. LeDoux, *Synaptic Self: How Our Brains Become Who We Are* (New York: Viking, 2002).

69. Joint Chiefs of Staff, "Psychological Operations."
70. Ibid., GL-7 (glossary). Some of the newer definitions are classified as secret.
71. The military definition changes often enough that many public information officers we interviewed are unfamiliar with the latest version, although the one quoted earlier is in widespread circulation.

Part II

# Media on the Brain

# 9 Mind Control in Hollywood

*Steven Gibson*

Although television shows and movies have depicted mind control and brainwashing for decades, such portrayals are often viewed primarily through the lens of entertainment value. When one looks closely at popular depictions of mind control, it is possible to explore questions of political and social trends and seek correlations with attitudes toward philosophies of mind. Numerous shows and movies suggest the human mind can be replaced or programmed to produce an obedient robot-like individual. Like a storehouse filled with memories, the mind can be induced to hold new thoughts or be replaced entirely, resulting in a servile, brainwashed minion. As Walter Bishop, the lead scientist in the television show *Fringe*, says in one episode, "the brain is a computer, it's an organic computer. It can be hijacked like any other."[1]

Fictional television shows such as *Dollhouse* (FOX), *Falling Skies* (TNT), and *Homeland* (Showtime) most often depict the mind as an isolated island that is hidden from the view of others, a point of view mirrored in movies like *The Manchurian Candidate* (1962). While the popularity of these shows is compatible with the expectations held by much of the targeted Western audience, cognitive research is demonstrating a more shared cognitive landscape than these shows imply. These shows most often show shared mental states after a mind has been taken over. In *Falling Skies*, when children are linked by a harness, they share their thoughts.[2] More famously, in *Star Trek: The Next Generation*, the fictional alien race the Borg subsumes those they conquer into a hive mind.[3] However, most researchers would also assert that normal individuals who are in social contact also share a great deal of cognitive information as well as their cognitive state with each other.

This chapter addresses the subject of shared minds by exploring the findings of cognitive research in theory of mind and applying some of those findings to evaluate mind control in fictional stories. A critical studies approach to movies and television shows that involve mind control and a review of relevant papers in cognitive science is employed along with a discussion of how a tool applied to Hollywood dramas might aid in testing cognitive theories. To begin to analyze the use of mind control in fiction, we will examine how theory of mind can be used to understand audience reading of these stories. Then we will lay the groundwork for future approaches to mind control fiction by employing a new tool based on theory of mind concepts. Initially, we will perform a brief critical examination of the history of mind control fiction in Hollywood. The learning outcomes for this chapter will include gaining an overview of scholarship in theory of mind branches of cognitive science and exposing the reader to one critical approach to popular media portrayals of mind control.

## MINDS IN FICTION

In *Why We Read Fiction: Theory of Mind and the Novel*, Lisa Zunshine expounds on how we respond to others' minds when we consume fiction. Zunshine's book builds a model of how we determine the state of mind of characters in novels drawing on theory of mind.[4] Alan Palmer, in *Fictional Minds*, also addresses the mind of characters in fictional portrayals. Palmer explores what information on the fictional minds of people in books can be obtained from those books.[5] David Seed conducts a review of literary and cinematic representations of brainwashing in the West during the Cold War period. Seed describes, "The basic argument of this study that the notion of brainwashing triggered and sustained an extended crisis of cultural self-examination."[6] This represents one aspect of how the ideas of mind control and brainwashing reflect on some of our deepest conceptions of ourselves and our minds. Mind control encompasses methods and tools which enable our friends, family, and fellow citizens to be transformed into enemies.

Some individuals doubt the existence or efficacy of mind control because they see a person's actions as an expression of a person's deepest beliefs. We conceive of special and steep requirements to explain successful cases of the conversion of people. These can vary from an acceptable change of conviction due to communication interactions to forms of coercive mind restructuring. When specifying a type of mind conversion, we are choosing among alternative interpretations of a person's behavior and responses to the person's social obligations. These choices might be explained by itemizing aspects of the change of mind or by showing some unexpected behavior by the affected character. Explanation of the changes can be structured in order to evaluate the appearance of mind control activity. In our everyday lives, we expect the people we know to stick to a consistent story, one composed of the aspects of their life as we see it. We expect them to be loyal to the same government, religion and family groups. We also expect that we can influence our friends and family members. But we take exception when strangers change the thinking or behavior of those individuals close to us.

## POLITICAL CONTEXT IN MIND CONTROL

A historical review of mind control in fiction will allow us to view the scope of our object of study, as well as show a non-cognitive approach to the field.

Numerous movies and television shows have been produced since the 1950s portraying the effects and results of mind control. One lens available to analyze these narratives is that of an expression of political context: society may articulate some political and social fears through depictions of mind control and brainwashing in mass media.

Depictions of mind control experienced an explosive growth in the 1950s, particularly during the Korean Conflict, when a number of captured American soldiers released statements that seemed to indicate that their internal belief structures had been altered. *The Manchurian Candidate*, released in 1962, was a fictional representation of the use of subliminal mental triggers to affect human behavior.[7] While the terms for mind control and brainwashing did not exist in the past, similar concerns were expressed in past cultural contexts. In religious texts, warnings are given against changes of faith, and fairy tales and folk tales feature stories of magic potions to make people fall into or out of love. In *A Midsummer Night's Dream*, William Shakespeare writes of Puck acquiring a magical flower, the juice of which makes a person fall in love with the first thing he or she sees upon waking.[8] In the retelling of *Pygmalion* by George Bernard Shaw, a woman is transformed into a completely and mostly unexpected new persona.[9]

In the early decades of the twentieth century in the United States and Europe, a cultural coding of drugs like opium took place so that political and social goals were accomplished by attributing extreme persuasive effects to illegal drug use. These techniques provided both demonizing of some individuals and forgiveness for others.[10] In the 1920s, Sax Rohmer introduced mind control drugs in a book which was made into a 1932 movie, *Fu-Manchu: The Mask of Fu-Manchu*, as a way of expressing some racial and prejudicial opinions of the times using pseudoscientific terminology.[11] While today the terminology is more sophisticated, some of the social impulses remain.

In subsequent decades political and social goals continued to be encoded into scares about mind control. Consequently, movies were made which expressed our societal fears and concerns, particularly throughout the 1950s and 1960s. In an article in 2011, Jonathan Leib and Thomas Chapman explain how the 1950s was the era of the emerging Cold War, when increased diplomatic tensions and "the accelerating nuclear arms race between the United States and the Soviet Union left most Americans uncertain about their future survival."[12] The movie *Invasion of the Body Snatchers* (1956), though not demonstrating mind control, portrayed the fear of the alien or other with the power to take over identity and personality.[13]

Popular press and scholarly works expressed views of the causes and effectiveness of mind control methods. In the 1950s, scholars and politicians asserted that Americans were subject to mind control because of weak will. Susan Carruthers explains that mind control can "exemplify America's collective failure of will."[14] Those views of mind control conceive of the enemy winning because of social or psychological techniques which destroy minds or will power. The enemy was seen as managing a systematic manipulation of dominated and controlled populations. These explications of mind control share a common inattention to the mechanics of brainwashing and ultimately deny the power of ideas to shape human behavior.

The 1970s saw the struggle over liberal versus conservative visions of the West, played out over contention about the efficacy of mind control and brainwashing techniques. The trial of Patty Hearst in 1976 involved a jury in California deliberating upon whether Hearst either was mentally transformed into another person or was acting on her own beliefs and desires. William Graebner in his book *Patty's Got a Gun* relates how an expert witness for Patty's defense offered explanations of coercive persuasion to account for altered thinking and her altered behavior after her kidnapping.[15] Other additional court cases and popular studies of the times disagreed over the occurrence of brainwashing by religious or cult groups, including the Unification Church and Hare Krishna movement. Shocking events like the Peoples Temple massacre in 1978 and increasing political violence around the world supported the desire for individual power and agency. Movies such as *A Clockwork Orange* (1971), *Solaris* (1972), *Star Wars* (1977), and *The Terminal Man* (1974) wrestled with the societal tension between independence of mind and action versus obedience to authority as expressed through the agency of mind control.

While the 1980s and 1990s saw a reduction in Hollywood's representations of mind control and brainwashing, there has been an increasing amount in the twenty-first century, when the reaction from 9/11 prompted not only fear of the other but also a fear of aspects of self. Terrorists are often feared to be able to "blend" in among us, and in some cases, were formerly "us" before undergoing conversion to the enemy. By "blending" in, they challenge our group identity and loyalty. Fear of terrorists is about the other and the self, and we see more of the mind control, mind game and altered reality themed material since 9/11 as paranoia rises and Hollywood pits groups against another with psychological elements heightening the stakes and drama.

This historical review has shown some of the fictional representations in the past decades in the West and pursued the line of political and social analysis to study those portrayals. Before we examine how cognitive science can offer answers to these questions, it will be helpful to tease out the myriad of concepts entangled in the term mind control. Attempting to outline categorizations and explications about types of mind control will assist in the understanding of the portrayal of mind control in fictional stories.

## TAXONOMY FOR MIND CONTROL

Fictional representations of mind control have transformed over the years and continue to change. In *The Manchurian Candidate*, the enemy uses Pavlovian techniques to plant beliefs and triggers deep in the minds of the brainwashed victims. Those victims are mostly unaware of what has been done to them and how they have been compromised.[16] In the television series *Homeland*, a more accurate portrayal of conversion is shown where the convert has adopted certain beliefs that change his loyalties.[17] In *Falling Skies* (TNT), *Continuum* (Syfy), *Star Trek* (CBS), *The Host* (2013), and *Puppetmasters* (1994), an external device or creature is introduced into the body or brain to exert control over the actions of the victim. In *Dollhouse* (FOX), *X-Men* (2000), and *Dark City* (1998), changes are made to the brain of the victim to alter ideas and memories. *Solaris* (1972), *Inception* (2010), *Memento* (2000), and *The Matrix* (1999) feature real and artificial memories that are manipulated to influence the behavior of the controlled subject.

These concepts might be valuable to sort mind control portrayals using the issues involved of self, identity, group loyalty, and memory. Individuals express these aspects of humanness through their actions; people likely act along a continuum of behaviors that others would interpret as showing they are in their "right" minds or have undergone mental alteration. There are alternate aspects of mind control, as some fictional stories present a person's mind being replaced completely, whereas in other scenarios, two minds exist simultaneously. In still others, types of persuasion or coercion are used to make the individual take action. In the movie *The Host*, the mind of the major character Melanie is set to be replaced by the alien Wander. Instead, both minds end up existing at the same time and struggle for control of the character's actions.[18] There are multiple examples of people being coerced into alternative behaviors through counterfeit memories, such as in *Blade Runner* (1982), *Dark City* (1998), and numerous television episodes: in the original series *Star Trek*, when an advance species carries out transferring minds into Spock and Kirk,[19] and in the television show *Continuum*, when the main character has her mind hijacked by a computer hack of her augmentation suit.[20]

Defining categories of mind control as a first step will aid in determining what aspects of a person's conversion should be addressed as a concern to the society, and to describing how relationships have changed in the context of narratives. Describing the mind alteration may include modeling views of external relations, such as those with family, friends and society as expressed through social interaction. Human consciousness, in this case, represents the demonstration of the mental state of the individual as shown by their physical behaviors toward the others in their group. This process of analysis, through the steps of labeling and explication, serves to assist in analysis of fictional mind control.

The structures of mind control and coercive persuasion displayed in modern fiction can be grouped and organized. Table 9.1 represents a taxonomy for mind control, and is derived by grouping the diverse types of coercion in different representations. Each element shows two aspects: the first is a title of the technique, and the second is a more detailed description.

The wide range of different types of coercion presented here is proposed to encompass fictional portrayals of mind control. Some shared elements

*Table 9.1*   Types of Mind Control

| Technique | Description |
| --- | --- |
| Persuasion | Behavior is changed through multiple methods |
| Brainwashing | Some contents of a mind are replaced by thoughts and beliefs |
| Conversion | A strongly held belief structure is replaced |
| Deception | Information fed to the subject leads to new beliefs |
| Environmental disguise | The environment is manipulated to change beliefs |
| Social control | Social pressure is put on the subject to make him comply |
| Chemical control | Drugs or chemicals are introduced into the subject |
| Physical hijacking | The body is controlled, sometimes without the mind |
| Biological control | An insect or animal takes control of the nervous system |
| Mental hijacking | All contents of the mind are replaced |

unite this body of fiction, such as transformation of strongly held opinions. A challenge to our understanding of what mind control represents in fiction today is the continual change in the portrayals and meanings that are employed. A first step is to explain how one human can appreciate what the group thinks or what other individuals think. A contested but valuable aspect of theory of mind is the potential ability to understand the mental states of other individuals, including their knowledge, beliefs and motivations. As a function of their mental processes, humans compose mental images or imaginations of the world around them as well as imaginary worlds. Interpreting the operation of the minds around us is being approached through theory of mind research.

## COGNITIVE SCIENCE AND THEORY OF MIND

Sciences of social cognition offer tools that can be turned to the effort to look at issues of mind control in fictional portrayals. There exist tools and models to assist in conceptualizing how we humans read other humans. For example one cognitive approach says that individuals build constructs of other minds around them. This construction of "other minds" allows us to understand our relation to these other people. Social cognitive tools and models attempt to explain how individuals often share mental pictures with other members of society. Uta Frith and Chris Frith state that the "social brain, for humans at least, has a 'theory of mind,' which enables us to predict what others are going to do on the basis of their desires and beliefs."[21]

A 1978 paper by David Premack and Guy Woodruff introduced the term *theory of mind* to address how thinking beings are able to work out the beliefs, desires, intentions and pretenses of other thinking beings.[22] Their paper embraces ideas that apply theory of mind to supporting distributed and social cognition. This is consistent with aspects of human cognition existing in order to serve social needs. Rebecca Saxe and Lindsay Powell carried out a neuroscientific study to determine brain regions in which an individual's theory of mind abilities might reside. Saxe and Powell describe how people are able to attribute to other people mental states that they themselves never—and some times could never—experience.[23]

Determining when the cognition system is used is an important factor in understanding how it functions. For individuals to understand other people's behaviors, they must identify the collection of acts and motivations that fit those behaviors. People act in multiple domains every minute of each day, and the picture formed by synthesizing these actions represents how we believe a person should behave. Theory of mind proposes that we have ideas of how other minds operate; the human mind goes through processes of making guesses about the physical and verbal behaviors of other humans. The field of cognitive science has explored how processes in the mind result in human behavior. Theory of mind is the umbrella term used to describe approaches to studying and reporting on humans reading the minds of other humans.

Cognitive science has embraced interdisciplinary approaches to theory of mind despite some disputes in terminology, meanings, and interpretations within the field. This field of study reflects findings from psychology, artificial intelligence, philosophy, neuroscience, linguistics, and anthropology. Identification of topics in the field involves laboratory work, in situ observation, data review, and hypothetical modeling. These approaches to exploration can be followed by a series of process tasks and steps, including gathering information, describing observed elements, and synthesizing patterns.

While many scholars agree that most people can read the intentions and aspects of the mental states of other people, how mind control should be studied in fiction remains to be more fully explored. This aspect of the field would involve views of the effect of mind control on humans and how to describe these influences. One aspect of mind control for future consideration is what the experience is like for the person whose mind has been compromised. Ben, a young character in the television series *Falling Skies*, says there's a feeling "like someone's thinking with you."[24] When there is a new consciousness and memory residing in the subject, they may experience very conflicted feelings and thoughts. After all, the premise of mind control is that an individual has given up loyalty to the group; thus, the subject's social relationship with the group is compromised. The subject must also confront the weaknesses or failures that allowed him or her to be controlled in the first place. Mind control causes individuals to betray friends and loved ones and leads to inappropriate behavior.

Theory of mind can supply tools and approaches for use in analyzing portrayals of mind control in fictional narratives. A new tool detailed below aims to systemize one aspect of describing mind control fiction. This tool uses theory of mind conceptualizations combined with a procedural process to tease out specific aspects of mind control as portrayed in the fictional representation.

## THEORY OF MIND IN MIND CONTROL FICTION

Challenges exist for understanding and communicating information about mind control in fiction, and a new tool for its explication can contribute to analysis. Applying an analysis tool may deliver results that aid in our understanding and offer explanations that map to our beliefs about mind control. It is proposed here that theory of mind can be a tool usable for analysis of mind control in movies and television fiction. The preliminary step involves outlining the tool in order to aid in framing the analysis, with future additional steps as yet undefined.

To build a procedural tool, we attempt to answer several questions out of numerous character and plot questions that could be asked. A six-step procedure is offered here that involves reviewing single scenes in a movie or television show and identifying the following factors: (1) in what scene in the narrative is mind control first revealed; (2) who is the mind-controlled character; (3) whether the scene reveals the mind control to other characters in the fictional narrative or only to the viewer; (4) if revealed to another character, identify one character; (5) what cues are offered in the narrative to reveal that the character has undergone mind control; and (6) if the mind control influence as revealed is a threat to other characters in the fictional portrayal.

We begin by examining three fictional dramas, first using the 2013 movie *The Host*, which portrays an alien invasion of Earth carried out by the insertion of small worm-like aliens into the back of the neck of target humans. The alien would then almost always succeed in completely taking over the mind of the human and using its body while the original mind withered. In the movie, the humans of Earth have been nearly entirely replaced by these hybrid, human-like aliens. There exists a remnant group of "wild" humans who know about the alien invasion and seek to live free with their original minds. In one scene, the body of Melanie has been captured by "wild" humans who knew Melanie prior to the alien insertion and who know an alien has been implanted. One of the captors, Melanie's uncle, protects her from the others because he wants to know if she can somehow be useful to the free humans in their fight against the aliens. He says to her, "Then I started thinking, when they put one of you in our heads, do we still exist? Trapped in there. If our memories are still alive, are we? You gotta believe some people wouldn't go down without a fight."[25]

Using the procedural tool, we ascertain that (1) the chosen scene is shortly after Melanie's capture, where Uncle Jeb speaks alone to her in the cave; (2) Melanie is the mind-controlled character; (3) the clues in the scene reveal the mind control to characters in the narrative; (4) Uncle Jeb is the character in this scene who knows Melanie is being controlled by an alien in her body; (5) in this movie, all mind-controlled former humans are identifiable by a shiny glow in the irises of their eyes; and (6) Uncle Jeb is directly addressing the issue of threat in this scene in that the other humans want to kill the former Melanie to protect themselves, whereas Uncle Jeb is waiting to determine if the body or mind of Melanie can help the humans.

In another case, we examine the Showtime drama series *Homeland*. This series follows the character of U.S. Marine Nicholas Brody, who is captured and held as a prisoner by the al-Qaeda-linked terrorist Abu Nazir. In a scene in the episode titled "The Weekend," viewers are introduced to a U.S. citizen named Aileen who has been converted into an al-Queda tool. She has been captured by the FBI and CIA after crossing into Mexico while trying to escape. One of the main characters, Saul, is a CIA manager and analyst who works in Washington, D.C. He has driven down to Mexico with FBI agents to bring Aileen back to Washington for imprisonment and questioning. While Saul is driving the prisoner Aileen back to D.C., they stop at a diner and have a private conversation. As they sit in a booth together, Aileen asks, "Why are you here? The FBI could have taken me back." Saul answers, "I am trying to help you get through this." He continues a previous conversation about her boyfriend, Faisal, by asking, "You were living in compound country." She answers, "There was something good there. I met him. My father saw us, riding that horse." Saul asks, "Is Faisal the reason you were shipped to boarding school?"[26]

We now have a scene we have identified and can compare to other example scenes in other fictional dramas. In this scene, Saul is talking to Aileen about when she was young. She was with her father living in Saudi Arabia, attending school with other American contractors' and politicians' sons and daughters. Saul figures out that Aileen somehow met a poor Saudi boy during that time. Saul is attempting to determine when and how Aileen was converted from being a loyal U.S. citizen to now serving the enemies of the United States. Our procedural tool allows us to abstract out a limited set of elements that may be shared between scenes in which mind control is in evidence. The procedure gives us that (1) the scene is shortly after Aileen's capture, when the caravan of agents is stopped during the drive back from Mexico, where Saul and Aileen are alone at a table in a diner without the other FBI agents; (2) Aileen is the brainwashed subject; (3) Saul is sure Aileen is controlled by al-Qaeda because of the trail of bodies and her suspicious actions since she entered the country; (4) Saul is the character in this scene who knows Aileen is being controlled by al-Qaeda; (5) Saul is aware of Aileen's betrayal; and (6) Saul is closely watching and communicating with Aileen in the hope of learning her secrets and converting Aileen into a CIA and FBI informant.

The third example involves an episode of *Falling Skies*. This TNT series, which began in 2011, features the story of an extraterrestrial invasion of

144 Media on the Brain

Earth and the capturing or killing of most of humanity. Tom Mason and his three boys are part of a small group of several hundred humans who are traveling from Boston toward Charleston. They are attempting to unite with other survivors while fighting the aliens, who have superior technology and weapons, along the way. In the episode "A More Perfect Union," a scene in the last few minutes shows Hal, the oldest son, who is recovering in a medical clinic room and regains consciousness. When he gets out of bed and examines himself in a mirror, a worm parasite crawls out of his eye and into his ear. Hal then begins to smile in a very disturbing manner as a calculating expression spreads across his face.[27]

This scene differs from the previous two, because no character in the drama witnesses what is occurring to Hal. Only the audience is privy to Hal being taken over by the alien mind control device. Regardless, our procedure allows us to select details about this scene: (1) the scene where mind control is revealed is the second to last scene in this episode; (2) Tom Mason's son Hal is the mind-controlled character; (3) this revelation is not made to any other character in the narrative, only to the viewer; (4) witnessing the eye worm and the change of expression on Hal's face reveals that he is now controlled by the aliens; and (5) audience members assume Hal is now a threat to the other group members, based on the context of the theme of alien invasion in the show and his facial expressions.

In each of these cases, there is evidence of the mind control that is a part of the plot of the drama. Cues are revealed which show, explain, and provide testing of relationships in the narrative. The camera shots utilized are close up and angled at characters in the action; the viewer is given some awareness of the mental states of characters in the action. At least one character within the narrative serves as a messenger to indicate mind control has occurred. The procedural tool consists of steps to aid in untangling the interaction between characters. It is hoped that this procedural tool might be useful for investigators who wish to examine fictional narratives that contain mind control scenarios.

## COGNITIVE SCIENCE AND MIND CONTROL

There are multiple approaches to mapping cognitive science views of mind control and brainwashing. These different approaches can be attributed to needs for different methodological fields within the study of the human mind. In differing fields, the conception of the human mind takes on slightly different aspects and foci. Mind control can be successfully studied by the employment of interdisciplinary methods. Some of the aspects of our previous understanding of mind control will undergo change as we build new models to explore these stories. The goal is to deliver usable concepts that have functionality for explaining the processes and results of mind control. Through studying mind control portrayals, the elements of how human mental states are shared can be interrogated and integrated into explanatory findings that will aid our research into human minds.

Discussions and fictional representations of mind control and brainwashing can offer fertile ground for the field of media studies. As proposed in this chapter, there are factors that are key to aid in reading and analyzing mind control stories. There may also be something to learn from mind control studies that can answer questions about the persuasive influence of media in general. Studies of mind control and brainwashing face challenges which differ from those in other areas of cognitive research, while some approaches can be shared across many different areas in the field.

Future steps in the understanding of mind control and brainwashing will involve addressing the issues of communication, identity, and socialization. Another area where interdisciplinary approaches may be helpful is within the social applications of social interaction and individual relations to the group. There are political and social implications and side-effects involved in exploring changes involving loyalty in social groups. There are formal and informal power relations and differences of communication competency, experience, and expectations. The areas of hierarchal power differences and communication expectations and behaviors are likely subjects for future research.

Current research is taking place that might address some challenges facing a fuller understanding of mind control in fictional narratives. Several paths that are being explored by researchers include the fields of social cognition and distributed cognition. Modeling based on computer methods holds promise, as does mapping of the human brain. Social and communication studies contribute to understanding by uncovering the roots of human behavior as socially dependent and influenced. Increased understanding of the complexity of mind control questions will be successfully accomplished through continual research, coordination between researchers and practitioners, and incorporating interdisciplinary scholarship.

A possible future direction of research is the question of individualism versus collectivism as highlighted in mind control fiction. Alex Pentland says, "The social networks containing the individuals are an important additional unit of analysis."[28] He also discusses frameworks that postulate human thought as a result of collective activity.[29] Similarly, Oscar Ybarra et al. state, "Social interaction is a central feature of people's life."[30] One aspect of political and cultural context is the expression of differences between individualism versus collectivism being addressed in mind control fiction. Harry Triandis says members of collective societies ". . . give priority to the goals of their in-groups, shape their behavior primarily on the basis of in-group norms, and behave in a communal way."[31] Ralph Adolphs says, "Our interactions with others is, I think, an important distinction of social cognition."[32]

Another question unanswered in this study is how consistent and accurate are fictional representations of mind control. Communication between fiction producers and audience members is difficult to achieve because audiences often identify and understand a different message other than what the media producers are attempting to convey. In addition, the articulated message changes over time as a result of changes in political and social philosophy and beliefs. Effective entertainment depends on audience understanding and appreciation of the medium and method. Several tools are employed by media producers to aid in communication with the audience; different tools of analysis can aid in systematic approaches to eliciting interpretations involving alteration of characters' minds in the narratives.

Another possible line of study brought to the foreground by this research is how we know someone has changed loyalty. In fictional narratives, markers usually are used to signal to the audience that a person has been brainwashed. This directly entangles us in problems of identity in the characters on screen and how the audience detects those identity issues. Research could potentially look into these markers used in the shows and determine if they are relevant for cognitive science studies. Studies in fictional aspects of mind spotlight the intersubjectivity of human communication experiences and is fertile ground for future research.

## CONCLUSIONS: PUTTING MINDS IN MIND CONTROL

By using analysis based in Theory of Mind approaches to understand human cognition, this chapter addressed a core issue for explaining mind control in fiction. The sharing of mental states between humans depends upon foundations of communication process as well as cognitive systems. Another influence on human interaction is the likelihood that any new interaction will include modifications or transformations of existing beliefs. This chapter focused on the centrality of shared mental states through communication with an emphasis placed on the key role of theory of mind in understanding human mental behavior and action. Speaking, writing, and reading are how we determine the status and condition of our fellows; communication also plays a role in resolving problems, in relating to others, and in driving understanding of processes of thought and behavior. These issues of mind as expressed through fiction offer a rich subject for research.

This chapter presented a potential tool for analysis of mind control in Hollywood fictional entertainment. Developments in cognitive science enable the understanding of how humans make decisions and change them. Cognitive science can serve in the analysis of mental interaction and alternation and how this impacts the group. This chapter demonstrated how cognitive science contributes to knowledge about the controlling and responding of minds. In addition, this chapter reviewed current ideas of social cognition, introducing an approach to improving explanation of mind control in fiction. Future research will point to ways in which the field of cognitive science can help us understand more aspects of human behavior change.

Studying fictional representations of mental behaviors, involving mind control and brainwashing, contributes to the field of cognitive science as well as social narrative studies.

## NOTES

1. J. J. Abrams and Alex Kurtzman, "Of Human Action," *Fringe*, season 2, episode 7, directed by Joe Chappelle, November 12, 2009 (FOX).
2. Robert Rodat, "Live and Learn," *Falling Skies*, season 1, episode 1, directed by Carl Franklin, aired June 19, 2011 (TNT).
3. Gene Roddenberry and Maurice Hurley, "Q Who?," *Star Trek: The Next Generation*, season 2, episode 16, directed by Rob Bowman, aired May 6, 1989 (CBS).
4. Lisa Zunshine, *Why We Read Fiction: Theory of Mind and the Novel* (Columbus: Ohio State University Press, 2006), 25.
5. Alan Palmer, *Fictional Minds* (Lincoln: University of Nebraska Press, 2004), 12.
6. David Seed, *Brainwashing: The Fictions of Mind Control: A Study of Novels and Films since World War II* (London: Routledge, 1999).
7. George Axelrod, *The Manchurian Candidate*, directed by John Frankenheimer (Los Angeles, CA: United Artists, 1962).
8. William Shakespeare, *A Midsummer Night's Dream* (London: Routledge Press, 1991).
9. George Bernard Shaw, *Pygmalion* (New York: Brentano, 1912).
10. Jenny Clegg, *Fu Manchu and the Yellow Peril: The Making of a Racist Myth* (Staffordshire, UK: Trentham Books, 1994).
11. Sax Rohmer, *The Mask of Fu Manchu*, directed by Charles Brabin (Los Angeles, CA: Metro-Goldwyn-Mayer, 1932).
12. Jonathan Leib and Thomas Chapman, "Jim Crow, Civil Defense, and the Hydrogen Bomb: Race, Evacuation Planning, and the Geopolitics of Fear in 1950s Savannah, Georgia," *Southeastern Geographer* 51, no. 4 (2011): 579.
13. Daniel Mainwaring, *Invasion of the Body Snatchers*, directed by Don Siegel (Los Angeles, CA: Allied Artists Pictures Corporation, 1956).
14. Susan L. Carruthers, " 'The Manchurian Candidate' (1962) and the Cold War Brainwashing Scare," *Historical Journal of Film, Radio, and Television* 18, no. 1 (1998): 75–94.
15. William Grebner, *Patty's Got a Gun* (Chicago: University of Chicago Press, 2008), 100.
16. Axelrod, *Manchurian Candidate*.
17. Alex Gansa and Howard Gordon, "Pilot," *Homeland*, season 1, episode 1, directed by Michael Cuesta, aired October 2, 2011 (Showtime).
18. Andrew Niccol, *The Host*, directed by Andrew Niccol (Los Angeles, CA: Nick Wechsler Productions, 2013).
19. Gene Roddenberry and John Kingsbridge, "Return to Tomorrow," *Star Trek*, season 2, episode 20, directed by Ralph Senensky, aired February 9, 1968 (NBC).
20. Simon Barry and Andrea Stevens, "Playtime," *Continuum*, season 1, episode 8, directed by Paul Shapiro, aired July 22, 2012 (Syfy).
21. Uta Frith and Chris Frith, "The Social Brain: Allowing Humans to Boldly Go Where No Other Species Has Been," *Philosophical Transactions of the Royal Society, Series B* 365, no. 1537 (2010): 165.

22. David Premack and Guy Woodruff, "Does the Chimpanzee Have a Theory of Mind?," *Behavioral and Brain Sciences* 1, no. 4 (1978): 515.
23. Rebecca Saxe and Lindsey J. Powell, "It's the Thought That Counts: Specific Brain Regions for One Component of Theory of Mind," *Psychological Science* 17, no. 8 (2006): 692.
24. Robert Rodat and Joseph Weisberg. "Silent Kill," *Falling Skies*, season 1, episode 5, directed by Fred Toye, aired July 10, 2011 (TNT).
25. Niccol, *The Host.*
26. Alex Gansa and Howard Gordon, "The Weekend," *Homeland*, season 1, episode 7, directed by Michael Cuesta, aired November 13, 2011 (Showtime).
27. Robert Rodat and Remi Aubuchon, "A More Perfect Union," *Falling Skies*, season 2, episode 10, directed by Greg Beeman, aired August 19, 2012 (TNT).
28. Alex Pentland, "On the Collective Nature of Human Intelligence," *Adaptive Behavior* 15, no. 2 (2007): 197.
29. Ibid.
30. Oscar Ybarra et al., "Mental Exercising through Simple Socializing: Social Interaction Promotes General Cognitive Functioning," *Personality and Social Psychology Bulletin* 34, no. 2 (2008): 248.
31. Harry C. Triandis, "Individualism/Collectivism and Personality," *Journal of Personality* 69, no. 6 (2001): 907.
32. Ralph Adolphs, "The Neurobiology of Social Cognition," *Current Opinion in Neurobiology* 11, no. 2 (2001): 236.

# 10 "My Brain Made Me Do It!"
## Neuroscience, Criminal Justice, and Media

*Emilia Musumeci*

## THE RISE OF NEUROCRIMINOLOGY

In an article published by the *Wall Street Journal*, the leading psychologist and criminologist Adrian Raine argued that "the field of neurocriminology—using neuroscience to understand and prevent crime—is revolutionizing our understanding of what drives 'bad' behavior."[1] *Neurocriminology* is just one of the multifaceted sides of the "neuroscientific paradigm"—a model that considers thoughts to be the result of synaptic connections or mere brain images[2] that can be captured by fMRI—that is now permeating all areas of knowledge: from arts (*neuroaesthetic*) to economy (*neuroeconomy*) to even religion (*neurotheology*).[3] Despite the several heterogeneous scientific disciplines that are included under the term *neuroscience*, there exists an underlying idea that unites them all: that it is possible to explain all human behaviors, even the most complex, simply by understanding how the brain works. In other words, for neuroscientists "we are our neurons" because the mind is what the brain does. Nevertheless, is this approach typical of our age, pretentiously defined as a post-human era or, more emphatically, a *neurocentric age*?[4] When taking a closer look at this research, we can see that it is deeply rooted in the classical neuropsychology that developed in the early nineteenth century, with phrenological studies by Franz Joseph Gall and Johann Gaspar Spurzheim; neurological studies by Pierre Paul Broca, Carl Wernicke, and Ludwig Lichtheim; and the studies conducted by Moritz Benedikt in Austria, by Henry Maudsley in the United Kingdom, and by Lorenzo Tenchini in Italy. Most importantly, the aim to give a strong significance to biological aspects of crime and, in particular, to the innate diversity of brains and bodies of criminals, inevitably recalls the thesis of "born criminality" developed in Italy by Cesare Lombroso[5] in the second half of the nineteenth century. All of these studies show different historical backgrounds and different approaches, with their focus on investigating and studying the brain and the skull, and may be considered as foreshadowing modern neuroscience. Not by chance, still today neuroscientists[6] frequently refer to the nineteenth-century case of Phineas P. Gage. In this well-known incredible story, Gage miraculously survived a terrible accident in Vermont in 1848 that irreversibly damaged his brain with reported effects on his personality.[7] It is therefore not surprising that these techniques, far from remaining closed in aseptic laboratories, have now entered even the most austere courtrooms. So, faced with the disintegration of the power of psychiatrists and their expertise, now deemed less objective and less credible, in the courts judges are increasingly choosing to rely on techniques that appear more "certain" and "infallible" than others, like neuroimaging techniques and genetic screening, which have more and more frequently played an important role in assessing criminal responsibility. Therefore, in the courtroom there seems nowadays to be less black robes and more white coats: if once new technologies were mostly used during the investigating period preceding the trial, now the possibility of "reading the brain" of the accused seems to be a new and unsettling reality of modern trials. In other words, the burning issue is the possibility of being convicted or acquitted simply because of one's own neurons or genes, with the risk of creating the so-called *CSI* effect,[8] or rather, the perception of the omnipotence of forensic science to resolve through scientific evidence every cold case, as it happens in the episodes of the American crime drama television series *CSI*.

The use of neuroscience in criminal courtrooms has been emphasized and, in some cases, dramatized by media, and in particular, newspapers and magazines. It is necessary to analyze the role played by those means of communication in the creation of the so-called Neurocentric Era. For this purpose, after the analysis of the ambiguous relationship between neuroscience and criminal justice, this chapter will investigate how popular media represent the entrance of neuroscientists in courtrooms, paying specific attention to reactions after two Italian judgments where neuroscientific and genetic tools were used in assessing criminal responsibility.

## BRAINS ON THE STAND IN THE UNITED STATES

The burning issue related with the entrance of neuroscientists in courtrooms is the possibility of being convicted or acquitted based on one's own neurons or genes. For decades, in Anglo-Saxon countries, especially in the United States, neuroimaging techniques (functional magnetic resonance imaging [fMRI], positron emission tomography [PET], etc.) and genetic screening have acted more and more frequently as an aid in assessing criminal responsibility. If once new technologies were mostly used during the investigating period preceding the trial, now the possibility of "reading the brain" of the accused seems to be a new and unsettling reality.

Thanks to these techniques, it is possible, indeed, to see which brain areas are activated in response to certain stimuli: PET measures the activation of certain brain areas through the intensity of their metabolism, while fMRI examines blood flow, which is required to understand what kind of brain activity is in progress, like a more sophisticated version of a so-called truth machine.[9] Another controversial technique that is used to retrieve the memory traces of people's experiences is that of *brain fingerprinting*, developed in the 1980s by Lawrence Farwell, a neuroscientist at Harvard University. It consists of a device able to probe human memory in search of "brain fingerprints" that reveal memories of events experienced in the past: certain brain waves, called p300, are detected through electrodes placed on the skull of the person to be tested. The machine measures the electrical activity in the brain subject to external stimulations.[10]

In the United States neurotechnologies in criminal trials have been used since the early 1980s, with the first pioneering decisions in the famous *Hinckley*[11] and *Weinstein*[12] cases. The first case is the famous trial involving John Hinckley Jr. who in 1981, being obsessed with actress Jodie Foster, attempted to assassinate President Ronal Reagan with the aim of impressing the young actress. A CT scan of Hinckley's brain was presented in order to support the insanity defense for schizophrenia diagnosis. While the scan's role in the verdict was unclear, Hinckley was found not guilty by reason of insanity.[13]

Conversely, in the Weinstein trial the use of this kind of evidence was only attempted: although the court allowed the defense to use the technique of brain imaging, it did not go so far as to assert such loss of connection with a propensity for violence, since one of the witnesses of the prosecution, the forensic psychologist Daniel Martell, said that brain-scanning technologies were too recent and that they were not yet fully accepted by the scientific community. Hence, on October 8, 1992, Judge Richard Carruthers issued a Solomonic decision: he admitted the presence of an arachnid cyst in Weinstein's brain, but he did not say that the latter was necessarily associated with violent behavior. The prosecution, fearing that showing images of Weinstein's brain in the courtroom would shake up the jury and make them decide on an acquittal, negotiated a reduced sentence of manslaughter.

A more recent and debated case involved Brian Dugan, infamous not only for the public sensation that it aroused but also because it focused attention on the one hand on the issue of criminal liability of legal persons and psychopaths, and on the other hand on the issue of the admissibility of neuroscientific evidence in court.[14] Dugan was accused of having raped and brutally murdered a twenty-seven-year-old woman and two girls aged ten and seven between 1983 and 1985. In an attempt to spare him the death penalty,[15] his defense tried to use the data from an fMRI of Dugan's brain as a mitigating circumstance, showing how the brain of the accused, a psychopath, differs from that of "normal" people. Kent Kiehl,[16] a controversial neuroscientist at the University of New Mexico and defined by some journalists as "the new Lombroso,"[17] was heard in support of Dugan's defense. Similar to the replicants in *Blade Runner*, perfectly identical to humans from without but different from them because of their coldness and inability to empathize, Dugan, as well as all criminal psychopaths studied by Kiehl, seem to differ from other human beings because their brains, as those of serial killers, are missing the connection between the limbic system (seat of emotions) and the prefrontal cortex (which controls all types of instincts, including aggressiveness), or in other cases the paralimbic system (the group of brain structures involved in processing emotions) would be, as shown in an fMRI, too underdeveloped.[18] From this, a main feature results: a "lack of empathy."[19]

## CRIMINAL BRAINS IN ITALY

The use of neuroscientific tools in criminal trials is not just a typical phenomenon of the American courts, having "infected" Italian courts in recent times. An important example of this is provided by an Italian decision that has been defined as historical, scandalous, based on a scientific paradox, revolutionary, and Lombrosian. It is the first decision in Italy so far (and perhaps also in Europe) in which neuroscientists and geneticists have played a fundamental role. This is the recent decision of the Court of Assizes of Appeal in Trieste,[20] which granted a reduced sentence to a man who was already convicted of murder for having committed the crime in a mental state of semi-insanity because he was "genetically predisposed to an aggressive behavior." The case involved a forty-year-old Algerian citizen, Abdelmalek Bayout, who had been living in Italy since 1993. In 2007 he stabbed to death a thirty-two-year Colombian citizen named Walter Felipe Perez Novoa, one of a group of men who called Bayout "gay." In his first conviction, Bayout was sentenced to nine years and two months imprisonment, but in the appeal trial this sentence was reduced because of the new findings of neuroscience and genetics. The experts, Pietro Pietrini, a molecular biologist from the University of Pisa, and Giuseppe Sartori, a cognitive neuroscientist from the University of Padua, conducted a series of tests on the accused and found abnormalities in fMRI brain-imaging scans and in five genes that have been linked to violent behavior, including the gene encoding the neurotransmitter-metabolizing enzyme monoamine oxidize A (MAOA-A), also called the "warrior gene,"[21] which is involved in the metabolism of catecholamine (neurotransmitters that are responsible for the modulation of mood). Carrying a low-activity MAOA gene (MAOA-L), Bayout was considered "more inclined to aggressive behavior if provoked or socially excluded" and he suffered from a sort of "genetic vulnerability." The Court, agreeing with the findings of the report, argued that the presence of certain genes in the accused's DNA made him "particularly aggressive—and therefore vulnerable—in stressful situations."

In reality, according to Bayout's clinical history, he was affected by serious mental health diseases because he was suffering from episodes of delirium and paranoia and had to be treated with psychotropic drugs. It is likely that the anxious research of the experts for signs or stigmata attesting to abnormality and innate aggressiveness in the brain and in the DNA of the accused actually did not have the assumed nature of "scientific objectivity," being rather an *ad hoc* construction to show an already preset thesis: criminals are born, not made.

This approach, previously only sketched, appears to be more powerful after a new Italian case law. The polemics about the Bayout case had just calmed when another judgment, in some ways similar to that of Bayout, rekindled the discussion about the presence of geneticists and neuroscientists in courtrooms. It was the decision of the Judge for Preliminary Investigations at the Criminal Court of Como on May 20, 2011 (the motivation of which was made public on August 20, 2011), where methods developed by cognitive neuroscience and behavioral genetics were used to decide on the criminal responsibility of Stefania Albertani, a twenty-eight-year-old woman charged with multiple accounts of aggravated murder of her sister and the attempted murder of her parents. She was sentenced to twenty years imprisonment instead of thirty, because she was deemed partially insane. Also in this case, the presence of low-activity MAO-A was found in the genetic makeup of the accused. In addition to genetic screening and clinical interviews, the accused was subjected to a battery of neuropsychological tests to assess both general mental health conditions and individual mental functions. Furthermore, her brain was analyzed by Voxel-Based Morphometry (VBM), which showed a lack of integrity and functionality of the anterior cingulated cortex, linked to obsessive-compulsive disorder and aggressiveness. With this considerable amount of data and results, which were presumed to be objective, Albertani was found guilty but only partially responsible and was recognized as a "socially dangerous person." The partial insanity ruling was strongly influenced by the findings of neuroscientific evidence based on a masked determinism.

To conclude, in the cases of Bayout and Albertani it is easy to achieve similar results regarding the criminal responsibility through "traditional" methods used by psychiatry, without carrying out any brain scan or submitting the accused to complex genetic tests. These judgments assume a strong symbolic and ideological meaning because they represent the wish to impose, in a juridical field, the neuroscientific paradigm of reducing ideas and thoughts to a series of cerebral images, produced through synaptic connections among neurons with the inevitable consequence that everything an individual thinks and claims is not a demonstration of his or her own conscience and his or her own personality, but a mere product of the brain.

## DRAMATIZING CRIMINAL CASES: THAT'S THE PRESS, BABY!

Both of the American and Italian court cases examined would probably have remained relegated to academic legal journals for experts in criminal law if the media had not examined the problem of the relationship between neuroscience and law and, in particular, between crime and brain. Despite forensic neurosciences, which historically have been the ideal development of forensic science and psychiatry, the public interest in these issues is fairly recent. It is sufficient to analyze the trends in search terms used in the Google search engine in the past decade to recognize that only in recent years has the problem of the relationship between neuroscience and crime arisen for the general public. The phrase "neuroscience and law" was not the subject of research by Internet users before 2007 (see Figure 10.1a), and even the syntagm "crime and brain" was not the subject of attention from Internet users before 2006 (see Figure 10.1b). After these years, interest in these topics has shown a constant upward trend. This public interest has arisen because of the growing space that newspapers and magazines have given to research on the brain. Not by chance, the challenging "brain mapping project" advocated by Barack Obama that set brain research as the focus of future scientific research also has the effect of bringing the general public to scientific issues such as neuroscience.[22] In other words, for the public, it seems that "our brains hold the key to whom we are."[23]

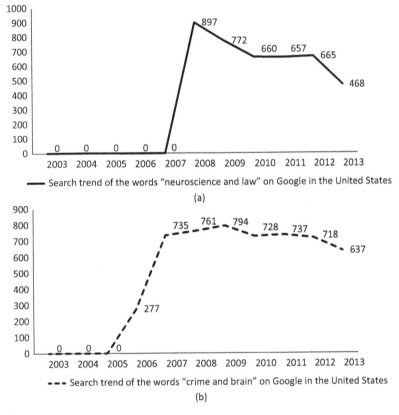

*Figure 10.1*   Search Trends: (a) "Neuroscience and Law"; (b) "Crime and Brain" (*Source*: data from Google Trend)

Therefore, there has been a proliferation in the past few years of articles and analysis on human behavior explained by neuroscience. The research on the human brain seems to be able to explain every action and every emotion; see, for example, articles such as "How Neuroscience Can Make You Kinder,"[24] "Zapping Your Brain Enhances Your Love of Classic Art,"[25] "Study Reveals Strong Link between Emotion and Financial Decisions,"[26] and even the creepy "Zombie Neuroscience: Inside the Brains of the Walking Dead."[27] In this sort of *neuromania*,[28] even criminal and/or antisocial behavior is not an exception,[29] but with a difference: while the articles referring to neuroscience research usually have either serious (concerning severe diseases or syndromes such as Alzheimer's or autism and possible new treatments) or jovial content (dealing with issues such as jealousy or love explained in a new, "neural" way), on the contrary, articles focusing on "neurocrime" are written in a rather alarmed or emphatic tone. Some of the first articles on this topic were published in the scientific journal *Nature* and were titled "Into the Mind of a Killer"[30] and "A Danger to Society"[31] (both in 2001), followed in 2007 by "Abnormal Neuroscience: Scanning Psychopaths"[32] and the special dedicated to Dugan's case in 2010: "Science in Court: Head Case."[33] Obviously, *Nature* is not consulted by the general public and the tone of the articles is much more scientific and "neutral." A more concerned tone is instead detectable in the chronicles of the Dugan trial in newspapers such as the article published on the BBC News website "Psychopaths: Born Evil or with a Diseased Brain?"[34]

This alarmist attitude is even more traceable in comments that arose after the two Italian cases discussed previously. In newspapers all over the world, the Bayout decision is referred to as a futuristic possibility of being convicted or acquitted by just "reading" one's genetic makeup or through brain scanning. In particular, many Italian[35] and foreign newspapers noticeably emphasized this case for its alleged "discovery" of the "murderer gene" or "violence gene." For example, the French *Libération*, in an article provocatively titled "Un Juge Italien Découvre le Gène du Meurtre"[36] ("An Italian Judge Has Discovered the Murder Gene") accused the Court in Trieste of issuing a verdict based on scientific nonsense, as the existence of a social and genetic predisposition to crime results from a strong racial prejudice that still pervades in Italy. The British newspaper *The Times*, with a very eloquent title "The Get Out of Jail Free Gene,"[37] wondered to what extent it is possible, scientifically and ethically, to use DNA as a defense in a criminal trial: "The Bayout trial is thought to be the first time that violent genes have been invoked to amend a sentence. It shows that, rather than being the stuff of some futuristic dystopia, the controversial field of behavioral genetics is having a dramatic effect in courtrooms today."[38] The sensation provoked by the Bayout case doesn't stop, however, with journalistic sensationalism. It also aroused the interest *Nature*,[39] which published an article titled "Lighter Sentence for Murderer with 'Bad Genes'" in which the journalist warned against the danger of the acceptance of genetic determinism in criminal cases. Similarly, *The New Scientist*[40] ran the article "Murderer with 'Aggression Genes' Gets Sentence Cut" that highlighted the "thorny question" related to this case: whether genes can absolve a person of responsibility for a particular act. In the same way, after the Albertani case many articles were published in newspapers and magazines around the world. For example, the *New Scientist* headlined "Brain Scans Reduce Murder Sentence in Italian Court"[41] and *Nature* titled an article "Italian Court Reduces Murder Sentence Based on Neuroimaging Data."[42] At the same time, many journalists portrayed Albertani as a "born criminal" and the decision as a result of a "new Lombrosianism."[43]

## CONCLUSION

In conclusion, the constant emphasis of newspapers on the few cases that use neuroscientific or genetic evidence in criminal trials is part of a wider framework that has been called the *"neurofication* of the humanities, social sciences, public policy, and the law."[44] Even the press and the media, reporting more and more "shocking" news on the entrance of neuroscientists in the courts, have contributed to the creation of a sort of myth around the neurosciences themselves. When the articles have been highly critical or worried about the new, or old, determinism, the continuous talk about the relationship between brain and crime has come to convey a clear message: neuroscientists are the only "experts" who today may hold the "scepter" of knowledge. Hence, brain science influences the practices of everyday lives so much that all human actions can be read through a sort of obsessive "brain-based healthism."[45] Many articles concerning neuroscience are accompanied by a picture of a brain scan with colored areas indicating regions such as "the locations of the functions of falling in love and resistance to smoking."[46] Consciously or unconsciously, by using these pictures to show the public "how the brain works," the media are contributing to the complex mechanism of "neuromanic imperialism"[47] that is grotesquely simplifying and degrading humanity to mere neuron movements. This is especially evident in the field of criminal law and criminology, where neuroscience seems to have the duty of distinguishing "bad" from "mad." In the trials we have analyzed, the opinion of the experts, though they were not binding on the court, became a sort of "legal evidence" influencing the judges' decisions. These judgments hide an aim that goes beyond case law and practical reason (i.e., to strengthen the thesis of defense against that of prosecution): they possess hegemony in the field of forensic evaluation of insanity. As we have seen, the role of expertise in courtrooms is today so crucial that it is possible to provocatively claim that the judges are bound to be supplanted by neuroscientists who would "write" the judgments of conviction or acquittal in their place. The new power of neuroscience, relying on a presumed objectivity, is undermining the older power of forensic psychiatrics, which for some decades has been in crisis. This is evidenced by the heated debate triggered on the one hand from the new edition of the *Diagnostic and Statistical Manual of Mental Disorders (DSM 5)*, the so-called bible of psychiatry, and, on the other hand, the recent polemics against so-called Big Pharma and the widespread "medicalization of normality." In other words, we are witnessing, as claimed by Nikolas Rose and Joelle Abi-Rached, a shift "from psy-disciplines to neuro-disciplines" resulting in the slow but inexorable de-legitimization of the first in favor of the latter or, rather, in the creation of a new way of "governing though the brain, and in the name of the brain."[48]

## NOTES

1. A. Raine, "The Criminal Mind," *Wall Street Journal*, April 26, 2013, http://online. wsj.com/article/SB10001424127887323335404578444682892520530.html.
2. C. Frith, *Making up the Mind: How the Brain Creates Our Mental World* (Malden, MA: Blackwell, 2007).
3. Cf. F. Vander Valk, introduction to *Essays on Neuroscience and Political Theory: Thinking the Body Politic* (New York: Routledge, 2012), 2.
4. P. Becker, "The Coming of a Neurocentric Age? Neurosciences and the New Biology of Violence: A Historian's Comment," *Medicina and Storia* 19–20 (2010): 101–28; J. F. Dunagan, "Politics for the Neurocentric Age," *Journal of Futures Studies* 15 (2010): 51–70.
5. On the Lombrosian legacy in neuroscience and law debate, see especially E. Musumeci, "New Natural Born Killers? The Legacy of Lombroso in Neuroscience and Law," in *Cesare Lombroso Handbook*, ed. P. Knepper and P. J. Ystehede, 131–46 (New York: Routledge, 2013).
6. See H. Damasio, T. Grabowski, R. Frank, A. M. Galaburda, and A. R. Damasio, "The Return of Phineas Gage: Clues about the Brain from the Skull of a Famous Patient," *Science* 264, no. 5162 (1994): 1102–5.
7. See M. Macmillan, *An Odd Kind of Fame: Stories of Phineas Gage* (Cambridge, MA: MIT Press, 2000); P. Becker, "New Monsters on the Block? On the Return of Biological Explanations of Crime and Violence," in *Cuerpos anómalos*, ed. M. S. Hering Torres, 270–82 (Bogota: Editorial Universidad Nacional, 2008).
8. J. E. Starrs, "The CSI Effect," *Scientific Sleuthing Review* 28, no. 2 (2004): 32–34.
9. In such a sense a recent judicial case in India is emblematic: thanks to an EEG, Aditi Sharma, a twenty-four-year-old girl accused of murdering her boyfriend by poisoning him with arsenic was sentenced because, according to the findings of the examination she was subjected to by a specific software called Brain Electrical Oscillations Signature (BEOS), the images of the murder were "contained in the memory" of her brain, not as a mere story, but as actually experienced. Cf. A. Saini, "The Brain Police: Judging Murder with an MRI," *Wired Magazine*, May 27, 2009, http://www.wired.co.uk/magazine/archive/2009/06/features/guilty.
10. See *amplius*, N. Levy, *Neuroethics: Challenges for the 21st Century* (New York: Cambridge University Press, 2007).
11. About this case see, at least, P. W. Low, J. C. Jeffries Jr., and Richard J. Bonnie, *The Trial of John W. Hinckley, Jr.: A Case Study in the Insanity Defense* (Mincola, NY: Foundation Press, 1986).

12. Cf. J. Rosen, "The Brain on the Stand," *New York Times*, March 11, 2007, http://www.nytimes.com/2007/03/11/magazine/11Neurolaw.t.html?pagewant ed=all&_r=0. The decision is Roper, Superintendent, Potosi Correctional Center v. Simmons, 543 U.S.—03-633 (2005), available online at http://supreme.justia.com/us/543/03-633/case.html.

13. Cf. H. T. Greely, "Neuroscience and Criminal Responsibility: Proving 'Can't Help Himself' as a Narrow Bar to Criminal Liability," in *Law and Neuroscience*, ed. M. Freeman (New York: Oxford University Press, 2011), 71.

14. Cf. G. Miller, "Investigating the Psychopathic Mind," *Science* 321, no. 325 (2008): 1284–86.

15. Dugan had been on death row until March 2011, when the governor of Illinois abolished the death penalty. His sentence was converted to life imprisonment.

16. Cf. J. Seabrook, "Suffering Souls: The Search for the Roots of Psychopathy," *The New Yorker*, November 10, 2008, 64–73.

17. F. Porciani, "Entra in Aula la Mente del Serial Killer. La Risonanza Magnetica Come Prova," in *Corriere della Sera*, March 28, 2010, 56.

18. K. A. Kiehl and J. W. Buckholtz, "Neuroscience Perspective on Psychopathy: Evidence for Paralimbic System Dysfunction," *Psychiatry Research* 142 (2006): 107–28.

19. Ibid.

20. Court of Assizes of Appeal in Trieste, 01.10.2009, pres. ed est. Reinotti, *Rivista penale*, 1, 2010, 70–75.

21. See *amplius*, D. P. Lyle, "Dangerous DNA: The Warrior Gene," http://writers forensicsblog.wordpress.com/2010/06/15/dangerous-dna-the-warrior-gene, and E. Yong, "Dangerous DNA: The Truth about the 'Warrior Gene,' " *The New Scientist*, April 12, 2010, no. 2755, http://www.newscientist.com/article/mg20627557.300-dangerous-dna-the-truth-about-the-warrior-gene.html.

22. Cf. G. Markus, "Obama's Brain," *The New Yorker*, February 18, 2013, http://www.newyorker.com/online/blogs/newsdesk/2013/02/obamas-brain.html.

23. N. Rose and J. M. Abi-Rached, *Neuro: The New Brain Sciences and the Management of the Mind* (Princeton, NJ: Princeton University Press, 2013), 1.

24. E. Svoboda, "How Neuroscience Can Make You Kinder," *The New Scientist*, October 23, 2013, http://www.newscientist.com/article/mg22029 390.300-how-neuroscience-can-make-you-kinder.html.

25. H. Cave, "Zapping Your Brain Enhances Your Love of Classic Art," *The New Scientist*, October 31, 2013, http://www.newscientist.com/article/dn24500-zapping-your-brain-enhances-your-love-of-classic-art.html.

26. L. Dagade, "Study Reveals Strong Link between Emotion and Financial Decisions," *Life*, October 29, 2013, http://www.international-adviser.com/news/life/standard-life-neuroscience-research-into-saving.

27. T. Lewis, "Zombie Neuroscience: Inside the Brains of the Walking Dead," *NBCNews*, October, 2013, http://www.nbcnews.com/science/zombie-neuroscience-inside-brains-walking-dead-8C11498311.

28. P. Legrenzi and C. Umiltà, *Neuromania: On the Limits of Brain Science* (New York: Oxford University Press, 2011).

29. The interest for this topic also among academics is witnessed by a number of recent publications: S. J. Morse and A. L. Roskies, eds., *A Primer on Criminal Law and Neuroscience: A Contribution of the Law and Neuroscience Project* (New York: Oxford University Press, 2013); A. Raine, *The Anatomy of Violence: The Biological Roots of Crime* (New York: Pantheon, 2013); N. A. Vincent, *Neuroscience and Legal Responsibility* (New York: Oxford University Press, 2013); M. S. Pardo and D. Patterson, *Minds, Brains, and Law: The Conceptual Foundations of Law and Neuroscience* (New York: Oxford University Press, 2013).

30. A. Abbott, "Into the Mind of a Killer," *Nature* 410 (2001): 296–98.
31. Ibid, 287.
32. A. Abbott, "Abnormal Neuroscience: Scanning Psychopaths," *Nature* 450 (2007): 942–44.
33. V. Hughes, "Science in Court: Head Case," March 17, 2010, http://www.nature.com/news/2010/100317/full/464340a.html.
34. M. Taylor, "Psychopaths: Born Evil or with a Diseased Brain?," *BBC News*, November 14, 2011, http://www.bbc.co.uk/news/health-15386740.
35. About Italian newspapers, see, at least, D. Fiore, "Pena Ridotta per Questioni di Geni: Non Dovrebbe Essere il Contrario?," *Il Piccolo–Trieste*, November 19, 2009, 22; M. Smiderle, "Sconto di Pena per l'Assassino: È Vulnerabile Geneticamente," *Il Giornale*, November 9, 2009, http://www.ilgiornale.it/news/sconto-pena-l-assassino-geneticamente-vulnerabile.html; A. Lavazza, "I Geni Costringono a Delinquere? No, il Riduzionismo è Già Superato," *Avvenire*, November 7, 2009, http://terzotriennio.blogspot.it/2009/11/i-geni-costringono-delinquere-no-il.html; G.O. Longo, "Dopo la Sentenza della Corte d'Assise d'appello di Trieste," *Avvenire*, November 7, 2009, http://terzotriennio.blogspot.it/2009/11/i-geni-costringono-delinquere-no-il.html; Redazione, "La Genetica Entra in Tribunale," *Il Sole 24 Ore*, October 25, 2009, http://www.ilsole24ore.com/art/SoleOnLine4/Italia/2009/10/tribunale-genetica.shtml?uuid=b6a25364-c198-11de-adc0; G. Surza, "Via Cernaia, Sconto di Pena per l'Assassino: È Geneticamente Predisposto alla violenza," *Messaggero Veneto–Udine*, October 25, 2009, 5.
36. M. Inizal, "Un Juge Italien Découvre le Gène du Meurtre," *Libération*, October 28, 2009, http://www.liberation.fr/monde/2009/10/28/un-juge-italien-decouvre-le-gene-du-meurtre_590482.
37. A. Ahuja, "The Get Out of Jail Free Gene," *The Times*, November 17, 2009, http://www.thetimes.co.uk/tto/science/genetics/article1844021.ece.
38. Ibid.
39. E. Feresin, "Lighter Sentence for Murderer with 'Bad Genes,'" *Nature*, October 30, 2009, http://www.nature.com/news/2009/091030/full/news.2009.1050.html.
40. E. Callaway, "Murderer with 'Aggression Genes' Gets Sentence Cut," *The New Scientist*, November 3, 2009, http://www.newscientist.com/article/dn18098-murderer-with-aggression-genes-gets-sentence-cut.html.
41. J. Hamzelou, "Brain Scans Reduce Murder Sentence in Italian Court," *The New Scientist*, September 2, 2011, http://www.newscientist.com/blogs/shortsharpscience/2011/09/brain-scans-reduce-sentence-in.html.
42. E. Feresin, "Italian Court Reduces Murder Sentence Based on Neuroimaging Data," *Nature–Newsblog*, September 1, 2011, http://blogs.nature.com/news/2011/09/italian_court_reduces_murder_s.html.
43. S. Bencivelli, "Restano i Dubbi, lo Spettro di Lombroso," *Alias–Il Manifesto*, October 2011, no. 38, 9.
44. M.J. Farah, "Endorsment," http://press.princeton.edu/titles/10023.html#reviews.
45. D.J. Thornton, *Brain Culture: Neuroscience and Popular Media* (New Brunswick, NJ: Rutgers University Press, 2011), 2.
46. Legrenzi and Umiltà, *Neuromania*, 25.
47. R. Tallis, *Aping Manking: Neuromania, Darwinitis and the Misrepresentation of Humanity* (Durham, NC: Acumen, 2012), 73.
48. Rose and Abi-Rached, *Neuro*, 8.

# 11 The Golden Voice of Neuroscience
## Fact Finding in Western Buddhist Media

*Jenell Johnson*

In the *Sutra [on Pure Realms] Spread Out in a Dense Array*, the Buddha advised his followers to examine his teachings the way a goldsmith examines gold—rubbing, cutting, and melting it—rather than simply accepting the teaching on his authority alone. This anecdote is one of many in which the Buddha advocated an empirical perspective nearly two millennia before Francis Bacon and his fellow revolutionaries began melting down the Idols of the Theater and reforming them into microscopes and telescopes. Among the world's major religions, Buddhism has long enjoyed a reputation as not just friendly to science but compatible to the point of collaboration.[1] In recent years, the perceived compatibility of Buddhism and science has only intensified in the wake of a number of high profile intersections between Buddhists and neuroscientists, who have taken an interest in contemplative practices such as meditation and mindfulness. In addition to identifying a number of health benefits associated with these practices, ranging from lowered blood pressure and stress levels to increased immunity and even genomic changes, researchers have also sought to map their neural correlates.[2] And in perhaps the most spectacular example of the intersection between Buddhism and neuroscience, in 2005 the Dalai Lama addressed the Society for Neuroscience in Washington, D.C., an event met by both praise and protest.

Intersections between Buddhism and neuroscience have drawn significant coverage in the mass media. The press stories I will examine in this chapter, however, are not essays like David Brooks's recent *New York Times* column "The Neural Buddhists," nor popular books like *Buddha's Brain: The Practical Science of Happiness, Love, and Wisdom*, which are written for a general public. Instead, this chapter explores how the intersection between Buddhism and neuroscience is presented for a Buddhist audience—specifically, a Western Buddhist audience—in popular Buddhist magazines like *The Shambhala Sun, Tricycle*, and *Buddhadharma*.[3] Science communication research has traditionally focused on mass media directed toward a general audience, or sometimes an audience explicitly interested in science, such as the readers of *Popular Science* or *Scientific American*. This chapter extends previous research by exploring an example of science communication for a specific public seeking information on something other than science. In addition, research on science communication for a general public tends to emphasize the importance of scientific understanding/engagement for healthy democracies. However, the form of specialized science communication explored in this chapter offers a new perspective on public engagement with science, raising questions not only about the purposes of that engagement but also its potential effects.

The Western Buddhist interest in neuroscience follows growing cultural and academic interest in neuroscience reflected in volumes such as the one you are currently reading. Following the much-hyped "decade of the brain," scholars from the humanities and social sciences have turned toward neuroscience for new insights into human behavior and cultural production, leading to the emergence of a number of "neuro-disciplines" like neurosociology and neurohistory.[4] Because many of these "neuroscholars" do not have formal training in neuroscience (or the natural sciences), they often draw on existing research instead of conducting new studies themselves. In a study of how neuroscholars use neuroscience as evidence, Melissa Littlefield and I found that scholars from the humanities and social sciences frequently cite books of popular neuroscience (like Antonio Damasio's *The Feeling of What Happens* or V. S. Ramachandran's *The Phantom in the Brain*) rather than primary scientific research and tend to incorporate findings into their arguments using rhetorical strategies we termed "fact finding" and "theory building."[5] Theory building positions neuroscience as one perspective on polysemic phenomena like consciousness, art appreciation, God beliefs, or reading. In theory building, insights from neuroscience are used to ask new questions and to open new avenues of research, and in so doing, theory building positions neuroscience as a coequal collaborator in the production of knowledge. Fact finding, in contrast, uses neuroscience to *answer* questions or to settle disciplinary debates (such as the origin of gender roles or the relationship between media violence and violent acts). Fact finding presents scientific research as the final word on a particular problem, keeping the "black box" of neuroscience firmly closed and tucking any disciplinary controversies neatly inside.[6] Rather than enrolling neuroscience as a true partner in transdisciplinary inquiry, fact finding reproduces an epistemological hierarchy in which neuroscientific knowledge is accorded more value than knowledge produced in the humanities and social sciences.[7]

The "neuroessentialism" found in some neuroscholarship is only amplified in science journalism, which has often been critiqued for exaggerating the certainty of primary research.[8] For example, Sandra Blakeslee's 2006 *New York Times* story on mirror neurons, "Cells That Can Read Minds," not only completely ignored the uncertain existence of mirror neurons in humans, but also made bold claims about how the research was being imported to other disciplines, writing that the discovery of mirror neurons was "shifting the understanding of culture, empathy, philosophy, language, imitation, autism, and psychotherapy."[9] While Blakeslee's collapse of philosophy into the sciences is troubling, her claim that mirror neurons "reveal how children learn, why people respond to certain types of sports, dance, music, and art, why watching media violence may be harmful and why men like pornography" reveals fact finding so breathtaking that one wonders what human activity mirror neurons *can't* explain. A story like "Cells That Read Minds" exaggerates scientific findings as well as their application and implications, and its use of words like "reveal," "how," and "why" not only reproduces deterministic ideas about human behavior but also reinforces a mythic image of science as a singular explanatory force. The effects on the *Times* readership largely remain in the abstract: a commentary on the relationship between science and the broader culture. However, what are the potential effects when a community's fact finding threatens the knowledge that gives rise to that community in the first place?

Western Buddhist magazines have run stories on suffering, illness, pain, and death for many years, often as a way to explore what a Buddhist perspective brings to these experiences. In Shinzen Young's 1997 article "Observing and Opening: A Practical Method for Transforming Physical Pain into Spiritual Growth," for example, the meditation teacher explains that although meditation may not be a "quick fix" for pain, it may allow practitioners to experience pain in a "new, empowering way." Other articles explored the question of whether or not taking Prozac might be cheating oneself of the suffering that leads to enlightenment.[10] In the late 1990s and early 2000s, however, Buddhist magazines began regularly featuring stories and columns about science and medicine. In 1999, for example *The Shambhala Sun* began running a regular column on health written by a physician who offered expert advice on nutrition and exercise as well as commentaries on scientific medicine.[11] Though the magazines clearly exhibited a growing interest in science and medicine, stories about neuroscience and Buddhism did not emerge until 2003, when *Tricycle* ran a special extended feature on Buddhism and science. Thereafter, stories on neuroscience began to appear with greater frequency and have now become a semi-regular feature in the magazines.

At first glance, many of the stories appear to use neuroscience to strengthen the authority of Buddhist teachings and practices. For example, an article titled "Buddhism and Pain Relief" begins by ruminating on the relationship between science and religion:

> While many religions value introspection, scientists often view it with skepticism. After all, if something is subjective and cannot be measured, how can you be sure it's true? The insights of the Buddha were produced by self-observation. Thus, until recently, they fell outside the realm of scientific verification. But with the development of brain imaging technology such as functional MRI, it is not possible to carry out introspection and scientific observation in parallel, and to assess how well self-observation stacks up with objective methods of inquiry.[12]

In the first two sentences, the story promises a critique, offering commentary on points of friction between scientific and Buddhist practices of knowledge creation. However, it then likens the collaboration between these perspectives as one of competition (how well Buddhist self-observation "stacks up" to fMRI). After providing a brief overview on the state of pain research, the story concludes that Buddhism comes out on top, stating that this research suggests "the Buddha's views on suffering associated with physical pain appear to be valid, and perhaps *more* advanced than those in the West" (italics in original). However, consider the implications of a phrase like "the Buddha's views on suffering associated with physical pain *appear to be valid*," which is also the article's main point. The claim is qualified with the word "appear." Its use of the word "valid," however, suggests two powerful implicit claims: first, that neuroscience is an appropriate instrument with which to measure the Buddha's views and second, that they were not valid to begin with. An essay titled "The Science of Mindfulness" makes a similar claim: "Wisdom traditions have for thousands of years recommended mindful practice in a variety of forms to cultivate well-being in an individual's life. Now science is confirming these benefits."[13] Again, consider the wording of the primary claim. In articles like these, neuroscience is used as a stamp to "validate" and "confirm" what contemplatives have been arguing for millennia on the basis of their own experiences—that meditation and mindfulness have significant physical and emotional benefits.

I want to pause here. By making this critique of the Western Buddhist media's representation of neuroscience, I am *not* saying that there is something inherently problematic about the studies themselves—making sense of contemplative experience from a scientific perspective is a fascinating and worthwhile endeavor, and I am hesitant to claim, unlike a number of other scholars critical of the neurosciences, that there are proper and improper objects of disciplinary inquiry. The question I raise is not whether neuroscientists *should* be studying Buddhist practice, but how this "collaboration" (as the intersection is so often described) is represented, and, more importantly, what claims are being made of it. My point, to put it another way, is that claims within articles like these are missing a small but crucial phrase: "The Buddha's views on suffering associated with physical pain appear to be valid *within a scientific framework*." Consider the shift in meaning if instead of declaring "Now science is confirming these benefits," the Siegel article had stated "Now a number of scientists agree."

Another story from *Shambhala Sun* about a study of the neural correlates of Shamantha meditation describes its goal as follows: "Is it true, as Buddhist contemplatives claim, that improvements in the voluntary control of attention and associated improvements in attention systems in the brain make it easier to recognize and overcome negative emotions, maintain resilience in the face of stress, and improve relationships with other people?"[14] Note the language here: the study's primary research question is said to be "Are the claims of Buddhist contemplatives *true*?" In this sense, Buddhist teachings are presented as falsifiable hypotheses to be tested rather than as guiding questions that might open up new venues of research. The dominant claim, then, in many Buddhist media stories about neuroscience is that science has finally proven what thousands of Buddhists have known for millennia. Yet in so doing, this kind of fact finding reveals a more troublesome implicit claim: Buddhist knowledge is not really knowledge at all.

Let's look at this question from another perspective: a point of perceived incommensurability between neuroscience and Buddhism. To put it simply, many Buddhists have a dualistic and transcendent understanding of the mind and consciousness. Neuroscientists do not.[15] This is a point not lost on Buddhists, as the Dalai Lama writes:

> There is a deep question about whether the mind and consciousness are any more than simply operations of the brain . . . though heavily contingent upon a physical base, including neural networks, brain cells, and sensory faculties—the mental realm enjoys a state separate from the material world. From the Buddhist perspective, the mental realm cannot be reduced to the world of matter, though it may depend upon that world to function.[16]

The dualistic perspective that undergirds much of Buddhist understanding of its own practices—the *episteme* undergirding the *techne* of contemplative practice—has proved difficult for neuroscience to stomach. According to philosopher Evan Thompson, "in Western science, there is a reaction against that kind of dualistic view. The stumbling block from science's perspective has been how to understand, conceptually, how there could be any kind of interaction between an autonomous consciousness, assuming this is what mind is, and the brain."[17] I won't delve too deeply into this issue due to space limitations, but I do want to use this issue to raise yet another question about how the "collaboration" between Buddhism and neuroscience is represented, or rather, to raise a point that is not being made in many of these stories. Simply put, the *techne* of meditation and mindfulness are being studied as objects in the lab, while the Buddhist *episteme* that explains that *techne* is often discarded as incommensurable if not altogether irrelevant.

The *Tricycle* article "The Lama in the Lab," for example, states that scientific studies of Buddhist practices aren't "trying to discover the neurological basis of nirvana but rather to investigate the brain mechanisms at work during various meditative states, and gain insight into the impact of meditation on our thoughts and emotions," which appears to position itself against a reductionist perspective. However, in the very next sentence the story suggests, "It may then be possible to objectively demonstrate the benefits of certain Buddhist contemplative practices—part of Mind and Life's ongoing efforts to explore how science and Buddhism, as equal partners, can help each other."[18] Here, then, is the key question: How do science and Buddhism help each other, as the article states? What does neuroscience give to Buddhism? We can see what Buddhism gives neuroscience—a flashy, interesting object with creative funding streams and clear, important, translational appeal, particularly in the development of mindfulness therapeutics—but what does neuroscience give back?

What the stories in popular Buddhist media suggest is that this intersection gives Buddhists, particularly Western Buddhists, a way to package ancient tradition to persons raised in a culture in which science is seen as the ultimate authority. According to one post on the *Tricycle* blog, reporting on a study that claimed that long-term meditators exhibited evidence of increased gray matter volume in the right orbito-frontal cortex, a positive effect may be "that meditation becomes ever more acceptable—and desirable—to the mainstream."[19] Buddhist Studies scholar Donald Lopez agrees, describing the Buddhism-and-science discourse as a rhetorical "weapon" to defend an ancient Eastern tradition against Western prejudices and predilection for positivism.[20] Yet for Lopez, there is a question that hangs over this discourse with a zen koan-like quality: how many Buddhist doctrines can be eliminated while allowing Buddhism to remain Buddhism? Lopez's question raises a larger one: while Buddhism may have something to gain from cultural perception that its teachings have been scientifically validated, what does it stand to lose?

While most stories in Buddhist media have been uncritically enthusiastic about the intersection between Buddhism and neuroscience, one recent article by Linda Heuman in *Tricycle* provides a trenchant answer to what Buddhism stands to lose. Writing about a retreat she had attended in which the health effects of meditation were being trumpeted over traditional Buddhist teachings, Heuman writes that she raised her hand and asked a question that made the room go silent:

> Given the depth of suffering in samsara and the possibility of a solution to it, and given that the very texts we study outline a path to that solution; given that we have a realized master right here who is, we believe, capable of leading us on the path to that solution—why would we devote our precious human lives to exploring whether meditation can lower blood pressure?[21]

Why, Heuman asks, do Buddhists feel compelled to reinvent a theory of a wheel that has worked for them for thousands of years? What's at stake when the dharma becomes "modern"? In some Buddhist circles, Heuman writes, to suggest that "the purpose of Buddhism is *exactly what the traditional texts tell us it is*—which is to say, that it is concerned with the transcendent—can be to come across sounding like a rube or to meet with condescension." *Like a rube*, that is to say, to come across as being unscientific and antimodern. Heuman then uses her questions to leverage a wider critique: however benevolent the intentions may be, what is said to be collaboration in theory often looks a lot like scientific imperialism in practice.[22]

We might ask, then, what is *lost* when Buddhism is represented as translatable, without remainder, into a scientific framework. And, more significantly, what is lost when Buddhist concepts of mind are seen to be translated, without remainder, into a materialist understanding of the brain, as the Dalai Lama points out. This, I believe, is the most salient critique that can be made of these press stories, and about the intersection of neuroscience and Buddhism more generally. Although the methods are acknowledged to be different, most of the stories seem to take for granted that neuroscientists and Buddhists are *looking at the same thing.* They take for granted that what Buddhists study through self-observation and what a neuroscientist measures using fMRI are one and the same. Yet although the maps may be in different languages, written at different times, and made of different colors, they are not maps of same territory.

In conclusion, I want to turn to a final point often raised about the intersection of Buddhism and neuroscience: praise for Buddhism's perceived lack of dogmaticism, which is reflected in my titular anecdote from the Buddha that his teachings should be seen as set in malleable gold rather than stone. According to Alan Wallace, Buddhism "presents many theories about the functioning and potential of human consciousness that can be tested empirically. . . . If many of these hypotheses are confirmed by sound and thorough investigation, we may need to radically alter our interpretation of both scientific and religious knowledge."[23] While scientific knowledge about the brain may be altered in the sense that it is revised or expanded, the scientific methods and epistemology used to generate that knowledge remain intact. However, as Heuman argues, it seems that Buddhist methods and epistemology *do not* remain intact, particularly for a Western audience. This point is repeated in an article in *Tricycle*, which describes the Dalai Lama as a "natural scientist" and concludes by describing a "principle that the Dalai Lama has repeated many times . . . if science can prove some tenet of Buddhism is untrue, then Buddhism will have to change accordingly."[24]

The problem is that in the "collaboration" represented between Buddhism and neuroscience in these magazines, only one voice is accorded the cultural authority to make factual pronouncements in the West; only one mode of observation is given the privilege to contribute to knowledge rather than serving as an interesting object of study. While the Buddhist resistance to dogmaticism and its openness to epistemological pluralism is to be rightly lauded in an age in which religious master narratives dominate public discourse, to return to the anecdote I used to begin this chapter, what I hope is that the authoritative voice of neuroscience would remain just as malleable to Buddhists as the golden voice of the Buddha himself.

## NOTES

1. The rich and complex relationship between Buddhism and science has been explored in a number of book-length studies that explore religious and epistemological terrain I haven't the space—or the expertise—to detail here. I feel

it necessary to note here that I am a rhetorician with an interest in the discursive circulation of scientific knowledge and the construction of authority and expertise and not a religious studies scholar of any stripe. For more thorough studies of the intersection of Buddhism and science, see Donald S. Lopez, *Buddhism and Science* (Chicago: University of Chicago Press, 2008); Lopez, *The Scientific Buddha* (New Haven, CT: Yale University Press, 2012).

2. See, for example, Richard J. Davidson et al., "Alterations in Brain and Immune Function," *Psychosomatic Medicine* 65, no. 4 (2003): 564–70; Jeffery A. Dusek et al., "Genomic Counter-Stress Changes Induced by the Relaxation Response," *PLoS One* 3, no. 7 (2008): e2576; Manoj K. Bhasin et al., "Relaxation Response Induces Temporal Transcriptome Changes in Energy Metabolism, Insulin Secretion and Inflammatory Pathways," *PloS One* 8, no. 5 (2013): e62817; Julie A. Brefczynski-Lewis et al., "Neural Correlates of Attentional Expertise in Long-Term Meditation Practitioners," *Proceedings of the National Academy of Sciences* 104, no. 27 (2007): 11483–88; Giuseppe Pagnoni et al., "Thinking about Not-thinking: Neural Correlates of Conceptual Processing during Zen meditation," *PLoS One* 3, no. 9 (2008): e3083.

3. *Shamabhala Sun* is the oldest of the three magazines and claims to have offered "the best of Buddhism in America" for more than thirty years. It features articles, fiction, poetry, art, book reviews, news on Buddhist celebrities, and classified advertisements—from funerary urns to personal ads—tailored for a Western Buddhist audience. *Tricycle* makes similar claims about its aims and readership and the stories are similar in tone and content. Founded in 1991, the magazine claims to be "the leading journal of Buddhism in the West, where it continues to be the most inclusive and widely read vehicle for the dissemination of Buddhist perspectives." *Buddhadharma: The Practitioner's Quarterly* is published by the Shambhala Sun foundation and is presented as an "in-depth, practice-oriented journal for everyone with a serious interest in Buddhism."

4. On the topic of neuro-disciplines, see Fernando Vidal, "Brainhood, Anthropological Figure of Modernity," *History of the Human Sciences* 22, no. 1 (2009): 5–36; Melissa Littlefield and Jenell Johnson, *The Neuroscientific Turn: Transdisciplinarity in the Age of the Brain* (Ann Arbor: University of Michigan Press, 2012); Nikolas Rose and Joelle M. Abi-Rached, *Neuro: The New Brain Sciences and the Management of the Mind* (Princeton, NJ: Princeton University Press, 2013); and David Gruber, "Mirror Neurons in a Group Analysis 'Hall of Mirrors': Translation as a Rhetorical Approach to Neurodisciplinary Writing," *Technical Communication Quarterly* 23, no. 3 (2014): 207–26.

5. Jenell Johnson and Melissa Littlefield, "Lost and Found in Translation: Popular Neuroscience in the Neurodisciplines," in *Advances in Medical Sociology*, vol. 11, ed. Martyn Pickersgill and Ira Van Keulen, 279–97 (London: Emerald, 2011).

6. Bruno Latour, *Science in Action: How to Follow Scientists and Engineers through Society* (Cambridge, MA: Harvard University Press, 1988).

7. See also Jordynn Jack and Gregory Appelbaum, "'This Is Your Brain on Rhetoric': Research Directions for Neurorhetorics," *Rhetoric Society Quarterly* 40, no. 5 (2010): 411–37; Joseph Dumit, "Twisting the Neurohelix," in *The Neuroscientific Turn: Transdisciplinarity in the Age of the Brain*, ed. Melissa Littlefield and Jenell Johnson, 233–40 (Ann Arbor: University of Michigan Press, 2012); Anne Beaulieu, "Fast Moving Objects and Their Consequences: A Response to the Neuroscientific Turn in Practice," in Littlefield and Johnson, *The Neuroscientific Turn*, 152–62.

8. Eric Racine, Ofek Bar-Ilan, and Judy Illes, "fMRI in the public eye," *Nature Reviews Neuroscience* 6, no. 2 (2005): 159–64.

9. Although research into the phenomenon has been around for nearly two decades in nonhuman primates, direct evidence of mirror neurons was only recently identified in humans. Neuroscientists are not only unsure about how mirror neurons work but they have also critiqued the translatability between monkey brains and human brains, and their existence and action in humans remains the topic of considerable discussion. For a more in-depth discussion of mirror neuron research, see the forum in the July 2011 issue of *Perspectives on Psychological Science*; Roy Mukamel, Arne D. Ekstrom, Jonas Kaplan, Marco Iacoboni, and Itzhak Fried, "Single-Neuron Responses in Humans during Execution and Observation of Actions," *Current Biology* 20, no. 8 (2010): 750–56; Gregory Hickok, "Eight Problems for the Mirror Neuron Theory of Action Understanding in Monkeys and Humans," *Journal of Cognitive Neuroscience* 21, no. 7 (2009): 1229–43.

10. Judith Hooper, "Prozac and the Enlightened Mind: Can Prozac Help or Hinder Waking Up?," *Tricyle*, Summer 1999, 39–41.

11. See, for example, Chris Stewart-Patterson, "In Defense of Western Medicine," *Shambhala Sun*, July 2001, 7.

12. Rick Heller, "Buddhism's Pain Relief," *Buddhadharma*, Fall 2010, http://www.thebuddhadharma.com/web-archive/2010/9/13/buddhisms-pain-relief.html.

13. Daniel Siegel, "The Science of Mindfulness," *Shambhala Sun*, March 2003, http://www.shambhalasun.com/index.php?option=com_content&task=view&id=3501&Itemid=0.

14. Adeline Van Waning, "Inside the Shamatha Project," *Buddhadharma*, Spring 2011, http://www.thebuddhadharma.com/web-archive/2011/5/16/inside-the-shamatha-project.html.

15. I might also note that "Buddhists" and "neuroscientists" are not necessarily two separate groups of people. Francisco Varela, for example, was a student of Chögyam Trungpa's, and James Austin is a longtime zen practitioner.

16. Dalai Lama, *The Universe in a Single Atom: The Convergence of Science and Spirituality* (New York: Random House, 2005), 126.

17. Sharon Begley, *Train Your Mind, Change Your Brain: How a New Science Reveals Our Extraordinary Potential to Transform Ourselves* (New York: Ballantine, 2008), 153.

18. Marshall Glickman, "The Lama in the Lab," *Tricycle*, Spring 2003, http://www.tricycle.com/special-section/lama-lab.

19. James Shaheen, "Meditators Have More Brains," *Tricycle* blog, June 10, 2010, http://www.tricycle.com/p/1884. For the original study, see Eileen Luders et al., "The Underlying Anatomical Correlates of Long-Term Meditation: Larger Hippocampal and Frontal Volumes of Gray Matter," *Neuroimage* 45, no. 3 (2009): 672–78.

20. Lopez, *Buddhism and Science*, 32.

21. Linda Heuman, "What's at Stake as the Dharma Goes Modern?," *Tricycle*, Fall 2012, http://www.tricycle.com/feature/whats-stake-dharma-goes-modern.

22. On this point, see Walter Mignolo, *The Darker Side of Western Modernity: Global Futures, Decolonial Options* (Durham, NC: Duke University Press, 2011).

23. Wallace, *Tibetan Buddhism from the Ground Up*, 25. See also Alan Wallace, *Contemplative Science: Where Buddhism and Neuroscience Converge* (New York: Columbia University Press, 2007).

24. Daniel Goleman, "The Natural Scientist," *Tricycle*, Spring 2003, 80.

# 12 Mindful Media
## Representations of the Effects of Mindfulness on the Brain in YouTube Videos

*Andrée E. C. Betancourt and Elise E. Labbé*

This chapter examines popular culture representations of the relationship between mindfulness and the brain through investigating short YouTube videos. In addition to providing analysis of specific YouTube videos, this chapter focuses on the ways in which YouTube users' comments about mindfulness videos provide insight on how online videos shape viewers' perceptions of the brain. A collaboration between a clinical health psychologist and a media studies scholar, this chapter offers fresh perspectives on mindfulness and the brain as well as provides an innovative model for transdisciplinary research. A discussion explaining what mindfulness is and a summary of recent research on the neuroscience of mindfulness is presented followed by a brief history of YouTube. We then provide both quantitative and qualitative data on the analyses of users' comments regarding the videos selected for this study.

## MINDFULNESS

Mindfulness is paying attention to the present moment with openness and curiosity.[1] Mindfulness can also refer to formal and informal practices. All formal practices involve meditation in various forms, from sitting to walking meditation. Informal practices are ones that help increase mindfulness in everyday activities such as eating mindfully or mindfully listening to someone speaking to you.

Mindfulness is a key component of Buddhism, although aspects of the concept can be seen in most varieties of religious and spiritual practices.[2] Mindfulness has recently become a hot topic in medicine and social sciences, and psychologists and neuroscientists have produced hundreds of studies on the effects of mindfulness and mindfulness meditation on all aspects of human functioning within the past decade.[3] In the process of this research, most researchers explore and define a secularized version of mindfulness.[4] Some researchers and practitioners of mindfulness have raised concerns about the different emerging definitions of mindfulness and believe that unless it is tied to its Buddhist roots, or at least an understanding of mindfulness within the context of Buddhism, it is not being understood and taught in its true nature. Therefore they warn that secularizing mindfulness may result in a less positive effect on human functioning.

Although mindfulness can refer to a way of being present in the moment, the term mindfulness can also be used in relation to meditation. Buddhist philosophy and psychology endorse the idea that to strengthen one's mindfulness, meditation practice is necessary. Within the meditation practices, there are many types of meditation styles that can be employed to enhance mindfulness. Some of these meditation practices involve concentration whereas with other practices the meditator does not focus on anything at all but "observes" his internal and external experiences including sensations, thoughts, and feelings. In concentration meditation the meditator focuses on a particular image, thought, bodily response, emotion, or an external object. One of the most commonly practiced meditations encourages the meditator to focus on the breath. The meditator focuses his attention on breathing in and breathing out. Eventually the mind begins to wander and the meditator attempts to notice the mind wandering and returns his attention back to the breath.

Owing to the efforts of several scholars and practitioners of mindfulness, including Jack Kornfield, Thich Nhat Hah, and Jon Kabat-Zinn, mindfulness and meditation have become popular in the West as a means of promoting physical and mental health.[5] Jon Kabat-Zinn created a program based on mindfulness that he called mindfulness-based stressed reduction (MBSR) to help people with chronic illness and pain cope more effectively with their symptoms.[6] Meta-analyses of the effectiveness of MBSR for a variety of physical and mental health problems support the conclusion that MBSR is an evidenced-based treatment for these problems.[7] Thus, mindfulness is becoming a "third wave" intervention in psychological interventions and is often integrated with first and second wave psychotherapy approaches, behavioral and cognitive therapies, respectively.

## NEUROSCIENCE AND MINDFULNESS

Significant technological advances have allowed neuroscientists the ability to explore how emotions, behaviors and cognitions can influence the structures of the brain as well as how neuronal systems become integrated or separated as a result of psychosocial experiences.[8] For example, Richard Davidson has used functional magnetic imaging (fMRI) to explore the effects of meditation on novice meditators compared to monks who devote their lives to the development of mindfulness through meditation.[9] In his studies he has found that through meditation training the neuronal pathways in the brain change. These new pathways have beneficial effects on your mind including better attentiveness while remaining relaxed and greater composure especially under stress.

The type of meditation a person uses may have different effects on brain structure as well as on emotional and cognitive functioning. For example, Lutz et al. studied the effects of a loving-kindness-compassion meditation in both novice and expert meditators.[10] They found that the limbic circuitry plays a role in emotion sharing. However, expert meditators compared to novice meditators demonstrated increased activation in the amygdala, the right temporo-parietal junction, and right posterior superior temporal sulcus during both meditations compared to rest in response to all sounds. These results suggested that experts were able to better detect emotional sounds, and enhanced mentation in response to emotional human vocalizations compared to novices during meditation. This research suggests the ability to cultivate positive emotions through meditation creates changes in the brain related to empathy and attention in response to emotional stimuli.

What is fascinating about these studies of the effects of meditation on the brain is that they clearly demonstrate that how we use our mind has a real and direct effect on brain structure and processing similar to medications that people consume to feel better. These studies support that there are many pathways to change, including practicing certain behaviors and ways of thinking about yourself and the world. We were interested in finding out if media is available to the general public to increase awareness of how meditation can affect one's mental, emotional and physical health.

## YOUTUBE: HISTORY, OBJECT OF STUDY, AND CURRENT STATUS

YouTube has come a long way from its official launch in June 2005, by founders Chad Hurley, Steve Chen, and Jawed Karim, as a service created to simplify the process of publishing, streaming, and sharing videos with the public. YouTube's "original innovation was a technological (but non-unique) one," and the company became a success story when Google acquired it for $1.65 billion in October 2006.[11] Tracing three myths about YouTube's mainstream popularity, Burgess and Green explain that these disparate narratives created three predominant ideas about what YouTube was: "another online fad, beloved by the tech crowd"; "a clever invention that people needed to be convinced to use"; "or a media distribution platform, kind of like television."[12] The initial "fog of uncertainty and contradiction around what [YouTube] is actually *for*" continues to be reflected in "the discomfort of" not only the general public but also corporate YouTube users.[13] Drawing on Jonathan Zittrain, Burgess and Green argue that "this uncertainty can also be interpreted as the source of YouTube's cultural 'generativity' which emerges from its multiple roles as a high-volume website, a broadcast platform, a media archive, and a social network."[14]

In outlining the challenges of studying YouTube, Kavoori asserts: "There is no reliable 'sample' of videos . . . no easily identifiable way to determine its dominant thematics; no way to evaluate 'quality'; no benchmarks for establishment of impact (beyond the questionable number of times a video has been watched), no seminal literature."[15] Like Burgess and Green, our approach involved treating YouTube in itself as an object of research, and like them we experienced YouTube as "a particularly unstable object of change marked by dynamic change (both in terms of videos and organization), a diversity of content (which moves with a different rhythm to television but likewise flows through, and often disappears from, the service), and a similar quotidian frequency, or 'everydayness.'"[16] Our study echoes Burgess and Green's assertion that "because there is not yet a shared understanding of YouTube's common culture, each scholarly approach to understanding how YouTube works must make choices among these interpretations, in effect recreating it as a different object of study each time—at this early stage in research, each study of YouTube gives a different understanding of what YouTube actually is."[17] Interested primarily in "how YouTube is structured and evolving as a media system in the economic and social context of broader media and technological change," Burgess and Green's book centers on participatory culture and, much grander in scope than our essay, surveys more than four thousand videos.[18] However, seeking to address "the missing middle between large-scale quantitative analysis and the sensitivity of qualitative methods" identified by Burgess and Green as problematic, we employed a method similar to theirs by conducting a close reading of media and cultural studies in combination with a survey of videos—though in our study the survey content was limited by specific search terms related to the relationship between mindfulness and the brain.[19]

Since Burgess and Green's 2009 study, YouTube has continued to gain popularity and the attention of academic researchers as well as the media. Explaining that "participation in YouTube can be highly seductive," Strangelove, referencing Seyward Darby, asserts that those who argue that "YouTube is more of an entertainment site than a venue for dialogue . . . overlook the high volume of conversation that takes place there."[20] In a 2011 cyberethnographic field study of the Banjo Hangout online music community of practice, Janice Waldron found that YouTube videos serve a dual purpose as "useful straightforward music teaching and learning aids" and "as vehicles of agency to promote and engage participatory culture through discourse in online community, thus also fulfilling a significant teaching role, albeit in a more nuanced manner then as a direct but informal music learning resource."[21] There are more than a billion YouTube users per month, and as announced on May 19, 2013, YouTube's eighth birthday, "100 hours of video are uploaded per minute."[22] According to Barclays its total value is between $15.6 billion and $21.23 billion, which "at the high end would make YouTube a third as valuable as Facebook."[23] Considering the growth and influence of YouTube, we turned to it for answers about popular conceptions of mindfulness, a practice that has also recently attracted numerous individuals and organizations. We are particularly interested in analyzing YouTube videos that focus on the effects of mindfulness on the function and structure of the brain.

## YOUTUBE RESEARCH IN PSYCHOLOGY

There has been increasing interest in studying the effectiveness of video for changing behavior and increasing the ability to learn new information and skills.[24] For example, Sacco and Bernstein evaluated the effectiveness of a video about psychological research on increasing psychology students' interest in participating in research studies as well as increasing their interest in research.[25] They showed the video in two of the introduction to psychology courses and did not show it to the two other introduction to psychology courses. They found that students viewing the video reported increased interest in research and completed more research participation hours compared to the students who did not view the videos. Sacco and Bernstein clearly showed that viewing a video changed participants' behavior and attitudes. An advantage of this type of study is that the researchers could randomly assign who saw the videos and evaluate for specific behavior and attitude change.

In studying the effects of YouTube videos on behavior and attitude change, it becomes more challenging to do quantitative research in the naturalistic setting of anyone who has access to YouTube and to evaluate the effects of what they are watching on behavior and attitude changes. First, one has to determine what types of videos are available on YouTube, how often they are accessed, and whether viewers can respond in some type of manner to what they viewed. In the current study we took a qualitative approach to determine what types of videos on the subject of mindfulness and the brain are available for viewers to watch and what kinds of responses they could make.

## OBJECTIVES AND HYPOTHESES

Our first objective was to search for YouTube videos that focus on the effects of meditation on the brain and to analyze the types of videos available and the content. A second objective was to determine whether viewers' comments provided insight on how the online videos shaped their perceptions of the brain. The first hypothesis was that most comments by viewers would be positive. The second hypothesis was that there would be comments regarding viewers' experience using meditation. In the following section, we describe how we created our data sample.

## METHOD

### Search Criteria

In identifying relevant YouTube videos, we used the search terms "mindfulness," "brain," "meditation," and "effect," after experimenting with numerous other combinations of terms, and we included videos with one or more terms in the title. The optional filters within the YouTube search feature that were applied to the data sample included (1) Upload date: This year; (2) Result type: Video; (3) Duration: Short (about 4 minutes); and (4) Sort by: Relevance. We did not apply the Features filter, an option that limits results based on the features: HD (high definition); CC (closed caption); Creative commons; 3D; Live; and Purchased. Many of the videos in our initial search were incorrectly tagged; in many cases the inaccurate association with the hot topic of mindfulness appeared intentional as an effort to attract viewers. Burgess and Green emphasize the naiveté of accepting user-assigned tags, titles, and descriptions as factual, and note that "misuses of tags may well turn out to be more interesting than their proper uses."[26]

Some of the YouTube videos do not allow comments. Because this study evaluated the comments made by observers of the videos we excluded from the (1) sample videos that had disabled comments; (2) videos in languages other than English; (3) videos that were clearly incorrectly tagged; (4) comments that had been flagged as spam; and (5) comments that had been temporarily or permanently removed. After reviewing more than seventy-nine YouTube videos that met the search criteria outlined above, we were left with a data set of twenty-three videos that can be accessed by opening the YouTube playlist links listed in Table 12.1.

## Results

There were a total of 6,841 views of the 23 videos we reviewed, with a mean of 297 views, and a range of views per video from 13 to 3,205. One challenge of researching YouTube videos is that our own views become added to the view count; also, view count numbers can be easily artificially inflated. The videos ranged in duration from thirty-one seconds to three minutes and fifty-two seconds. Table 12.1 features a summary of data on the twenty-three videos in our final sample including: video links; titles; channel; video duration; date uploaded; number of user comments, likes, and dislikes; and number of views. For all twenty-three videos, there were a total of twenty-five comments, with only five videos having user comments. Of these five videos, three had one comment each, one video had six comments, and one video had sixteen comments (eight comments were responses to the other eight viewer comments). The majority of the comments were positive; one featured a grammatical correction. Only one of the comments specifically mentioned the brain. Examples of the comments include BigAlx's "SWEET!!!," which was the sole comment on the "Mindfulness—how it effects the brain" video; Edsky's "just the qoute by thich nhat hanh said it all. your comparsion said some but less" was one of six comments (and the only negative one) on the "2013—Meditation—Drunk on Energy?" video; EnthusiasticBuddhist's "This is so wonderful! Thank you for bringing together meditation and social action to make a better world! Great animation too—definitely brings home the point! Sharing this now:)" was

Table 12.1 Summary of YouTube Video Data in Sample

| ID | Link to YouTube video | Title | Channel | Video duration (minutes: seconds) | User comments, likes, or dislikes[a] | Upload date | Views |
|---|---|---|---|---|---|---|---|
| 1 | http://www.youtube.com/watch?v=UBpJP_vQU5o | Mindfulness—how it effects the brain | MyFrikkinOpinion | 3:15 | 1 Comment 1 Like | 4/9/2013 | 262 |
| 2 | http://www.youtube.com/watch?v=j7zj2_nea5o | Mindfulness and the Brain—Going Beyond the Mind | Ruth Buczynski | 3:04 | 5 Likes | 11/9/2012 | 3,205 |
| 3 | http://www.youtube.com/watch?v=qFNpfuF1m-Y | About Meditation Effects of Meditation and Mindfulness Training | NaturalMindSolutions | 1:49 | n/a | 6/11/2013 | 24 |
| 4 | http://www.youtube.com/watch?v=5XEUzNRwBZU | Introduction to Mindfulness Meditation | TheGardenofNOW | 3:50 | n/a | 1/18/2013 | 211 |
| 5 | http://www.youtube.com/watch?v=TsxX25EVojU | Mindfulness—Doko talks about our brain's bias towards negativity | Mudita Institute | 2:40 | n/a | 12/13/12 | 241 |
| 6 | http://www.youtube.com/watch?v=4flLfN9jtTM | Mindfulness-Based Stress Reduction in Mind-Body Medicine | G Ross Clark | 1:22 | n/a | 4/4/2013 | 32 |
| 7 | http://www.youtube.com/watch?v=hfqKHOXOY4k | Why Meditate Benefits of Meditation Explained | NaturalMindSolutions | 1:21 | n/a | 7/11/2013 | 19 |

(Continued)

*Table 12.1* (Continued)

| ID | Link to YouTube video | Title | Channel | Video duration (minutes: seconds) | User comments, likes, or dislikes[a] | Upload date | Views |
|---|---|---|---|---|---|---|---|
| 8 | http://www.youtube.com/watch?v=wKEbykuMOFY | Music, Art, and Your Brain | S'eclairer | 2:15 | n/a | 4/22/2013 | 27 |
| 9 | http://www.youtube.com/watch?v=XJcBSXsoh5g | Guided Health Meditation | Yufang Lee | 3:03 | n/a | 10/22/2012 | 55 |
| 10 | http://www.youtube.com/watch?v=XkuGaNNzmt4 | October 2009 Dan Siegel and Pat Ogden | LifespanLearning LA | 2:05 | n/a | 8/21/2013 | 112 |
| 11 | http://www.youtube.com/watch?v=29Li_nMC0NQ | Alpha Theta Meditation with Neurofeedback | yourbraintraining | 3:19 | 1 Like | 7/17/2013 | 110 |
| 12 | http://www.youtube.com/watch?v=YgVs399yKVY | 2013—Meditation—Drunk on Energy? | Matti Freeman | 2:20 | 6 Comments 40 Likes 1 Dislike | 1/14/2013 | 596 |
| 13 | http://www.youtube.com/watch?v=nc5uS3-0d6Q | Meditation Health Benefits | informationwarfare | 1:16 | 1 Comment (not visible) 3 Likes | 10/16/2012 | 89 |
| 14 | http://www.youtube.com/watch?v=4BEuN-tZP9g | Has the course changed your ideas about Meditation? | OnlineMeditation | 2:40 | 1 Comment 1 Like 1 Dislike | 1/16/2013 | 68 |
| 15 | http://www.youtube.com/watch?v=OUD3Tv05b04 | What a Simple Meditation can do to your Life | Plainly Simple Studios | 2:30 | 16 Comments (8 are uploader comments that respond to the other 8 viewer comments) 22 Likes | 4/15/2013 | 789 |

| # | URL | Title | Channel | Duration | Comments/Likes[a] | Date | Views |
|---|---|---|---|---|---|---|---|
| 16 | http://www.youtube.com/watch?v=0wKNrnOgSg8 | How could MBSR have an effect on my life? | dukeintegrative | 1:15 | n/a | 2/5/2013 | 116 |
| 17 | http://www.youtube.com/watch?v=Z73rByDMOEw | Benefits From Meditation | MeditationMindSource | 3:52 | n/a | 7/8/2013 | 31 |
| 18 | http://www.youtube.com/watch?v=pFY_nqLpUrw | Mindfulness & Attention Deficit Disorder | NourFoundation | 1:56 | 8 Likes | 2/25/2013 | 663 |
| 19 | http://www.youtube.com/watch?v=3f5So9Xdi-M | Mediated meditation | TheOfficialACM | 0:31 | n/a | 6/7/2013 | 13 |
| 20 | http://www.youtube.com/watch?v=i_yDSItJ31I | How to Meditate—Preparation, About Meditation | NaturalMindSolutions | 1:56 | n/a | 6/11/3013 | 13 |
| 21 | http://www.youtube.com/watch?v=ctj1AAKvEP4 | NY Insight Meditation—Feeling about coming to the center | New York Insight | 1:34 | n/a | 10/23/2012 | 21 |
| 22 | http://www.youtube.com/watch?v=0fLUEDZAMIM | Binaural Beats Meditation (BBM)—Deep Meditation | BBMeditation | 2:01 | n/a | 10/6/2012 | 24 |
| 23 | http://www.youtube.com/watch?v=dCJrJRgum9U | Has MBSR been helpful to you? | dukeintegrative | 0:37 | n/a | 2/5/2013 | 120 |

*Note:* Approximately 196,000 results for "mindfulness" and approximately 16,600 results for "mindfulness brain meditation effect." Added filters: video, 852 results; short, 305 results (long was 155); this year, 79 results (long was 76); sorted by relevance. Twenty-three videos met the final criteria. The twenty-three videos are featured in the YouTube playlist: http://www.youtube.com/playlist?list=PLNS62gc_EdG5VvISG6oCG9ZP0IGSwovbh. Results from 9/15/2013 search.

[a]Value of zero unless otherwise noted; n/a indicates no comments, likes, or dislikes.

one of six viewer comments on the "What a Simple Meditation can do to your Life" video.[27]

For all twenty-three videos, there were eighty-one Likes. Eight of the twenty-three videos had Likes: three videos had one Like, one video had three Likes, one video had five Likes, one video had eight Likes, one had twenty-two Likes, and one had forty Likes. Dislikes were found for only two videos, each of which had one Dislike. The "2013—Meditation—Drunk on Energy?" video that appears on Matti Freeman's channel received one of the Dislikes; the About section features a link to Freeman's related blog post, which reveals his membership in the Destini Research Group, a group considered by many to be a dangerous cult—an identity the group contests on its homepage. Given the tactics associated with the group, we might question if the five positive comments on Freeman's video are genuine or if they were added by fellow Destonians primarily in an effort to spread the group's philosophy.

All of the videos appeared on different channels except for three that were featured on NaturalMindSolutions's channel, and two that were featured on dukeintegrative's channel. The majority of the videos appear to be created primarily for marketing purposes by individuals, corporations, or nonprofit organizations. Many aim to educate the viewer, and contact information for those interested in more information or products is usually featured in the videos, in the About section that accompanies the video, or in both locations. The majority of the videos appear to be created by the individual or group behind the channel. MyFrikkinOpinion's "Mindfulness—how it effects the brain" video, however, is a recording of a television screen featuring a *Daily Planet* story on mindfulness meditation. In the About section she asserts: "Mindfulness meditation and the science showing why it works . . . Everyone needs to learn this, it's the only way to overcome life's stresses. This is legitimately how I ended my depression! It works! And it keeps working! You rewire your brain to choose its reaction."

We were surprised, and admittedly disappointed, that there were so few comments on the videos, and that the majority of the comments did not explicitly address the relationship between the brain and mindfulness meditation. It was interesting to discover that by delving deeper into media related to the channels, it became evident that despite the lack of comments on the YouTube videos the site remains an important resource for those seeking to learn more about mindfulness. For example, an article online in the "Teachers Blog" section of the *Guardian* about Mind Space, the U.K.-based organization behind the channel OnlineMeditation, is followed by two comments.[28] L. L. Turner, the author of one of the comments, explains: "I myself am a professional writer and illustrator who after many months of CD's, books, workshops and youtube videos found that it is NOT about DOING . . . it's about NOT doing. . . ."[29] A flyer for the Mindful Chocolate Eating Workshop that is featured on the Mind Space homepage promotes the event by noting that "major companies like Google, Facebook, Deutsche Bank are now offering Mindfulness and Meditation to their employees with great results."[30] Considering that Google owns YouTube, it is interesting to find these circular references between the videos and channel-related media that extend beyond the YouTube website.

## DISCUSSION

### Implications for Future Research

Our findings suggest that there are indeed some YouTube videos that present empirically based information on how the brain is changed through meditation and how these changes can be beneficial to both physical and mental health. The next step in researching this topic would be to take a quantitative approach to find evidence that viewing these videos affects behavior and cognitive changes. Based on our findings it would be useful to propose a study that elicited potential viewers to watch a selection of empirically based videos on the topic of mindfulness and the brain. Using an online survey, one could then determine if the videos affect viewers' understanding of how the brain changes through meditation and whether they would be willing to practice meditation after seeing the videos. A software system could be used to integrate the videos and survey which could then be accessed through a variety of social media.

Taking a step in a different direction, a step that could perhaps be taken in collaboration with the research described above, an ethnography of a mindfulness-oriented YouTube community could yield fascinating results. Referencing Patricia Lange's two-year ethnography with the YouTube community, Burgess and Green note that "her work insistently reminds us of the need to consider fully the lived experience and materiality of everyday cultural practice," and they explain that the importance of Lange's work is that "it asks us to think about the *uses* of YouTube by real people as part of everyday life and as part of the mix of media we all use as part of our lives, rather than thinking about YouTube as if it is a weightless depository of content."[31] Through our focus on user comments, we hoped to gain more insight into the role YouTube plays in everyday practices of mindfulness ranging from novices seeking an introduction to experienced practitioners desiring to strengthen their practice; however, since comments were so few and relatively unsubstantial, an ethnographic approach would potentially better address these challenges.

Considering YouTube's recent emphasis on channels versus individual videos, an ethnography could also consider how channel subscribers function as subcommunities. Janice Waldron's cyberethnographic field study of the Banjo Hangout online music community of practice provides a model that could be used for researching the integration of on-and offline mindfulness communities.[32] YouTube continues to grow and make national headlines, most recently for "An Interpretive Dance For My Boss Set To Kanye West's Gone," a viral video created by and starring Marina Shifrin. Through text captions, Shifrin explains why she quit her job in the video, and her creative effort led Queen Latifah to offer her a job on *The Queen Latifah Show*.[33] As mindfulness meditation practice also grows, and new discoveries are made about its relationship with the brain, it is important to continue examining how this knowledge is shared and understood in popular culture contexts including YouTube and beyond.

Further research is needed to explore the possibilities of sharing empirically based videos through distribution platforms such as YouTube. We found that the overwhelming prevalence of commercial and other promotional appeals on YouTube made it more difficult to find empirically based videos about mindfulness and the brain. Recent backlash over YouTube changes implemented after we completed our study, such as requiring users to comment on videos through the Google identity platform, further problematizes possibilities for more democratic communication on the site.[34] It is arguably now more challenging to comment anonymously on YouTube videos, and the impact of comments being marked by Google+ identities will need to be considered in future studies. According to Strangelove, "a single video on YouTube can engender over 500,000 comments and more than 2.5 million words."[35] The association of users' Google+ identities with their comments may result in users commenting less or not at all; users may also restrict the visibility of their comments. It could also lead to more accountability for one's comments and ideally to more generative exchanges and even greater communitas. Helft and Mansour highlight YouTube's investment in jumpstarting original channels ("more than 130 channels and a reported $200 million in total funding") as well as changes it made to the user interface in order to put channels, rather than individual videos, "front and center."[36] It remains to be seen if this shift to channels will promote or hinder public dialogue on YouTube.

Suggesting that we view YouTube as "much more than a website," Kavoori asserts that "it is a key element in the way we think about our on-line experience and (shared) digital culture."[37] Although "videos create words, engender dialogue, and foster interpersonal relations," Strangelove cautiously reminds us that "the outcome of this age of the image remains uncertain."[38] As other sites and forms of social media challenge YouTube's dominance and reach, we are hopeful they will increase public communication among researchers and practitioners of mindfulness. TED is an example of a nonprofit organization that features videos about mindfulness, among many other topics, on its official website as well as on its YouTube channel. As individuals and other organizations with the resources to do so follow this model, new and overlapping spaces for public dialogue about mindfulness and its effects on the brain will develop.

# NOTES

1. Jon Kabat-Zinn, *Full Catastrophe Living: Using the Wisdom of Your Body and Mind to Face Stress, Pain, and Illness* (New York: Delacorte Press, 1990); Elise E. Labbé, *Psychology Moment by Moment: A Guide to Enhancing Your Clinical Practice with Mindfulness and Meditation* (Oakland, CA: New Harbinger, 2011).
2. Daniel Goleman, *The Varieties of the Meditative Experience* (New York: Irvington, 1977).
3. Benjamin D. Hill and Elise E. Labbé, "Measuring Mindfulness," in *Psychology of Meditation*, ed. Nirbhay N. Singh (New York: Nova Science, 2013), 11–28; Labbé, *Psychology Moment by Moment*.
4. Elise E. Labbé, Melissa Womble, and Jessica Shenesey, "Evaluating the Relationship between Mindfulness and Resilience," in *Handbook on Spirituality: Belief Systems, Societal Impact and Roles in Coping*, ed. Cleveland A. Stark and Dylan C. Bonner, 303–12 (New York: Nova Science, 2011).
5. Labbé, *Psychology Moment by Moment*.
6. Jean Kristeller and Lobsang Rapgay, "Buddhism: A Blend of Religion, Spirituality, and Psychology," in *APA Handbook of Psychology, Religion and Spirituality: Vol. 1, Context, Theory, and Research*, ed. Kenneth I. Pargament, 635–52 (Washington, DC: American Psychological Association, 2013).
7. Labbé, *Psychology Moment by Moment*.
8. James McAbee, Elise E. Labbé, and Kelley Drayer, "Mindfulness-Based Interventions: Evaluating the Biopsychosocial Effects for Patients with Cancer," in *Psychology of Mindfulness*, ed. K. Murata-Soraci (New York: Nova Science, 2013), 87–105.
9. Richard J. Davidson and Sharon Begley, *The Emotional Life of Your Brain* (New York: Plume, 2012).
10. Antoine Lutz, Julie Brefczynski-Lewis, Tom Johnstone, and Richard J. Davidson, "Regulation of the Neural Circuitry of Emotion by Compassion Meditation: Effects of Meditative Expertise," *PLoS ONE* 3, no. 3 (2008): 1–10, doi:10.1371/journal.pone.0001897.
11. Jean Burgess and Joshua Green, *YouTube: Online Video and Participatory Culture* (Boston: Polity Press, 2009), 1.
12. Ibid., 3.
13. Ibid., 3, 5.
14. Ibid., 5.
15. Anandam Kavoori, *Reading YouTube: The Critical Viewers' Guide* (New York: Peter Lang, 2011), 1.
16. Burgess and Green, *YouTube*, 6.
17. Ibid., 6–7.
18. Ibid., 9.
19. Ibid.
20. Michael Strangelove, *Watching YouTube: Extraordinary Videos by Ordinary People* (Toronto: University of Toronto Press, 2010), 47.
21. Janice Waldron, "Locating Narratives in Postmodern Spaces: A Cyber Ethnographic Field Study of Informal Music Learning in Online Community," *Action, Criticism, and Theory for Music Education* 10, no. 2 (2011): 31–60, http://act.maydaygroup.org/articles/Waldron10_2.pdf.
22. Miguel Helft and Iris Mansour, "How YouTube Changes Everything," *Fortune* 168, no. 3 (2013): 52–59.
23. Ibid.
24. Beverly A. Bondad-Brown, Ronald E. Rice, and Katy E. Pearce, "Influences on TV Viewing and Online User-Shared Video Use: Demographics, Generations,

Contextual Age, Media Use, Motivations and Audience Activity," *Journal of Broadcasting and Electronic Media* 56, no. 4 (2012): 471–93, doi:10.1080/08838151.2012.732139.
25. Donald F. Sacco and Michael J. Bernstein, "A Video Introduction to Psychology: Enhancing Research Interest and Participation," *Teaching of Psychology* 37, no. 1 (2010): 28–31, doi:10.1080/00986280903425995.
26. Burgess and Green, *YouTube*, 8.
27. Comments and user names are quoted from YouTube directly without any correction made to spelling or grammar.
28. Liese Stanley, "Teaching Meditation at School," *Teacher's Blog* (blog), *The Guardian*, November 10, 2011, http://www.theguardian.com/teacher-network/2011/nov/10/teaching-meditation-at-school.
29. L. L. Turner, comment on Stanley, "Teaching Meditation."
30. "The Mindful Chocolate Eating Workshop at Warwick University," *Mind Space*, October 2013, http://www.mindspace.org.uk/2013/10/the-mindful-chocolate-eating-workshop-atwarwick-university/.
31. Burgess and Green, *YouTube*, 8–9.
32. Waldron, "Locating Narratives."
33. Lesley Savage, "Kanye West and YouTube Help Woman Very Publicly Quit Job," *CBS News*, October 1, 2013, http://www.cbsnews.com/8301-504784_162-57605459-10391705/kanye-west-and-youtube-help-woman-very-publicly-quit-job/.
34. Alex Hern, "YouTube Co-founder Hurls Abuse at Google over New YouTube Comments," *The Guardian*, November 8, 2013, http://www.theguardian.com/technology/2013/nov/08/youtube-cofounder-why-the-fuck-do-i-need-a-google-account-to-comment.
35. Strangelove, *Watching YouTube*, 193.
36. Helft and Mansour, "How YouTube Changes."
37. Kavoori, *Reading YouTube*, 3.
38. Strangelove, *Watching YouTube*, 193.

# 13 Selling the Brain
## Representation of Neuroscience in Advertising

*Celia Andreu-Sánchez and Miguel Ángel Martín-Pascual*

## NEUROSCIENCE IN THE MEDIA

That neuroscience is constantly present in the media is a reality today. And it is understandable. In recent decades, neuroscientific knowledge has advanced as it has never done before. Over the past few years, the number of scientific articles related to neuroscience published in the most prestigious scientific journals has increased significantly. If we conduct a search of the topic "neuroscience" in Thomson Reuters's database Web of Knowledge, we find that in the early 1990s, 1,149 neuroscientific articles were published, whereas in the first decade of the century, 2,916 were published (more than double); in turn, between 2011 and 2013 (up to July 10), more items were published than in the entire decade of the 1990s: 1,188 (Figure 13.1).

In addition, some of the knowledge generated in the scientific field is being transmitted with greater ease by the media to non-expert audiences as popular science. Sometimes, however, we encounter a problem: the journalist does not understand (or believes that the public will not) what has been discovered, what has been learned about the brain, and simplifies the content of disclosure, turning it into controversy in order to sell more.[1] As a result, the audience receives mistaken information.

Several researchers in Quebec, Stanford, and Vancouver[2] have carried out some interesting research on how contemporary neuroscience is depicted in print media. Since recent technological innovations in neuroscience have opened new windows to the understanding of the brain, researchers study how public interest and support for neuroscientific research have increased in recent years. Their research involves the analysis of newspaper articles in the United States and the United Kingdom between 1995 and 2004 to find patterns of use and citations of neuroscience in print media. Once they identified 1,256 articles about neurotechnology, they started working with this sample divided into 335 articles related to positron emission tomography (PET) and/or single-photon emission computed tomography (SPECT), 284 articles on electroencephalography (EEG), 235 on neurostimulation techniques, 223 on functional magnetic resonance imaging (fMRI), and 179 on neurogenetics. Some of the most important conclusions reached in this

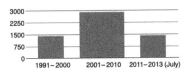

*Figure 13.1*  Neuroscientific Papers Published in Most Prestigious Scientific Journals, 1991–2013 (*source*: compiled from Thompson Reuters)

study are that the majority (68 percent) of published articles on neuroscience in print media had one clinical or non-clinical benefit for the population, and only 28 percent of them discussed a delicate scientific or ethical issue. Except for the articles on neurostimulation, the rest did not provide explanations of neuroscience technology. Most of the items were optimistic or neutral, with few critical items, in the area of neurogenetics. Among the articles related to the results of scientific research, many did not provide important data for specification of the number of subjects or funding sources. In short, the authors argue, among other ideas, that reports on neuroscience in the media are so lax and scarcely critical that they serve as a basis for activities and business practices. And this is what happens with the direct-to-consumer advertising (DTCA). The DTCA is used quite frequently in the drug market in the United States by offering pharmaceutical products to the user based on the increase of their technical knowledge of science. Therefore, audience's learning of a particular scientific progress can be used, as explained by Zuckerman,[3] for commercial purposes. And the mass media help it, providing coverage of medical records in response to pharmaceutical and economic interests.

In the 2011 edition of the *International Behavioral Neuroscience Society (IBNS) Annual Meeting*, scientific journalists were invited to give a talk about how the media disseminate scientific knowledge.[4] Science journalist Mariette DiChristina, eighth editor-in-chief of *Scientific American*, participated in the meeting. DiChristina confirmed the increased consumption of information related to scientific knowledge in recent years and the general positive attitude toward it. However, the lack of understanding of scientific results, she said, is also very high. The renowned science writer Sandra Blakeslee also gave a presentation at that meeting titled "Journalists Are from Venus, Scientists Are from Mars." Blakeslee advised that scientific content writing in general newspapers should be done in a more casual manner that is more understandable to non-specialist readers.[5] Somehow, the situation is this: scientists are accurate in their content and believe that non-specialist readers do not understand the scientific progress that is being made. Conversely, journalists make this scientific progress understandable at a price: the loss of specific details. Headlines sell.

Another issue that was addressed in the *IBNS Annual Meeting 2011* was the change that has occurred in the world of science journalism since the emergence of bloggers. Scientific blogs are experiencing great success, as Paul Raeburn, journalist, broadcaster and author, recounted. Raeburn explained that blogs and online news sites are changing the nature of science. According to him, behavioral neuroscientists are not immune to criticism and public challenges and, therefore, Raeburn advises them to pay special attention to what the public sphere debates.[6]

## NEUROSCIENCE CREDIBILITY

At the same time, we know that neuroscience brings credibility. Recently, the prestigious journal *Neuron* published a study on how neuroscience is seen in the public sphere.[7] O'Connor, Rees, and Joffe have developed the idea, already raised previously by several authors,[8] of how credibility is linked to neuroscience. They note that brain-based information possesses rhetorical power, so that irrelevant neuroscience information is used as an argument with authoritative and scientific credibility for a non-specialist audience.

McCabe and Castel[9] conducted some interesting research on the effect that brain images have on judgment and veracity of content. Based on the idea that brain images are persuasive to the general understanding of neuroscience research, they conducted different experiments in which neuroscientific results were accompanied by bar graphs and by brain images. The result is that subjects believe that articles presenting brain images accompanying the text are superior in scientific argumentation, compared to articles with simple bar charts. In agreement with the authors, we can say that part of the fascination and credibility that is being given to neuroscientific knowledge today lies in the power of persuasion that brain images have on the public. This is crucial because, if it is proven that the same message is more credible and better valued if it is accompanied by a brain image, advertising, as discussed below, uses this fact to make more believable and, supposedly, more scientifically supported messages.

In the same vein, several researchers from Yale University[10] have studied the seductive allure of neuroscience explanations. Authors presented explanations of psychological phenomena accompanied with neuroscience or a lack of it, to skilled and unskilled subjects in neuroscientific knowledge. It turned out that non-experts judged that explanations with logically irrelevant neuroscientific information were more satisfying than those explanations without neuroscience. Thus, the researchers conclude that explanations of psychological phenomena generate more interest and credibility when they contain neuroscientific data.

As mentioned, *Neuron* has published a research on how neuroscience is seen by the public. O'Connor's team conducted an analysis of neuroscientific research articles between 2000 and 2010.[11] The sample of 2,931 articles selected was confined to six national newspapers in the United Kingdom: *Daily Telegraph, Times, Daily Mail, Sun, Mirror*, and *The Guardian*.

According to their research, they found three major themes of neuroscience representation in the media: "the brain as capital, i.e., a resource to be optimized; the brain as an index of difference, using neuroscience to delineate boundaries between categories of people; and brain research as biological proof of the legitimacy of particular phenomena or beliefs."[12] The research concludes that during the first decade of the twenty-first century, the media coverage of neuroscience research has been intensified and has been applied to a wide variety of topics. Neuroscience has been incorporated into the everyday repertoire of topics in the media. And, as neuroscience has been assimilated into the cultural register, it has been appropriated by a society structured by diverse interests.[13] Also, in recent years, many popular science TV shows have devoted significant resources to reflecting how neuroscience research advances. And the fact is that people are interested in science. When European Union citizens are asked what news-related issues interest them, scientific research is mentioned by 31 percent, and whereas 57 percent of European Union citizens are interested in scientific research, 93 percent of them use the media for information on science.[14]

So, the media and science are very connected. Hence the fact that there are now many journalists who write books with scientists, like Sandra Blakeslee, mentioned earlier, who has published books with neuroscientists. Such is the case of *Phantoms in the Brain*, written with Vilayanur S. Ramachandran, or *On Intelligence*, written with Jeff Hawkins. However, in recent years, most of the best popular books on science are not created by journalists who translate scientific knowledge to readers, but are written directly by scientists.[15] This fact is the result of the popularization of science (and neuroscience) in the media. In this way, neuroscientists Oliver Sacks, Antonio Damasio and David Eagleman, among many others, show the most informative character of neuroscience. Their books reveal to the masses the more dramatic knowledge (though not necessarily relevant) obtained in recent years.

Oliver Sacks has several publications that have been important for the dissemination and understanding of neuroscience for the non-expert audience, among them *The Man Who Mistook His Wife for a Hat* (1985). The book, which includes a cluster of curious cognitive deficit medical cases, far from becoming a work to share medical knowledge among colleagues, is already a classic neuroscientific disclosure. It is common to find this book on neurological disparities that occurred in anonymous patients in unspecialized bookstores such as in airports and train stations. Neurological disorders are explained with an air of popular science, avoiding the complex knowledge of researchers and specialists. Antonio Damasio, in his book *Descartes' Error*, published in 1994, shows the somatic marker hypothesis as a mechanism that rules the emotions in decision making. This work has been postulated as a modern work of popular science. Following this publication, the *New York Times* called him one of the world's leading neurologists. David Eagleman is a current example of a neuroscientist who is dedicated to the dissemination of neuroscience and succeeds. In 2012 the author published the book *Incognito: The Secret Lives of the Brain*. On his website, Eagleman is described as a neuroscientist and a *New York Times* bestselling author. With him, popular science is assured: his Facebook fan page has more than 40,300 followers, and his Twitter account has more than 16,500.

With this background, we can understand that the public has access to a fairly high knowledge (compared to decades ago) of neuroscience. In this context, advertising is no stranger to this new situation, and it uses what we know about the brain to encourage and convince customers to buy their products.

## REPRESENTATION OF NEUROSCIENCE IN ADVERTISING

At present, advertising is very accustomed to making use of neuroscience and the perception of it to sell products. In general, the representation of neuroscience in advertising lends credibility to the brand and the advertised product. Advertisers tend to use images of brains with two aims: to appeal to clients' reason, inviting them to make use of it to purchase the product, or to appeal to their emotions, because we know that these are not in the heart.

Today, we find that several trends exist in this regard. We highlight some in the following.

### The Brain as Synonymous with Creativity

In many cases, creativity is represented through brains. Many advertising agencies and advertising schools promote themselves using brain images as proof of their creativity. It is easy to find examples of advertising and communication agencies and schools that make use of an image of a brain to demonstrate and defend their creativity. An example of this is the original release made by the Drive Communication advertising agency, in which a jump rope creates the shape of a brain.[16] The slogan says "Keep your brand in shape," and then the advertising agency's contact details are displayed. This is a clear use of the image of the brain linked to creativity for the sale of an advertising and communication agency. At the same time, there is wordplay between "brand" and "brain."

Very similar examples may be found in art, advertising, and communication schools. An example is the project Wherecreativitygoestoschool. com, owned by the Canadian strategic marketing company Big Clic Inc.[17] The website provides an interesting test of creativity with the image of two brains. The test appears once you are in the respective websites of art centers such as the Art Institute of Vancouver or the Art Institute of Pittsburgh, among others, in which creativity is a highly valued skill. Another example can be found in the College for Creative Studies in Detroit.[18] They created a campaign with a fried egg in a frying pan. The fried egg yolk creates the face of the well-known painting *The Scream*, by the Norwegian painter Edvard Munch. The text accompanying the image says, "This is your brain on art" and "Talk to your kids about art school: College for Creative Studies." Again, creativity and brain concepts are linked to the sale of a product: an art school. Following this same line, it is also worth mentioning the Brother Creative School, based in Barcelona, Bogota, Buenos Aires, Caracas, Mexico, Montevideo, Santiago, and Santo Domingo.[19] The school conducts a campaign to promote itself using a drawing in which a doll's brain is used as a parachute. The slogan is a quote from Frank Zappa: "A mind is like a parachute. It doesn't work if it is not open."

We should note that creativity is directly linked to the brain in neuroscience research. An example of this is the Brain and Creativity Institute at the University of Southern California. This institute was established by neuroscientists Antonio Damasio and Hanna Damasio and currently has more than fifty researchers working to find the neurological basis for mental functions such as emotion, decision making, and creativity expressed in the arts, sciences, and technology.

## Brain Hemisphere Specialization

Another trend widely used in advertising is abusing the theory of hemispheric specialization of the brain to give the message that both reason and emotion are represented in a product. A good example is the Mercedes Benz campaign of 2012, in which a brain divided into both hemispheres appears.[20] The left side, beige with thin black lines, shows the following: "Left brain. I am the left brain. I am a scientist. A mathematician. I love the familiar. I categorize. I am accurate. Linear. Analytical. Strategic. I am practical. Always in control. A master of words and language. Realistic. I calculate equations and play with numbers. I am order. I am logic. I know exactly who I am." In the right hemisphere, colored with red, pink, orange, green, and blue, the text says: "Right brain. I am the right brain. I am creativity. A free spirit. I am passion. Yearning. Sensuality. I am the sound of roaring laughter. I am taste. The feeling of sand beneath bare feet. I am movement. Vivid colors. I am the urge to paint on an empty canvas. I am boundless imagination. Art. Poetry. I sense. I feel. I am everything I wanted to be." In this case, the advertiser, Mercedes Benz, has used simplifying knowledge of brain specialization to appeal to both reason and emotion, to convince the buyer that both of them are in its product: a car. The brand introduced this idea back in 2006 with another campaign that included a commercial with the slogan, "Beauty is nothing without brains," in which it appealed again to beauty and intelligence.[21] In 2011, Mercedes Benz launched another campaign with two images of the scientist Albert Einstein. In one picture, Einstein seems serious, and the text says "Left Brain." In the other picture, he is smiling with his tongue out; the text says "Right Brain."[22] It would appear that the 2012 campaign is following the same line.

Another example is Brock University in Canada. The university has had for years a campaign with the slogan "For Both Sides of the Brain." This campaign emphasizes their dedication to develop both the personal and the academic sides of students' brains.[23]

## The Brain as Reason

In addition, the brain is used in advertising as a synonym for logical reasoning or authority within the discourse. It appears as biological proof. There are many cases in which, as mentioned, advertising appeals to reason by showing a brain between their images or texts. For example, we find the campaign Pango Mobile Parking, an application that manages payment of parking through a mobile phone.[24] In the campaign that launches Pango, the main image is a brain parked on a street, as if it were a car. The ad asks the consumer to use reason and use this service. The image of a brain parked using the product represents that reason.

Another example is the campaign for Colgate dental floss with the slogan "So you can think of something else."[25] For this campaign, Colgate used the image of a white brain with its fissures as clean as if the brand's dental floss had passed between them. Somehow, Colgate tells us to use our head, be practical, and use its dental floss, as the ad's brain does. A similar idea can be found in the following example. In 2007, Coke Zero launched a funny commercial in which a tongue, an eye, and a brain talk about the product.[26] The narrative is as follows: the eye talks to the tongue saying that what is in front (a glass bottle of Coke Zero) is not Coke, it is something else, and the tongue tastes it and argues that, therefore, it is Coke. In this discussion, the brain enters the scene, with a deeper voice placing an order, and reports that it is Coke Zero with the slogan "Real Coke taste, zero sugar." Reason has come to tell the viewer that although the flavor is like Coke, this is another product. The brain (representing reason) has said it is Coke Zero, and that must be the truth.

A similar case is found in EVO Bank.[27] This is a new bank that has launched on the market in Spain, where the financial market has suffered the greatest crisis in its history. Spanish customers have a real lack of confidence in the banking system and do not believe that any bank can guarantee their savings. In this context, the advertisement of the EVO Bank launch campaign says the following: "Why do you need to change to EVO? Because there is a part of your brain where financial concerns are concentrated and this intelligent new account takes away that problem forever." Meanwhile, in the image we see how a doll's concerns are removed with an iron hand while a hat is put on his head and a bird perches on it. Again we have a case in which the presence of a brain to endorse the product makes the consumer understand that it is reasonable to choose that product. The brain is the proof.

Nintendo goes one step further to promote its product Brain Training.[28] It launches a visual campaign in which we can see excited neurons in constant motion. It launches the idea that if you use its product you will exercise your brain. The allusion is more direct.

## Brain-Shaped Advertising

Another use of the brain is found in advertising campaigns that show brain-shaped images. This happens in the campaign that *The Economist* released in 2012, directed by Ogilvy and Mather, where several magazines of *The Economist* create the shape of a brain.[29] This is a practice that is not innovative, because there are many objects that are advertised forming a brain. For example, the Mercedes Benz campaign made in 2010 creates brain forms with various old car models dating back to 1890.[30] Or consider the campaign launched in 2013 by the Holy House of Mercy of São Paulo, in which a brain appears as if it were a map.[31] Sanyo did the same in 2005, forming a brain with garments to advertise washing machines.[32] More recently, Trivial Pursuit created a brain-shaped maze with the campaign slogan "You know more than you think," where the destination is a game response.[33]

## Other Ways of Representing Neuroscience in Advertising

Lastly, we have found other recent advertising campaigns that, while they do not follow any of these particular trends, do use neuroscience and the brain in advertising. In 2013, Virgin Mobile launched a campaign with the slogan "Retrain your brain."[34] Using a brain, the commercial tries to convince the target audience that it is time to retrain the brain, with the brand insisting on telling the brain to wake up and switch mobile phone carriers. The commercial begins, "You deserve Virgin Mobile, but something in your brain is afraid to switch." From there, the commercial reportedly justifies reasons with characteristics of the product, such as price and service, that "it's time to retrain your brain."

In a 2012 campaign, the travel search engine Kayak launched the campaign "Be the brain of your own travel operation."[35] In the commercial, a neurosurgeon is shown operating on the brain of his patient. During the operation, the surgeon controls the patient's arms by manipulating his brain to have the patient type on a laptop computer and search travel sights. The nurse, who sees the practice as unethical, tells the doctor to save time by using Kayak.

Bimbo, a Mexican bread and sweet company with a strong presence in Europe, used in its 2011, 2012, and 2013 campaigns an image of the most renowned science writer in Spanish, Eduard Punset.[36] Punset's campaigns starring a new product are enjoying great success among the Spanish public. Punset presents the most important Spanish-language science TV program, with major neuroscientific content. The use of celebrities in advertising has been studied in a neuroscientific way.[37] The presence of the scientist aims to guarantee the quality, credibility and rigor of the product presented, in this case, sandwich bread. The explanation of the success of Bimbo's approach is found in an investigation conducted by Klucharev, Smidts, and Fernández to determine the persuasiveness of what is known as "expert power."[38] One of the most interesting conclusions reached is that the presentation of objects followed by famous people with high expertise or experience in the subject causes greater activation in brain regions associated with semantic processes than objects presented by non-experts. Experts mean that the attitude toward presented objects is 12 percent more favorable and increases the probability of recognizing an object by 10 percent. This helps to understand the successful sale of the advertised product by renowned science writer Punset for Bimbo's campaigns.

## CONCLUSIONS

We conclude that, despite not having quantitative data revealing the specific amount of advertising that is being carried out using the brain and neuroscience as tools of persuasion, these discussed examples show that there is a notable tendency in this regard.

The image of the brain has a strong influence on the consumer. We can find multiple ads that consistently have used the image of the brain as well as its appeal through text to lend more credibility to their messages. The goal is to sell, and it is clear that by using brain images the target audience will give more scientific merit and, with it, more fascination and reliability to the ad. It is therefore understandable that brands and agencies make use of the representation of neuroscience in their advertising messages. If, as we have seen, the public judges that explanations with neuroscience are more satisfying than explanations without, it is also normal that advertisers use them.

If the brain and neuroscience are used to sell more and better, it is because its persuasive effectiveness on the consumer is crucial. The role of both neuroscience disseminators and the media is still essential for advertisers to find new ways of appealing to feelings. The image of the brain is very important to the public. The brain seems to be the new heart of the consumer, not always protected from authoritarian reasoning, which with pseudo-scientific coverage appeal to feelings. Today, consumers also know that these feelings are in their brains.

In short, neuroscience is used by ads to validate an opinion or thought as scientific, but in many cases it requires an act of faith. The paradox is in justifying advertising arguments with logic and reason that supposedly come from neuroscience. Just by providing some references to the brain, scientific truth saves advertising lies.

## NOTES

The reader can obtain all the examples explained in this chapter, as support material, on the website http://www.neuroscienceandmedia.com.

1. Giovanni Carrada, *Communication Science: A Scientist's Survival Kit* (Luxembourg: Office for Official Publications of the European Communities, European Commission, 2006).
2. Eric Racine, Sarah Waldman, Jarett Rosenberg, and Judy Illes, "Contemporary Neuroscience in the Media," *Social Science and Medicine* 71, no. 4 (2010): 725–33, doi:10.1016/j.socscimed.2010.05.017.
3. Diana Zuckerman, "Hype in Health Reporting: 'Checkbook Science' Buys Distortion of Medical News," *International Journal of Health Services* 33, no. 2 (2003): 383–89, doi:10.2190/pmm9-dput-hn3y-lmjq.
4. Sandra Blakeslee, Mariette DiChristina, Paul Raeburn, and Kelly Lambert, "Behavioral Neuroscience and the Media," *Physiology and Behavior* 107, no. 5 (2012): 617–22, doi:10.1016/j.physbeh.2012.04.012.
5. Ibid.
6. Ibid.
7. Cliodhna O'Connor, Geraint Rees, and Helene Joffe, "Neuroscience in the Public Sphere," *Neuron* 74 (2012): 220–26, doi:10.1016/j.neuron.2012.04.004.
8. David P. McCabe and Alan D. Castel, "Seeing Is Believing: The Effect of Brain Images on Judgments of Scientific Reasoning," *Cognition* 107 (2008): 343–52, doi:10.1016/j.cognition.2007.07.017; Deena Skolnick Weisberg et al., "The Seductive Allure of Neuroscience Explanations," *Journal of Cognitive Neuroscience* 20, no. 3 (2008): 470–77, doi:10.1162/jocn.2008.20040.
9. McCabe and Castel, "Seeing Is Believing."
10. Weisberg et al., "Seductive Allure."
11. O'Connor et al., "Neuroscience in the Public Sphere."
12. Ibid., 221.
13. Ibid.
14. European Commission, *Special Eurobarometer 282: Scientific Research in the Media* (European Union: European Commission, 2007).
15. Carrada, *Communication Science*.
16. We Love Ad, "Drive Communication. Drive. Brain fitness. WE LOVE AD," http://www.welovead.com/en/works/details/6b6wnovC (accessed July 10, 2013).
17. Wherecreativitygoestoschool.com, "Where Creativity Goes to School—Art and Design School Offers Design, Media Arts, Culinary Arts, Fashion Programs in 35 Locations," http://www.wherecreativitygoestoschool.com (accessed July 19, 2013).
18. We Love Ad, "College for Creative Studies. Team Detroit. Your Brain. WE LOVE AD," http://www.welovead.com/en/works/details/ac2Ehsuz (accessed July 10, 2013).
19. We Love Ad, "Brother. Parachute. WE LOVE AD," http://www.welovead.com/en/works/details/7d4Bilwv.
20. We Love Ad, "Mercedes-Benz. Y&R. Left Brain–Right Brain, Paint. WE LOVE AD," http://www.welovead.com/en/works/details/117Cfptw (accessed July 10, 2013).

21. "Funny Comercial Beauty Is Nothing without Brains Mercedes-Benz Class E," YouTube video, posted by "3dana," http://www.youtube.com/watch?v=dFAe Bb2QvYU.

22. Great Ads, "Mercedes Benz 'Einstein' Print Ad Is a Genius Idea," http:// great-ads.blogspot.com.es/2011/03/check-out-brain-on-einsteins-mercedes. html (accessed July 19, 2013).

23. Sharpshooter, "Sharpshooter and O+—Case Studies—Brock University Ad Campaign—Print, Outdoor, and Cinema," http://www.sharpshooterinc.com/ casestudies/brock-university-ad-campaign-print-outdoor-and-cinema.html (accessed July 19, 2013).

24. We Love Ad, "Pango. No, No, No, No, No, Yes. Smart Parking. WE LOVE AD," http://www.welovead.com/en/works/details/954Emqqz (accessed July 10, 2013).

25. We Love Ad, "Colgate. Tempo Advertising, Brain. WE LOVE AD," http:// www.welovead.com/en/works/details/15dBmmrv (accessed July 10, 2013).

26. We Love Ad, "Coca-Cola. Wieden+Kennedy. Brain. WE LOVE AD," http:// www.welovead.com/en/works/details/97ezepsy (accessed July 10, 2013).

27. "Con EVO ¡¡Bye Bye preocupaciones financieras!!," YouTube video, posted by "Evo Banco," http://www.youtube.com/watch?v=Q7eX061Y-_k (accessed July 2, 2013).

28. We Love Ad, "Nintendo. Ogilvy. Achterbahn. WE LOVE AD," http://www. welovead.com/en/works/details/6b1BnpoC (accessed July 10, 2013).

29. We Love Ad, "The Economist. Ogilvy. Brain. WE LOVE AD," http://www. welovead.com/en/works/details/696wisrx (accessed July 10, 2013).

30. We Love Ad, "Mercedes-Benz. Y&R. Left Right 72_5. WE LOVE AD," http:// www.welovead.com/en/works/details/1cfCnrxx (accessed July 10, 2013).

31. We Love Ad, "Santa Casa de Misericórdia. Y&R. Invasions 3. WE LOVE AD," http://www.welovead.com/en/works/details/425Eipuw (accessed July 10, 2013).

32. We Love Ad, "Sanyo. GMSCO. Sanyo Brain. WE LOVE AD," http://www. welovead.com/en/works/details/7cdBmlxx (accessed July 10, 2013).

33. Dabriodabriodabrio, "Trivial Pursuit: You Know More Than You Think," http:// www.dabriodabriodabrio.com/2012/04/trivial-pursuit-you-know-more-than-you-think/#!/-1/ (accessed July 19, 2013).

34. "Funny Commercial 'Retrain Your Brain' Virgin Mobile TV Ad," YouTube video, posted by "amazing24hours," https://www.youtube.com/watch?v=40Mg3Tad760.

35. We Love Ad, "Kayak.com. Barton F. Graf 9000. Brain Surgeon. WE LOVE AD," http://www.welovead.com/en/works/details/3b6Elutw (accessed July 10, 2013).

36. "Spot Pan Bimbo 100% Natural, con Eduardo Punset 2011 (España)," You-Tube video, posted by "CanalBimbo," https://www.youtube.com/watch?v=iCE5qXqvS7A; "Spot Pan Bimbo 100% Natural, con Eduardo Punset 2012 (España)," YouTube video, posted by "CanalBimbo," http://www.youtube. com/watch?v=h6_nREeux2o; "NUEVO Spot Pan Bimbo 100% Natural, con Eduardo Punset 2013 (España)," YouTube video, posted by "CanalBimbo," http://www.youtube.com/watch?v=B1iDvlzo7c8.

37. Mirre Stallen et al., "Celebrities and Shoes on the Female Brain: The Neural Correlates of Product Evaluation in the Context of Fame," *Journal of Economic Psychology* 31, no. 5 (2010): 802–11.

38. Vasily Klucharev, Ale Smidts, and Guillén Fernández, "Brain Mechanisms of Persuasion: How 'Expert Power' Modulates Memory and Attitudes," *Social Cognitive and Affective Neuroscience* 3, no. 4 (2008): 353–66, doi:10.1093/ scan/nsn022.

# 14 Braining Your Life and Living Your Brain

## The Cyborg Gaze and Brain-Images

*Alexander I. Stingl*

## THE POLITICS OF TANGIBLE IMAGES

Images have tremendous power. What kind of power? That depends. Sometimes images can be extremely coercive. The images of his exposed nether regions can coerce a politician to step down from office when they reach the public, they may also coerce him into paying money when somebody threatens to make them public; that is, when he is blackmailed. Images have, therefore, tangible consequences.

But coercion implies a strong and usually not very subtle use of force, wherein the interrelations between the image, the decisions, and the consequences are quite explicit. There are, however, many more tacit and "softer" power-plays that images are enmeshed in. Images, as part of knowledge regimes and techno-scientific practices, are persuasive—they legitimize, they justify, and they *make* knowledges and their objects. In other words, they have the property of possessing *epistemic authority*.

Regardless of which precise definition of power one follows—between sociology, political science, history, media studies, there are many different ones—I think that we can safely say that nearly everyone should be willing to agree with the following position: images, because they can be *powerful* (i.e., have/exert power) as much as they can *be* power, are therefore political, make politics, and/or are made by politics. I don't think that one can still genuinely hold the belief that images are (politically) innocent.

Here, I am concerned with one particular type of image, a type of image that is produced and put to use in biomedical and health care contexts: the techno-image that is the result of the techno-scientific practices around medical imaging technologies in expert-lay, expert-expert, and lay-lay interactions, that involve publication of research results or health care policies, clinical interactions and decision making, and doctor-patient interactions, as well as situations of everyday life that have become "bio-medicalized." Images that are products of medical imaging technologies, I posit, obtain epistemic authority that functions as a persuasive technology to the point of working like propaganda. The subject depicted in the images in question is the human brain, and since images are media and since images are used in other media *to do* things, I propose that we must interrogate critically both the *matters of fact* and the *matters of concern* that are inscribed in those images and that are engraved into the media contexts that the images are produced and used in; we must, furthermore, trouble the situations where their power is constituted and brought to bear, where their epistemic authority is obtained and unfolded, and when they re-assemble the past, present, and future; that is, the realities, of actual people—in other words, we must account for *matters of care*.[1]

In this chapter, I will try to accomplish the gesture of a *troubling*[2] of a regime of established techno-scientific practices; that is, of practices that reify norms of gender, illness, and ageing through the involvement of medical images in social interactions. I will *trouble* them by *interrogating* how images work as affective-persuasive technologies through narrative empathy that takes seriously the effect of what I have called *narrative dialectics of techno-scientific seeing*.[3]

The pictures that imaging technologies produce of the human brain, pictures that media outlets as well as medical research and clinical experts reproduce, make a (truth-)claim of representing objectively the nature of the human brain. And yet, we may challenge this "objectivity" by countering: What is this Nature, but "[a] metonymic series [that] becomes a metaphor. [. . .] 'Nature' is a Pandora's box, a word that encapsulates a potentially infinite series of disparate fantasy objects."[4]

## CYBORGING GAZES, DECOLONIALIZING PRACTICES, DISOBEYING EPISTEMIC AUTHORITIES

In the long and complicated history of the modern idea of scientific objectivity that emerges in between visualization and seeing as a complex of depth and transparency, medical imaging technologies are merely a chapter; but they are an immensely significant one, because they seem to allow us a look into the body without having to open it: they take the eye to places where it cannot itself go, and to see what it cannot see immediately or without further action or help.[5] But in doing so, this technology allows for (re)constructions of the bodies that the eye is gazing upon and into. Bodies are (re)assembled in space and time: they are (re)articulated, (re)spatialized and (re)temporalized.

### The Clinical Gaze

In the analysis of the history of medicine, the productive power of the modern mode of visualization has been called the *medical* or *clinical gaze* by Michel Foucault, denoting the effects of the learned way of looking and gazing at the body by specialists; that is, medical experts such as physicians, particularly in the clinical context. It obtains as a way of knowing as well as a way of *making* the body gazed at. The act of "seeing something" is an act of seeing it in a particular and formative way: the amorphous mass in an opened skull is *made* into a tumor and surrounding brain tissue *is* healthy by seeing it as such, the brain structures that make one person male and another female are *made real* by seeing them through a learned gaze. Tissues, structures, and entities therefore exist as a historically and locally situated standpoint that is part politics, part economy, an epistemology, and an ontology. That does not mean, as some positivist or naïve naturalist critics would have it, that this analysis is a "mere postmodernist constructionism" that denies the reality of observed differences and would conclude that all truths are just made-up stories. What it means is, actually, that our practices have an effect on what truth itself can possibly mean. "Practices" means how we come to know something (epistemology), our understanding of what it is that we can come to know something about (ontology), and the negotiations that we make between these two levels as well the negotiations we have with others in interactions about what to do with that knowledge (political), why to do something with that knowledge (politics), and how to accomplish the goal (economy).

The visual mode is one mode of techno-scientific practice. The relation between the medical mode of visualizing[6] and the medical mode of seeing is what we call the medical or clinical gaze that forms the human body normatively in the medical/clinical context. But for the body to become subject to this gaze, features and properties had to be identified in a manner that suggested that it should be subjected to a gaze in medical/clinical context in the first place. This process was critiqued, first, as *medicalization*.

## Medicalization

The concept, introduced and disseminated by Irving K. Zola and Peter Conrad, refers to the process that renders issues, problems, processes, and entities that were previously not subject of the discourse of medicine into such.[7] The concept is usually used critically; that is, as a mode of interrogation into the conditions of possibility that offered potential for a specific subject to become subject of the discourse of medicine and an evaluation of whether or not this subjectivation was substantially and normatively justified[8] and an evaluation of the options derive from this interrogation in order not to be mindlessly governed by this subjectivation.[9] Sometimes, the concept is used polemically,[10] in claiming that medicalization is the process by which neoliberal agents "invent" diseases and disorders to suppress individual freedom, to rule over populations, and to maximize profit (of Big Pharma). It is true, however, that there are strong social trends and currents—although a product of complex social, affective, and material forces rather than "evil conspiracies"—to "enforce" and "reify" cultural norms and imperatives of "normalcy," and to *medicalize* a range of behaviors, bio-physical attributes, and processes. The lines between mere sadness and clinical depression,[11] between stressful lives or hairspray-induced headaches or having migraine, between ageing and menopause,[12] between children being children (i.e., in development) and ADHD or bipolar disorder, are constantly contested and re-negotiated, presently more often toward *medicalization* and pharmacological treatment than in the other direction. However, that does not mean that this is or would need to be a mono-directional trend.[13] In short, *medicalization* is the process that makes things a concern of medicine that were not before.

## Biomedicalization[14]

In recent decades, medicalization was turned up a notch and critiqued as *biomedicalization*, the transformation of self and identity-forming process, extending Foucault's discussion of biopower and biopolitics, between the molar and the molecular gaze in the creation of neuronal and molecular selves[15] from biosociality.[16]

Clarke et al. understand *biomedicalization* as a process that constitutes what they call techno-scientific identities; these are identities people are "frequently inscribed upon" in a process of production.[17] As "production," they understand the "application" of techno-scientific practices involving both bodies and products that harbor or infringe the body; they specifically cite images that are produced by medical imaging technologies as an exemplary techno-scientific practice. Techno-scientific identities are therefore "new genres of risk-based genomics-based, epidemiology-based or other techno-science-based identities."[18]

Identities such as the neuronal self appear as particular cases of techno-scientific identities.[19] In investigating these identities, *biomedicalization*[20] is not just a categorization but also a research program:

> Although we can conceptually tease apart organizational, clinical, and jurisdictional axes of change and their situatedness within a politico-economic and sociocultural sector-however vast-the ways in which these changes are simultaneous, co-constitutive, and nonfungible inform our conceptualization of biomedicalization. That is, a fundamental premise of biomedicalization is that increasingly important sciences and technologies and new social forms are co-produced within biomedicine and its related domains. Biomedicalization is reciprocally constituted and manifest through five major interactive processes: (1) the politico-economic constitution of the Biomedical TechnoService Complex, Inc.; (2) the focus on health itself and elaboration of risk and surveillance biomedicines; (3) the increasingly technoscientific nature of the practices and innovations of biomedicine; (4) transformations of biomedical knowledge production, information management, distribution, and consumption; and (5) transformations of bodies to include new properties and the proauction of new individual and collective

technoscientific identities. These processes operate at multiple levels as they both engender biomedicalization and are also (re)produced and transformed through biomedicalization over time.[21]

In his work on the molar and the molecular perspective[22] and the *neuromolecular gaze*,[23] Nikolas Rose understands the notion of the gaze with Michel Foucault as a dynamic that mutually shapes perception, expression, and the perspective or style of thought, which Foucault understood to be an *ethos*. More than even Clarke et al. or Rose (with Abi-Rached), other writers have pointed out the dialectical connection between the emergence of a conception of self, and technologies of the self that are rooted in biomedicalization, its neuromolecular gaze and a neoliberal ideology. A dominant perspective foresees the future of medical sociology as a discipline being busy with technology[24] and subjectivities[25] in continuing to ask questions about the paradoxes of economy and morality, others propose that empowering patients is not enough if they are not provided with skills and knowledge to appropriate decision-powers to their life circumstance[26] and some argue that neoliberal governance has subjected us to/in politics of lifestyle and risk, which lead us to adapt our everyday technologies of self-making to the paradox of biological determinism and neuronal plasticity.[27] These perspectives construe a notion of biological citizenship, which appears delimited by neoliberalism, but which can however be critique by notions of bio-civics, solidarity and empathic integration.[28]

## Cyborg Visualization

Among other things, the biomedical gaze is a gaze that medicalizes while it re-spatializes what it sees—it is not only displacing the "medical" into the body interior; that is, it is constructed by the "myth of transparency" that constructs the discourse of medical imaging,[29] and it succumbs to the "myth of depth" of going deeper or magnifying and bringing into focus more particulars.[30]

When bringing subjectivities, technology, and the biomedical gaze together in the main mode of biomedical inquiry underlying research and clinical techno-scientific practices, we encounter a novel regime of representational practice that is, nonetheless, determined by an uncanny primacy of perception, which has consequences for how it produces scientific and clinical evidence, for the resulting research and clinical interventions, and for the decision-making processes that affect publics, policy makers, health practitioners, and individual patients.

Amit Prasad describes this mode in his argument

> . . . that visualization produced by technologies such as MRI has some similarities with nondigital visuality. Moreover, it continues to depend on other visualization technologies and diagnostic inputs in fixing

biological reality and detecting pathology. Nonetheless, a change in the nature and status of the image radically alters the mechanics and architecture of the medical gaze, shifting it to a new visual regime that should be appropriately called cyborg visuality.[31]

*Cyborg visuality* in this account both "extends the medical gaze" *and* "reconfigures the body." But this mode does not emerge out of nowhere as a socially accepted practice. Prasad and others show that processes of "disciplining," "domestication," "standardization," "normalization," and "institutionalization" of both the particular visual *form* and the sets of practices have to occur before they can unfold their power as a visual *regime*. But once it has attained such a status, this mode extends to take part as a constitutive process in producing scientific models of the inner workings of organisms, bodies, and, in particular, the human brain. In *becoming* constitutive and in producing/confirming models, this mode of visuality is treated *as if* it was unconditional. It has been pointed out[32] that this myth of unconditioned visuality is based on the perception by those who are not directly involved in the actual production of medical images through imaging technologies, that these technologies produce images *as if* they were photographies.[33]

The real problem arises, when the *as if* of images, extends into one's life course (its temporalities), and the narrative of one's life begins to be in-formed and governed by an image produced in cyborg visuality, in other words, once someone begins to live *in this image*. Cyborg visuality, I argue, must be understood as an even more complex process: the extension-reconfiguration of medical gaze and body is both intertwined and mutually reinforcing, producing not *transparency* but *vitreousness*. Thereby the interlocutors involved adopt the gaze, even for purposes of "navel-gazing" so to speak, and reconfigure not only their body and not only their illness narrative, but they reconfigure their entire set of intertwined temporalities, the narrative of their relational self—future, past, and present. In adopting the mode of cyborg visuality—not only as a technology in clinics and research facilities, in the technological adoption of machines, such as fMRI or PET scanners, but—as a technology of selves, cyborg visuality becomes more than a mode of visuality. It turns into a gaze: it affects spatializing, temporalizing, and (re-)configuring of bodies as well as embodiment and enactment, perception, and conceptualizations, and the very ways of individual and social world and kind making. Rooted in cyborg visuality, primacy of the anthropic brain, and the Western colonial matrix of power, this gaze obtains and exerts practical authority that colonizes knowledge-making and knowledge-deploying practices in culture, politics, and medicine.

The task of the mode of critique that I am proposing through my work is an agonistic pluralism and decolonial, epistemic disobedience that allows and requires the exploration of different possibilities, however, within a scape of options that are actually possible.[34] I insist that critique cannot simply mean that we deny the efficacy of Western medicine, nor that we can simply "go back" to a status before biomedicalization and cyborg visuality. I aim to uncover the modes of production and create epistemic responsibility for the practices and subjectivties they make possible. Here, I aim to show how imaging technologies can function as (propaganda-like) persuasive technologies. To make this inquiry tangible, I will unfold some of the practices of images and the cyborg gaze that work to focalize issues of the chronicity of illness, ageing, and gender around the brain as a matter of both politics and poetics that lead to the assemblage of *braining lives and living the brain*.

## BRAINING LIVES, LIVING THE BRAIN

Despite scientific practice and evidence pointing to the contrary, two myths about causality are still widely given credence among the lay public, among many scientific experts, and among those intermediate actors that we can summarize under the terms science commissioners and regulators; that is, those who decide on policies, funding, ethics, and bureaucratic governance of science: the myth that genes have direct determinative power and the myth of the primacy and imaging-induced transparency of the brain. These myths lead to simple binary concepts and dichotomous worldviews of the kind where "gay-genes"[35] are talked about as *factoids* in *truthiness*, and where brains *are* male or female, where ADHD *is* a hormone imbalance *in the brain*, and where thoughts can be read and even implanted.[36] In the brain myth, sometimes the brain is equated with mind and consciousness, other times it is afforded separate agency besides the mind, and sometimes the brain is given primacy over, even against, the mind.[37] In the latter case, the argument "my brain made me do it (against my will)" is both legally and ethically sensitive, but then requires the following question regarding the effects of pharmaceutical interventions, which David Karp so eloquently posed: *is it me or my meds?*[38]

Some of these "science stories" we encounter seem like caricatures, but we often find that, even though they have all the markers of being naive or fictitious and that no scientist or science commissioner could possibly take them seriously, they still appear to drive scientific research policies, funding, and implementation. We do meet researchers and clinical practitioners who, even though they are not ideologues, find themselves persuaded (*tangibly*) by stories about or accompanied by images that clearly do no justice to the complex reality that researchers and clinicians actually try to tackle. They seem to hold two opposing views simultaneously. What has been widely dubbed as *brain research* is very much part of this kind of dynamic. People believe that brain-images show "like a photograph what is going on inside your brain and mind," and that this was allowing diagnosis and prognosis about developments that affect and steer individual life and show how events in individual biographies[39] can affect and change the brain. In assigning the brain this much importance (and even agency), in coming close to equating it with human existence or localizing it *in the* brain,[40] I want to speak of an assemblage that I call *braining life and living the brain*. I also posit that once this assemblage is established, its two sides cannot be separated, because for all their affects and effects, they constitute a dialectical relationship. In other words, once you have bought into an image to "show you your brain," you cannot but "live your life as if you were your brain," and once you find yourself convinced by popular science that people "are their brains," you cannot but accept whatever a person vested with scientific authority tells you "about your brain as a definition of who and what you are and are not."

## When Is the Brain? The Issue of Chronifying Illness and States of Being

The assemblage *braining life/living the brain* reveals a particular caveat I find in both current biomedical and biopolitical regimes that concern the question of the body/brain and the state equally. Both discourses, which from a point of view of academic discipline could not seem farther apart, are however both constrained by the same set of conceptualizations.[41] Both the body/brain and the state remain constituted by territorial boundaries and a linear concept of time. Biomedical research and clinical practice, it seems, have remained within the concept of (historical) time, which "ultimately rests on a 'Hegelian' conception of time, which has two mutually reinforcing defining characteristics: 'the homogeneous continuity of time' and 'the contemporaneity of time.'"[42] While much research in neuro-cognitive science, biology, and biomedicine, as well as in political science and sociology, seems to point out the necessity of deterritorialization of both concepts, of unhinging the temporal frameworks to be less mono-linear,[43] and to depart from the focus on the actor-perspective in favor of network, relational, or practice-oriented approaches, only a few researchers and scholars actually try to do so. The shift in both lines of inquiry must be to not only ask "what is a state or body/brain?," "where is a state or body/brain?," and "where is that state function or bodily/brain function located?"; the meshwork of inquiries must also interrogate the troubling questions "when is the state?," "when is a body/brain?," and "when is this embodiment/enactment being practiced, what is its duration, and what are entangled temporalities?"

It seems to me that the most controlled and governed variable in clinical and research practice is time. To situate human agency in the body and the brain, to locate (mal)functions in the brain, the (temporal) *presence* of the brain must be constructed: the brain must be *present* and *in the present*. To be *in the present*, time must be controlled, normalized, imagined in a spatialized way of a timeline. The varying temporalities that the brain and its human are enmeshed in are being made to succumb to a temporal regime of a singular, mono-linear time. The question "when is something happening in relation to other, different temporalities,"[44] it seems, is hardly ever asked.

The paradigm is that of a present state of the brain that is compared to an idea of normalcy, and constructed into linear past/future-and before/after-schemas. The goal is to rebuild the brain as a fixed normality in a future present to make it be like its normal/before: the ageing brain must be made younger, the dopamine-imbalance must be normalized, and so on. At the same time, the present state becomes fixed in time, rewriting past and future: MS, Alzheimer's, ageing itself, are progressive over (linear) time: they are a chronic illness, the brains and their humans belong to the *new chronic*, and the brain's illness must be managed by trying to keep it as close to the normal/before as possible: (almost) frozen in time. This process of re-rendering temporalities of individual people (e.g. patients) and of the brain as an epistemic object of research, reconfiguring them as subject to the *cyborg gaze* and the regime of the *new chronic*, aligned to a mono-linear time continuum, is what we can call *chronification*.

*Chronification* means a process of reconfiguring biomedicalized entities, in re-making their present state as a being static over time, fixing their future and re-narrating their past, ruling out different temporal alignments, fixing epistemic patterns of development pre-set into the timeline, discontinuing processes of individuation, and replacing them with individual variations of the same, shared present.

This *chronification* of the brain in medical imaging happens, because brain states are "imaged" by use of technologies such as PET, MRI, (BOLD) fMRI, and SPECT, which do not directly take a picture (like a photograph), but they take measurements of where particular molecules are concentrated. These molecules can present from the use of radiotracer solutions that subjects are injected with or they can involve hydrogen, spin-changes, or hemoglobin as oxygen-carrying and non-carrying molecules, allowing to show where blood flows are directed in the brain, for example in relation to an event experienced, which however occurs with a certain time-lag. Imaging machines are subject to intricate calibrations by technicians (thickness of the slices, contrast, etc.). Measured data are compared to a standardized atlas/model, "white noise" is filtered, and computer programs *calculate* an image. One can see the many steps, influences, filters, and decisions that are necessary to produce an image, which is not a direct representation but a construct; in other words, its production spans an *inferential distance*.[45] And one can see that in each of these steps, a unique temporal organization is at play, to which the temporalities of the original brain have little direct relation. To function, these steps in the process of cyborg visualization must be aligned by one linear biomedical time—however imaginary—and escond the actual brain's real temporalities, to become *chronified*.[46]

## Gender

The issue of gender and sex obtains a particular importance for an investigation into the complex issues relating cyborg visuality, biomedicalization, media, and the brain and creating the assemblage *braining life/living the brain*.

To begin with, there is the matter of political contemporaneity, where brain research is deployed in both actual policy making and the (deadly) game of politics that involve, among others, the discourses of sexual identity or women's health. Second, most of the relevant issues emerge from the assemblage *braining life/living the brain* in the intersection of ageing, illness, race, and gender. Finally, assemblage, political deployment, and intersection describe the deeply intertwined, chaotic reality that is subject to emerging myths and phantasms that human actors use to make sense of their situation, to communicate with others, or to negotiate boundaries and solution strategies in organizations and institutions.

We can identify ageing and, ultimately, old age as a process that is re-written into a chronic illness through biomedicalization in general, and by cyborg visuality in *braining* it in particular. Yet, the biomedical construction[47] of ageing must be viewed as differentiated where it intersects with gender. A common perspective on female ageing is visualized in the image of *Menopause Lane*, which inherently prescribes the linear progress of female ageing as a biomedicalized timeline captured in a phantasmic visualization.[48] Despite the work of cultural anthropologists like Margaret Lock and others, who interrogate the Western temporal and biomedical normativities of menopause, medical imaging technologies are deployed[49] to make Menopause Lane visible in the brain and establish the brain (our central neural system), for example in showing women that "this is what experiencing a hot flash looks like"[50] in fMRI images of a woman's brain, and, therefore, as one blogger duly quoted, "identifying the neural origins of hot flashes in menopausal woman."[51] Other research groups claim to have demonstrated[52] that sexual arousal in menopausal women is lower. When showing ten menopausal and ten premenopausal women non-erotic and erotic short films, the researchers found that "the overall [brain] activation ratios of the premenopausal women were greater than those of the menopausal women by approximately 8% on average."

Of course, with such a small sample size and the consideration of what 8 percent in average means here with regard to the inferential distance (i.e., the number steps the subject's brain is separated from the researcher's interpretation), and adding that there may be generational effects as to what counts as "erotic," not to mention whether "erotic" was perhaps defined from a male perspective (*male gaze*) and the arousal measured in younger participants may have been a mere transference effect onto the researchers rather than a direct stimulation,[53] and so and so on. Again, this is not intended to create a pejorative criticism and deny the importance of these kinds of studies. My aim is to point out that the value of this research should be viewed with a critical appreciation for its severe limitations and the persuasive power it holds when transferred to other contexts.

In short, research on menopause that is informed by biomedicalization and cyborg visuality tends to create research with too little reflection on individual and cultural variations, presupposes the existence of a male/female binary of the brain, and constructs in particular sexuality along an axis of heteronormativity uncritically.[54] In *braining* menopause, researchers construct a *menopausal life of the brain* that emerges through images, that have a direction of fit with the binary concepts and linear model they posit in the creation of these images.

There are several disorders that have proliferated the deployment and reification of the male/female binary, the history of migraine is a good example of stereotypes that influence the gendering of the discourse on migraine. "The notion that sex differences involve both brain structure as well as functional circuits, in that emotional circuitry compared with sensory processing appears involved to a greater degree in female than male migraineurs."[55]

There are Western social elements that persuade us that migraines are 'something' that is in the brain, and that something is female, which is why research is geared to begin with these assumptions as they are reported by doctors and patients alike.[56] But here, the technology used for studying and diagnosing is primed to actively see the gender binary into the brains it studies, and dialectically narrate migraine as a gendered disorder.

Finally, in contemporary Europe, people seem to hold a multicultural view on sex, gender, and sexual lifestyle. At the same time, there seems to be a widespread belief that, at least for the brain, there exists a clear-cut bifurcation into male and female brains. Within "social telemedicine" resources that are accessible to the wider public, such as WebMD, we find the following summary statement: "Recent studies highlight a long-held suspicion about the brains of males and females. They're not the same."[57]

Reiterating supposedly novel "hormone influences fetus" studies, which have actually been around for decades and are filled with ambiguities,[58] articles such as found on WebMD fuel and reify the male-female binary in endocrinology. At this point, medical imaging enters the picture and is turned into stereotype-reifying technologies for generations to come: for example, the executive director of the Center for Sensorimotor Neural Engineering at the University of Washington maintains an "innocent" educational website on Neuroscience for Kids.[59] And even though, in his conclusion, he states that the science is still inconclusive, that individuality may yet trump gender, his language and the images he uses continuously reify the standard male-female binary: while reinforcing his supposedly neutral "scientific authority" as a neuroscientist by posting pictures of brains, he titles the page "He Brains, She Brains."

From research to clinical practice, with regard to establishing and asserting scientific authority and the mantle of objectivity and neutrality in the eyes of the public, the use of brain-images has become necessary and is often treated as sufficient in acts of persuasion.[60] This is consequential for the reification of the cultural pattern of the sex/gender binary into ontologicalized and medicalized knowledge regimes that constitute baseline parameters for clinical practice and research.[61]

Make no mistake, neuroimaging is used in the biomedicalization of sex and gender in the reification of the binary and, therefore, part of the gender politics of the construction of disease and disorder entities, such as for example migraine, which has previously been socially stigmatized through linking it to gender issues and for a long time not been taken seriously in the medical community.[62] More importantly, "imaging technology"–related research can be used in politically and ideologically controversial issues such as intersex decision making or the American anti-abortion discourse.

The sexing of brains by way of medical imaging technology is prone to be abused to reify the claim that women are "more emotional," and even though in the scientific discourse itself, "being emotional" may have a variety of different meanings from being more sensual to being more attuned to judge the emotions of others (emotional intelligence), this scientific image-enhanced talk about the "emotionality of women" can be used to justify structural-conservative positions of any ideological agenda, such as by the Religious Right on the issue of abortion: women, it is argued, are too emotional to make such decisions, and the emotional impact of an abortion after the fact is too much to bear and cannot be adequately understood before, because women are considered too emotional. A woman, an American literature professor and her psychologist husband state in one article, "may reason her way to the decision to terminate the unwanted pregnancy,"[63] but she is supposedly unprepared for the emotional trauma after aborting her baby, because, these authors argue, women are more vulnerable to depression. In their words:

> Men's and women's brains also work differently in handling memory and memories. Men are more apt to recall facts of all kinds, on the one hand, and a global picture of events, on the other. By contrast, women remember people (for example, faces), details of all kinds, and emotion-laden narratives—and they may return to them obsessively.
>
> Women are more vulnerable to depression and anxiety than men, perhaps because they have a lower level of serotonin, an important neurotransmitter. In addition, women are twice as likely as men to suffer from post-traumatic stress disorders. Men suffer more than women from other mental pathologies, such as autism, dyslexia, and Narcissistic Personality Disorder; the two sexes suffer about equally from yet other mental problems, such as bi-polarity.

What do these differences add up to, practically speaking? Let's walk quickly through an unplanned pregnancy and abortion. A woman may reason her way to the decision to terminate the unwanted pregnancy. Her abortion decision may seem, and may indeed be, rational in terms of her long-term goals and interests, and her chosen values. But afterward, a woman may experience several powerful reactions, which are rooted in the structures and basic chemistry of her brain.[64]

In this case, braining women's lives and life choices become a deeply political matter. By *braining* women's health choices and in reifying the male-female brain binary, women's choices are rendered questionable, their moral agency is re-told as a fiction that states that women should not make reasonable choices. Women's lives are reconfigured as 'more emotional, because of their "brains." Are we not led to infer as a consequence of this logic that men are more rational, less emotional, and that women should not be allowed to make health choices, including the choice to terminate a pregnancy?[65]

In an ironic twist, the reification of the male-female brain, as part of the cyborg gaze, can be abused to justify taking away women's choices about their health through acts of epistemic paternalism. The deployment of technologies like imaging devices is never politically innocent because it constructs and stabilizes ontologies that become tangible and matters of both freedom of choice and of life and death. When imaging technologies are already imbricated in media discourses to show that voters are swayed by emotions not reason,[66] what is to stop a political extremist to claim that women should not be allowed to vote or hold political office because brain research shows that they are too emotional? After all, a serious contender for the Republican nomination for the presidential election and former state senator, Rick Santorum, is quoted saying in an interview with CNN:[67] "I do have concerns about women in front-line combat. I think that could be a very compromising situation, where people naturally may do things that may not be in the interest of the mission because of other types of emotions that are involved. It already happens, of course, with the camaraderie of men in combat, but I think it would be even more unique if women were in combat."[68]

## IMAGES OF THE BRAIN AS PERSUASIVE TECHNOLOGIES

I have elaborated here an account of what kinds of relational modes— biomedicalization and cyborg visuality—shape the narratives of techno-scientific practices that emerge as the assemblage *braining lives/living the brain* in practice and in media discourses. I have illustrated a dialectical generative relation with this assemblage to turn our focus to the mechanisms of how medical imaging technologies and their products obtain persuasive functions. In a nutshell, people understand their own situational dynamic in the form of narratives. These narratives are never fully complete, and people need to make decisions between alternative ways of completing a narrative. Images provide "vivid descriptions" of how narratives can be completed, in ways easy to decide on.

### The Hole in the Picture

I distinguish my parsimonious use of the word *narrative* from story, plot, or fiction, all of which refer to more rich and detailed accounts. Barbara

Tversky originally suggested to understand *narratives* to be no more but also no less than *the representation of at least two events with a temporal ordering between them.*[69] With regard to the two issues of narratives of selves and techno-scientific practices, this leads to an inquiry into the ways of how we know ourselves narratively, because narratives stand in a mutually (re)configurative relationship[70] with *how* practices are connected into sequences. Because these narratives and practices involve *what* we can know *that is* (ontology) and *how* we come to *know* (epistemology), we run into a number of problems that together constitute a logical gap, which has many descriptions and names that come with it, but I personally prefer *hiatus irrationalis*—the gap "between irrational reality and rational concept."[71] For example, what lies *in between* ontology and epistemology or in between subjectivity and objectivity is something that one can actually conceive by inter-mediacy or inter-*esse* (on this issue in ecomimesis, i.e., writing of nature).[72] In practice, we cannot forget that there are interests that are vested and relations that are medial. And the formative powers of interests and media that are inherent to them are something we should not discount: media in particular have material and vital agency in this process, and this agency establishes *ekphratic* force as its emergent property, because the media and articulation of interests themselves are techno-scientific practices—what else could they be? For any theory of human agency that involves narratives of selves, the notion of narrative, while not fictitious, still requires (political) imagination.[73] Imagination is not a process, however, that emerges in a vacuum, nor does it produce only one possible option to complete fragments to a totality (Simmel): our imagination builds alternatives in the interplay of myths and phantasms that it has acquired (1), and decides between the emerging narratives affectively as a process of empathy (2).

*Phantasms*
Ernst Boesch shows that a "myth of lurking chaos" is an integral social-psychological component of human civilization and, as a consequence, in the development of each individual child. He understands a *myth* to be a pre-structural guiding pattern. That means that it is not even as elaborate as a theory or a precise idea. It exists on a deeper affective level as an "unspecified 'mould' of receptivity and evaluation."[74] The myth of lurking chaos is one of the most primal and most influential myths, but it is not the only one, and there are different ways of dealing with myths. In the concept of *phantasms*, Boesch describes one of these ways: phantasms emerge during the individual development of children through processes of selection and amalgamation. Phantasms are individual or collective patterns that deal with myths. What we call phantasms are the perceiving, transforming as well as anticipating images, bound up with the acting party (or actor), whereas myths are the situational problems actors perceive. A narrative is the practice set that emerges from the interplay between a myth and a phantasm.

Boesch warns that phantasms are "over-determined."[75] They provide a way in which

> culture certainly influences the way we think and evaluate, shapes our action interaction. However, it acts no less below the surface, in those mythical dispositions, which we now hardly notice. Culture, then, makes us form phantasmatic orientations of which we recognize the more 'rational' manifestations—our goals and fears, affections and antipathies—but which nonetheless act at a depth that we will hardly ever be able to reflect on.[76]

### Narrative Empathy

Decision making on which narrative affects seem plausible follow a concept of empathy. When we are shown brain research or interact with a doctor who discusses an MS diagnosis, we field potential narratives about the narratives the interlocutors are actually involved in. Fritz Breithaupt has argued, and recent cognitive research[77] supports this—and arguments on the temporality, spatiality, and integration of narratives[78] make this clearer—that this can be recast as a problem of empathy.[79] Breithaupt acknowledges the existence of (at least) three credible standard accounts for empathy, which he calls different "cultures of empathy."

First, the mirror neuron account that is established in theories from neuro-cognitive science (involving, of course, medical imaging technology, directly). This idea posits that brains include neural formations that "fire" when another actor is observed performing an action that is identified *as if* oneself was performing it. The idea is often illustrated on the example that yawning is contagious. Proponents of this theory claim that empathy can be explained by the existence of mirror neurons. Second, the theory of (theory of other) mind or simulation account, assumes that empathy emerges in a person's developing in their mind a simulation of another mind. Finally, the coercion or Stockholm syndrome account, assumes that actor's are thrust into a situation where they must decide between (at least) two alternatives and adopt it as one's own, whereas one alternative, that is adopted as one's own, exerts coercive power, similar to the situation of a hostage psychologically siding with the hostage taker. This form of empathy, however, reveals an important step forward: actors do not decide based on dyadic interaction. Instead, the possibility arises that situations of narrative decision making involve at least three parties—the actor who decides, and the two narrative positions, neither of which is in and of itself created sui generis by the actor.

Breithaupt identifies empirical and theoretical problems in each of these three accounts, revealing an underlying structural-theoretical gap they share. The reduced but still viable explanatory power leads Breithaupt to speak of them as three separate modes or *cultures of empathy*. In his triadic approach, an actor decides between two (or more) opposing (actor) narratives that he is presented with or fields; that is, between two or more different options for the (temporal) ordering of events. In addition, Suzanne Keen distinguishes between three *spatializing* types of narrative empathy—*bounded, ambassadorial*, and *broadcast narrative*:[80]

> In narrative fiction, authorial strategic empathizing takes three forms. The first is *bounded* empathy, on behalf of members of one's own group (here it would be highly unusual not to find other people, but one might also discover an honored object, such as the flag, or a location such as the homeland) . . ., *ambassadorial* empathy, attempts to move more distant others on behalf of those represented empathetically, often but not exclusively other human beings . . ., and *broadcast* strategic empathy: it calls upon every reader, and most often evokes compassion for universal objects of concern, like infants and victims of disasters.

Which narrative prevails to sequence the actual relations of practices that follow is subject to different forces, materialities, and affectivities (so each cultural variant can come into play, but is not enough to account for empathy itself). The case of coercion is certainly very strong; too strong in fact, as I have argued in the introduction to this chapter. But sometimes the persuasive power of one narrative alternative obtains a force, through the (institutional and organizational) interests vested in it and the media deployed to communicate knowledge about it: When practices that obtain and wield *ekphratic force*, the force that closes the epistemic gap that emerges when narratives are being decided *and* reflected upon, become institutionalized along with other practices into forms of knowing (epistemic), this force obtains authority—*epistemic authority*—which it exerts to the point of turning into hegemony—*epistemic paternalism*.

*Epistemic authority* covers the increasing inferential distance[81] between the "black box" of the construction of a medical image and the patient's integration of this image into his or her narrative: while most patients or lay audiences are unaware of the "actual inferential distance," they do assume an "apparent inferential distance."[82] These distance relationals describe the *epistemic gap*[83] measurably: "Neuroimages are inferentially distant from brain activity, yet they appear not to be."[84]

While inferential distance is the measure of the epistemic gap, it is the increase of the gap between actuality and appearance that is the persuasive power of images: the wider the distance between the actual inferential distance from the apparent inferential distance, the higher the persuasive power it wields. When the apparent inferential distance comes close to zero, where as the actual inferential distance is large, we might even speak of *propaganda*. Cyborg visuality and biomedicalization also co-produce an apparent distance shorter than the actual one. They reach the level of *propaganda*, when the modes of *narrative empathy* presents as a culture of narrative empathy that can be characterized a *coercive broadcast culture of empathy*.

Once broadcast culture and the persuasive power of images infects the (political) ontology of medical production—the poetics and politics of tangible images—it can be argued that technology itself becomes the "inventor" of disease.[85]

## THE NARRATIVE DIALECTICS OF TECHNO-SCIENTIFIC SEEING

The switch in modern Western health care to a "patient-centered" approach, focusing on communication and empowerment, combined with digitalization, accountability, and management practices was considered a *medico-ethical* step forward in diminishing structural paternalism and installing patient autonomy.[86] With new power relations emerging, we must however trace their actual influence on real patients: techno-scientific practices that involve new technologies (re)configure how biomedical research and clinical medicine are practiced, including the relations of practitioners and their patients/audiences, through reconstituting epistemic objects and media of communication.

To account for the relations between technology and illness in this process, Hoffman has provided a comprehensive description for to the role of technology in the "invention of disease." This leads us to question the ambiguous status of disease entities as being either clear or vague:

> In this way technology has not only influenced the concept of disease, but also the status of the disease entities. Acute high-tech diseases, for example myocardial infarction, enjoy a higher status than chronic low-tech diseases in the same way that heart and brain surgery gain a higher position than geriatrics. Malaria, tuberculosis, and cancer are conceived as clear cases of disease, whereas colour blindness, senility, and depression are vague cases. In addition, as already noted, whiplash, and fibromyalgia are low-status diseases because they are not technologically detectable or treatable. Thus, there is a technological influence on the status of the disease entities.[87]

This conclusion is arrived at by separating the influence of technology on the concept of disease in three distinct ways, according to Hoffman.

1. Medical practice, at the very latest since the nineteenth century, has become dependent on technology in the production of data; therefore, technology provides the physiological, biochemical, and biomolecular entities that are applied in defining diseases.
2. Technology constitutes medical semiotics in establishing the procedures of the attainment of knowledge of disease in theory and the forms of practical disease recognition in the constitution of the signs, markers and end points that define disease entities and it strongly influences the

explanatory models of disease as well as medical taxonomy.[88] Before the nineteenth century, medical semiotics was largely defined by procedures originating in the juridical discourse.

3. Technology establishes actions and reactions that are embedded in the process of the constitution of disease by diagnosis and treatment technologies. "Content and configuration" of modern medical knowledge have been become effectively changed with the introduction and evolution of technology. Most importantly, technology-dependent semiotics, in defining and detecting disease, rely on "paraclinical signs" (such as detection via imaging technologies, X-ray, PET, CAT, or fMRI). A main criterion for the constitutive role of these paraclinical signs is *reproducibility.*

However, in the establishment of this technological knowledge regime within the actual institutions of care, *the patient* becomes paradoxically reconfigured into a passive object because of technological path-dependencies within illness trajectories and patient-career management regimes, rather than being considered as a person with a subjective experience and individual life course. This process of detachment of medical knowledge regime from actual patient subjectivities through the technological construction of disease,[89] results in a neglect of subjectivities and experience of suffering, reduction of illness to a mere registration of the existence of disease as an entity and (possibly) pain, and, as a further consequence, underestimation of the influence of suffering on the real progression of illness which may deviate from the trajectory.[90] "It's just in your head" is a sentence that many patients have come to loathe, particular in situations that concern women's health. Female patients' individual problems are often enough whisked away by relocating a physical suffering's causality into the brain, thereby making it at the same time clinically less real. From famous examples such as an allergy to onions to depression, differences in the experience of menstrual cycles or orgasms, and so on, the technological invention of disease as a paradoxical hot mess is at the same time strikingly male oriented and brain oriented.[91]

We can now forward a (tentative) definition of the process of *the narrative dialectics of techno-scientific seeing*: we accept a situation, involving practices between human actors, has a character of a certain vagueness of concepts (epistemic deficiency), knowledge and information asymmetry, and at least one party presents as more *epistemically vicious,*[92] resulting in a situation of *epistemic disagreement.* Epistemic disagreements are not arbitrary and incommensurable in practice, but they can, instead, be made reasonable and, in (medical and health care) practice, lead to the construction of realist ontologies. It is this pragmatic construction that establishes the need to accept epistemic responsibility for practices. The dialectics of seeing[93] is the notion that seeing is a mediated inter-relationship that affects both sides in iterative ways. Tools that constitute technological kinds of

seeing can be conceptualized as social actors with respective agentic properties that change the way we know and experience these affective relations.
Medical imaging technologies, for example, and their final, visual products
*enable* a cyborg gaze, a visual regime that presents only a partial image,
which is superimposed on the body of the patient in differential analysis, de
facto extending and augmenting the body by *and* into the image. The connection between image and patient body is reconfigured both dialectically
and iteratively in the individual temporalities of image, patient, and clinical,
wherein the practice of articulation of the image becomes narrativized as an
event in this fashion. The epistemic disagreement is overcome paternalisti-
cally by an *agnotological* stance toward the difference between the individual inferential distances assumed, evoking narrative cultures of empathy
that constitute a *merely* dyadic relationship of persuasive power beyond
the boundaries of an epistemic in-group. In short, techno-scientific seeing
changes, therefore, in the *event* of the articulation of the image both (1) the
temporal sequence of the image itself and (2) the temporal configuration of
body and narrative of self of the patient.

## The Western Colonial Matrix and Decolonial Options

In arguing that there is a valid theoretical point of view that can describe
the situation, and allow important insights into the use of medical imaging
technologies and the gaze that they allow, which enables the assemblage
of *braining your life/living your brain*, we find also options for resistance
that make it possible to engage techno-scientific practices politically seriously and ontologically realistically.[94] This approach consists in the exercise of *epistemic disobedience*. In unraveling the coloniality of power[95] and
the Western matrix of power,[96] we understand that the problem with brain
research is not the brain, but the *braining of our lives* that leads us to *live our
brains* which then *reifies the brain into our lives* even further. Decolonizing
the Western matrix means to understand on the one hand, that the braining
of our lives is the outcome of the Western history of the search for the seat
of the soul, which picked up before Descartes and led from the *sensus com-
munis* as an organ to the centrality of the brain. It means to understand that
this history was enmeshed in binaries that it helped reify and that helped
stabilize it in turn, including ideas about race, gender, sex, and ableism.
On the other hand, it means to understand that brains are not (universally)
lived, and that there is no universal brain or biology, no universal self, nor
a universal culture; lives are lived differently and diffractively individuated.

The research of Hustak and Myers[97] unravels the Western language of
neo-Darwinism and shows that biological knowledges must be and also
can be far more than we allow for, whereas Gilbert et al.[98] break with the
universalizing dogma of biomedical research, that we can be analyzed as
individuals, and that individuality as a research principle allows to infer
universal, unconditional concepts. Henrich et al.[99] show that behaviors that

are assumed both rational and universal are not, and that experiments that have been conducted to explore and proof universality and rationality of behavior patterns, such as game-theory and neuro-economics, have been biased in favor of Western culture. Instead, Henrich et al.'s experiments on decision-making behavior show that behaviors and rationalities vary across cultures. Additionally, research involving animals as well as investigations of non-human agency in biology and physics is beginning to show that in the sciences the Western matrix of power is unraveling. None of these developments means that we must abandon the brain as an important object of research and clinical practice, nor that medical imaging is useless. It means to challenge any deployment of the assemblage *braining live/living the brain* or of imaging technology practices that result in acts of epistemic paternalism. It means to take epistemic disagreement seriously, and to create epistemic agreement not only reasonably but most of all responsibly.

## CONCLUSION

### "I'm Telling It Like It Really Is": Making Things Tangible and the Imperial Politics of Epistemic Authority

"I am telling you, how it really is." Epistemic paternalism is widely accepted both within expert-discourses and in expert-lay interactions. It describes the primary attitude in what Kelly Joyce on the example of medical imaging has aptly called the mode of *authoritative production of knowledge.*[100]

The enterprise of the social sciences, particularly the sociologies of science, knowledge, and technology, and science studies aka STS, despite calls and provocations to the contrary—that is, from feminist theories, new materialists, and others—has utterly failed to react critically to epistemic paternalism in situations, wherein negotiations over epistemic differences run the danger of being pre-emptively and deterministically decide by epistemic authorities. This failure is partially (con)founded in the uncritical and acquiescent acceptance of external circumstances, such as explicit knowledge regimes of neoliberalism and post-democracy stemming from the Western colonial matrix of power. More importantly, there is a tendency to uphold a "mandarinate" paternalism—pace Fritz Ringer—within the social sciences themselves, especially at their core, sociological theory: epistemic paternalism is, above and below all, a political issue. Against this logics from the Western colonial matrix of power, one can defend only through gestures of *decolonial option* and *epistemic disobedience.*

The construction of our livelihoods, our bodies, and our identity narratives (specifically regarding ageing, chronic illness, and sex&gender), as those belonging to neuronal selves and biological citizens—in other words, we as *brainified* political beings—depends on persuasive justifications through *a poetics and politics of tangible images.* Mass media and popular culture are full of such constructions, myths, and phantasms. Countless articles on ageing, gender, chronic illness are accompanied by brain-images. Television shows like *House, M.D.* feature brain scans as their secret lead-actors. Small wonder an fMRI hasn't already won an Emmy, Golden Globe, or Oscar.

The popular, neoliberal account of the body as "fully transparent" treats the "technological image" as if it were an unconditional concept. However, it is easy to see how various deployments of concepts as "unconditional" are *epistemically defective*. To resolve this recalcitrant problem toward a genuine *practical philosophy of knowledge and understanding*, we need to introduce distinctions between fact-meaning and meaning-entitlement in epistemic practices that constitute biomedical images in diagnostics and research. Both biomedical clinical and research practices include constructions of age, illness, and gender that inform and are informed by imaging technology. The actual social actor role of the imaging technology as a persuasive technology, therefore, lies in the (social) construction—not of facts—but of *entitlements*. Facts, as such, derive in the form of the practices we decide upon in further interaction; for example, forms of therapy. In other words, a technology is revealed as a social actor only in the actions that follow, thereby it is constitutive of practices because technology as a tool is inherently persuasive.

We must understand and account for what I have called the *narrative dialectics of techno-scientific seeing*, as an engine of "making up kinds," because images of the brain in research and clinical practice are being actively persuasive with regard to making illness chronic, to gendering, and to aging. Media outlets on recent research "breakthroughs" are accompanied by photos of doctors studying brain-images, television shows feature doctors practicing the art of divination while gazing onto a tapestry of brain snapshots. *Public* research on "this is your brain-disorder, really," "this is your brain on age, really," and "this is a male vs. a female brain, really" are legion. In exposing the mechanisms behind the persuasion, critique is possible and so is *better* medical and scientific practice. We must simply understand that the brain isn't everything; it is certainly not your life, nor is it unconditional. To put it in one of the most powerful terms: the brain is necessary but it is not sufficient.

## NOTES

The present chapter has profited from audiences of talks I gave between 2011 and 2014 at annual meetings of the American Sociological Association (ASA), the Society for the Social Study of Science (4S), the Society for the Study of Symbolic Interaction (SSSI), and the Northeastern Pop-Culture Association (NEPCA), as well as students in a gender course of the STS department of the Rochester Institute for Technology. I also thank my students and TAs (*Tutoren*) at Leuphana University Lüneburg who engaged and discussed literatures and knowledges with me and happily challenged my conventional views and my provocations alike over the past few years. I am indebted to Nance Cunningham and panelists for their insightful comments at 4S in Cleveland, 2011, and to Hans Bakker for reminding me of semiotics and for serving as the "image of a woman" at SSSI in New York City in 2013. I want to thank Kelly Joyce, Linnda Caporael, Nancy Campbell, Ron Eglash, Gareth Edel, Deborah Blizzard, Sebastian Deterling, and Michael Dellwing, among many others, for discussion, comment, and/or advice. I am, as always, indebted to the deterritorializing and detemporalizing dialogue with my partner in life-and-crime Sabrina M. Weiss.

1. Alexander I. Stingl and Sabrina M. Weiss, "Making Trouble," in Psychology instead of Ethics? [working title: Proceedings BMBF Wrokshop], Cordula Brand et al., eds. (London: Springer, 2015 forthcoming).
2. The mode of "interrogation" I have adopted from my collaborator Sabrina Weiss; the figure of "troubling a concept" I recently heard in a presentation by Tom Gerschick at ASA 2013 on gender and disability.
3. Wherein techno-scientific seeing is merely a case of the narrative dialectics of techno-scientific practices.
4. Timothy Morton, *Ecology without Nature* (Cambridge, MA: Harvard University Press, 2009), 14.
5. The second part of this story of visualization and seeing is the story of magnification, i.e., the story of microscopy.
6. Visualization here refers to several dimensions, the two most important of which are (1) visual representations that are materially produced and studied by experts in learning how something is supposed to look (ideal-typically), for example, anatomical illustrations, and (2) how experts imagine in the form of mental maps.
7. Irving Kenneth Zola, "Medicine as an Institution of Social Control*," *The Sociological Review* 20, no. 4 (1972): 487–504; Peter Conrad, "Medicalization and Social Control," *Annual Review of Sociology* 18 (1992): 209–32; Conrad, *The Medicalization of Society: On the Transformation of Human Conditions into Treatable Disorders* (Baltimore: Johns Hopkins University Press, 2007).
8. This is how I understand the concept of critique.
9. Peter Conrad is one of many typical representatives of the critical rather than polemical use of the concept.
10. In my view, polemics is almost always a bad tactic and counter-productive. It promotes the polemic individual's prestige but not the matter of concern. In rare cases of political deadlock and in the face of dominating powers (here I mind the difference between antagonism&domination as one side, and agonism&hegemony on the other), it is an extreme measure that can prove effective to create new room to maneuver, usually not for polemicist but her allies. In terms of Michel Foucault and Michel deCerteau, I would stress that polemics is always a tactic; it never works, i.e., it misfires as a strategy.
11. Both migraine and depression are highly "gendered" issues as well as subject to the deployment of medical imaging technologies and brain scanning.
12. An issue of gender as well as culture. Emma K. Jones, Janelle R. Jurgenson, Judith M. Katzenellenbogen, and Sandra C. Thompson, "Menopause and the Influence of Culture: Another Gap for Indigenous Australian Women?," *BMC Women's Health* 12, no. 1 (2012): 43, doi:10.1186/1472-6874-12-43; Margaret M. Lock, *Encounters with Aging Mythologies of Menopause in Japan and North America* (London: University of California Press, 1993); M. Lock and P. Kaufert, "Menopause, Local Biologies, and Cultures of Aging," *American Journal of Human Biology* 13, no. 4 (2001): 494–504, doi:10.1002/ajhb.1081.

13. At the 2013 meeting of the American Sociological Association, a panel on the creation and implications of the newest, fifth edition of the influential *Diagnostic and Statistical Manual of Mental Disorders* (*DSM 5*) revealed an interesting paradox in a several anecdotes that were shared and discussed by the presenters. Since the American National Institute for Mental Health (NIMH), dissatisfied with the *DSM 5*, decided to create its own dialog of criteria for mental illness instead, sociologists inquiring about the impact of this decision for both research and clinical practice encountered a puzzle. Many researchers seemed of the opinion that the *DSM* was used by clinical practitioners and had little value for research, meaning that they only used its categories for grant proposals, IRBs, policy consulting, and other administrative rather than practical purposes. Clinical practitioners, it was reported, largely did not use the *DSM* for diagnosing and treating patients but only for administrative purposes, such as dealing with health care insurance providers, journalists, and so on, and we are told that otherwise clinical practitioners were of the opinion that it was researchers that use the *DSM*. Now if these anecdotes have a basis in fact, and from the discussions it seems they do, but we would need genuine sociological research on the matter, the curious question arises, who actually used (and uses) this "curious artifact" called the *DSM*? We can assume that involved political, administrative, and public/lay agents circulated constructions that have unfolded an intriguing "kind-making" power that obtains while being detached from the agents of clinical and empirical research practice.

14. The difference between critique and polemical use applies equally to the concept of biomedicalization as it does to the entire argument presented here.

15. Victoria Pitts-Taylor, "The Plastic Brain: Neoliberalism and the Neuronal Self," *Health* 14, no. 6 (2010): 635–52; Nikolas S. Rose, *Politics of Life Itself: Biomedicine, Power, and Subjectivity in the Twenty-First Century* (Princeton, NJ: Princeton University Press, 2007).

16. Rabinow in Sahra Gibbon and Carlos Novas, *Biosocialities, Genetics and the Social Sciences: Making Biologies and Identities* (New York: Routledge Press, 2008).

17. Adele Clarke, Laura Mamo, Jennifer Ruth Fosket, Jennifer R. Fishman, and Janet K. Shim, eds., *Biomedicalization: Technoscience, Health, and Illness in the United States* (Durham, NC: Duke University Press, 2007).

18. Ibid.

19. In the research work that I am conducting with Sabrina M. Weiss, we are pointing out, however, that techno-scientific practices include both categories that we distinguish as high-tech and low-tech practices; and one of our main caveats regarding STS discourses on biomedicalization and related fields is in their focus on high-tech practices, these discourses are reifying the distinction high-tech/no-tech imperially.

20. On origins of the concept *biomedicalization*, C.I. Cohen, "The Biomedicalization of Psychiatry: A Critical Overview," *Community Mental Health Journal* 29, no. 6 (1993): 509–21; C.L. Estes and E.A. Binney, "The Biomedicalization of Aging: Dangers and Dilemmas," *The Gerontologist* 29, no. 5 (1989): 587–96; Karen A. Lyman, "Bringing the Social Back In: A Critique of the Biomedicalization of Dementia," *The Gerontologist* 29, no. 5 (1989): 597–605, doi:10.1093/geront/29.5.597.

21. Ibid.

22. Rose, *Politics of Life*.

23. Joelle M. Abi-Rached and Nikolas Rose, "The Birth of the Neuromolecular Gaze," *History of the Human Sciences* 23, no. 1 (2010): 11–36.

24. Monica J. Casper and Daniel R Morrison, "Medical Sociology and Technology: Critical Engagements," *Journal of Health and Social Behavior* 51 (2010): S120–32.

25. João Biehl, Byron Good, and Arthur Kleinman, eds., *Subjectivity: Ethnographic Investigations* (Berkeley: University of California Press, 2007).

26. Stuart J. Murray, "Care and the Self: Biotechnology, Reproduction, and the Good Life," *Philosophy, Ethics, and Humanities in Medicine* 2, no. 1 (2007); Alexander Stingl, "The Virtualization of Health and Illness in the Age of Biological Citizenship," *TeloScope*, http://www.telospress.com/author/stingl/.

27. Pitts-Taylor, "Plastic Brain"; Catherine Malabou, *What Should We Do with Our Brain?* (New York: Fordham University Press, 2008); Bernard Stiegler, *Taking Care of Youth and Generations* (Stanford, CA: Stanford University Press, 2010).

28. Sabrina M. Weiss, Sal Restivo, and Alexander I. Stingl, *Worlds of Science-Craft: New Horizons in Philosophy, Sociology, and Science Studies* (Surrey, UK: Ashgate. 2014).

29. Kelly A. Joyce, *Magnetic Appeal: MRI and the Myth of Transparency* (Ithaca, NY: Cornell University Press, 2008).

30. This combination of transparency and depth (myth of total interiorization), and the opportunities of intervention it supposedly empowers its users to wield (myth of total control), I have described elsewhere in the two notions of *hyper-differentiation* and *hyper-universalization*, which combine into a process of ongoing *virtualization*. Alexander Stingl, "The ADHD Regime and Neuro-chemical Selves in Whole Systems. A Science Studies Perspective," in *Health and Environment: Social Science Perspectives*, ed. Helena Kopnina and Hans Keune, 157–86 (New York: Nova Science, 2010); Weiss et al., *Worlds of ScienceCraft*; Alexander Stingl, "Digital FairGround," *Current Perspectives in Social Theory* 32 (2015): 53–93.

31. Amit Prasad, "Making Images/Making Bodies: Visibilizing and Disciplining through Magnetic Resonance Imaging (MRI)," *Science, Technology, and Human Values* 30, no. 2 (2005): 292.

32. Hannah Fitsch, "(A)e(s)th(et)ics of Brain Imaging. Visibilities and Sayabilities in Functional Magnetic Resonance Imaging," *Neuroethics* 5, no. 3 (2012): 275–83; Adina L. Roskies, "Neuroimaging and Inferential Distance," *Neuroethics* 1, no. 1 (2008): 19–30; Laura Perini, "Truth-Bearers or Truth-Makers?," *Spontaneous Generations: A Journal for the History and Philosophy of Science* 6, no. 1 (2012): 142–47; Stephen M. Downes, "How Much Work Do Scientific Images Do?," *Spontaneous Generations: A Journal for the History and Philosophy of Science* 6, no. 1 (2012): 115–30.

33. It must be noted that the notion of "objectivity" and of representing/mediating visual reality "as it really is" does not and has never held true for even photography itself.

34. With Peeter Selg, [Peeter Selg, "The Politics of Theory and the Constitution of Meaning," *Sociological Theory* 31, no. 1 (2013): 1–23, doi:10.1177/0735275113479933.] I distinguish three normative frameworks for politics of theory and methodology: consensual mainstreaming, antagonistic exclusivism, and agonistic pluralism. But I do reject naive absolutist stances such as bald naturalism/physicalist reductionism or hyper-constructivisms, precisely because absolutism leads to antagonism and can only be resolved through a meager synthesis of irreconcilable positions that are then mainstreamed, or through polemical destruction of alternative positions. Neither is an attractive, scientifically sound alternative, even though the latter tactic is often chosen by some actors who claim to speak "in the name of science."

35. Christine Hsu, "Gay Gene" Survived Evolution As It Is Carried by Mothers Who Have More Children, Study," *Medical Daily*, 2012, http://www.medicaldaily.com/gay-gene-survived-evolution-it-carried-mothers-who-have-more-children-study-240813; Andrea S. Camperio Ciani, Lilybeth Fontanesi, Francesca Iemmola, Elga Giannella, Claudia Ferron, and Luigi Lombardi, "Factors Associated with Higher Fecundity in Female Maternal Relatives of Homosexual Men," *Journal of Sexual Medicine* 9, no. 11 (2012): 2878–87; Alexandra Sifferlin, "New Genes IDd in Obesity: How Much of Weight Is Genetic?," *Time*, http://healthland.time.com/2013/07/19/news-genes-idd-in-obesity-how-much-of-weight-is-genetic/; Liuyan Zhang, Suhua Chang, Zhao Li, Kunlin Zhang, Yang Du, Jurg Ott, and Jing Wang, "ADHD Gene: A Genetic Database for Attention Deficit Hyperactivity Disorder," *Nucleic Acids Research* 40 (2012): D1003–9; Steven Reinberg, "Shared Genes May Link ADHD, Autism, and Depression," http://www.webmd.com/add-adhd/news/20130227/shared-genes-may-link-adhd-autism-and-depression (accessed September 13, 2013); Josephine Elia, Joseph T Glessner, Kai Wang, Nagahide Takahashi, Corina J. Shtir, Dexter Hadley, and Patrick M. A. Sleiman, "Genome-Wide Copy Number Variation Study Associates Metabotropic Glutamate Receptor Gene Networks with Attention Deficit Hyperactivity Disorder," *Nature Genetics* 44, no. 1 (2011): 78–84.
36. Steve Ramirez, Xu Liu, Pei-Ann Lin, Junghyup Suh, Michele Pignatelli, Roger L. Redondo, Tomás J. Ryan, and Susumu Tonegawa, "Creating a False Memory in the Hippocampus," *Science* 341 (2013): 387–91.
37. Ilana Singh, "Brain Talk: Power and Negotiation in Children's Discourse about Self, Brain and Behavior," *Sociology of Health and Illness* 35 (2013): 813–27.
38. David Allen Karp, *Is It Me or My Meds? Living with Antidepressants* (Cambridge, MA: Harvard University Press, 2006).
39. "Events" is here taken to mean a variety of things, including the commitment to a pharmacological regime, such as treating a child with ADHD medication.
40. Although thought-experiments in the philosophy of mind and neuro-cognition involving a "brain in a vat" are often based on this ideology. This position, however, cannot really hold up when challenged by a view called enactivism. Alva Noë, *Out of Our Heads—Why You Are Not Your Brain, and Other Lessons from the Biology of Consciousness* (New York: Hill and Wang, 2009). Enactivist arguments show convincingly that conception and perception are linked together through practice and that any brain in a vat necessarily depends on "helping" parts to maintain itself. These parts, when accounted for, functionally resemble a body in an environment up to the point where there is no more difference to a human being with an actual body interacting in an environment. In short, you can't *have* "just a brain" to *be there* at all.
41. Uli Linke, "Contact Zones: Rethinking the Sensual Life of the State," *Anthropological Theory* 6, no. 2 (2006): 205–25; Alexander Stingl, "How to Map the Body's Spaces: Using Foucault's Heterotopology for the Cartography of Corporeal Myths," in *Proceedings of the Conference Held at the University of Bucharest, 6–8 October 2011*, http://www.unibuc.ro/n/resurse/myth-maki-and-myth-brea-in-hist-and-the-huma/docs/2012/iul/02_12_54_31Proceedings_Myth_Making_and_Myth_Breaking_in_History.pdf; Renee Marlin-Bennett, "Embodied Information, Knowing Bodies, and Power," *Millennium–Journal of International Studies*, online first (May 2013).
42. James Read, "The Althusser-Effect: Philosophy, History, Temporality," *Borderlands* 4, no. 2 (2005): http://www.borderlands.net.au/vol4no2_2005/read_effect.htm.

43. Of course, that the idea of a singular timeline can be critiqued is not itself a novelty item. Althusser, for example, produced a critique of historicism that famously argued that history cannot be measured against such a monolinear time-stream. "Althusser somewhat cryptically states that the origins of this conception of time are to be found in 'the false obviousness of everyday practice.' . . . Hegel is instructive not as the originator of a particular understanding of time and history, but as the one whom perhaps first rendered it explicit" [read "the Althusser-effect"]." What we are currently discovering, however, is that temporalities can and must be diffractively negotiated, and that (or because of) the realization that the (political) nonhuman agency, i.e., things/ materialities, must also be accounted for, where Althusser and others focused on immaterial social structures.

44. One might like to call this, evoking Barad and Haraway, a *temporal diffractive perspective.*

45. Adina L. Roskies, "Neuroimaging and Inferential Distance," *Neuroethics* 1, no. 1 (2008): 19–30.

46. Owing to constraints of space, a section on ageing had to cut from this chapter. Also, the original was referencing four times as much literature. I apologize for what may seem as obvious omissions. I may either really be ignorant of them or was lacking space here.

47. There are, of course, also class [C. J. Gilleard, *Contexts of Ageing: Class, Cohort, and Community* (Cambridge: Polity, 2005); Alex Dumas and Suzanne Laberge, "Social Class and Ageing Bodies: Understanding Physical Activity in Later Life," *Social Theory and Health* 3, no. 3 (2005): 183–205, doi:10.1057/ palgrave.sth.8700056]; race/ethnicity [Jan E. Mutchler and Jeffrey A. Burr, "Race, Ethnicity, and Aging," in *Handbook of Sociology of Aging*, ed. Richard A. Settersten and Jacqueline L. Angel, 83–101 (New York: Springer, 2011), 83–101, http://link.springer.com/chapter/10.1007/978-1-4419-7374-0_6.], cultural, and post-colonial [Louise Racine, "Implementing a Postcolonial Feminist Perspective in Nursing Research Related to non-Western Populations," *Nursing Inquiry* 10, no. 2 (2003): 91–102] constructions of ageing.

48. Jay Stevens (EHwell), "Menopause Lane . . . The Unknown Path for Many!," http://ehwell.com/patient-info/easyblog/entry/menopause-lane-the-unknown-path-for-many.html (accessed September 16, 2013)

49. Victor W. Henderson and Michael D. Greicius, "Functional Magnetic Resonance Imaging and Estrogen Effects on the Brain: Cautious Interpretation of a BOLD Finding," *Menopause*, May 1, 2010.

50. Shaunancy Ferro, "This Is What Experiencing a Hot Flash Looks Like," *Popular Science*, http://www.popsci.com/science/article/2013–07/what-experiencing-hot-flash-looks.

51. Neurosciencestuff, "Scientists Identify Neural Origins of Hot Flashes in Menopausal Women," *Neuroscience*, http://media.wayne.edu/2013/07/15/wayne-State-University-Scientists-Identify-Neural-;http://neurosciencestuff.tumblr.com/post/55640319218/scientists-identify-neural-origins-of-hot-flashes-in.

52. Gwang-Woo Jeong, Kwangsung Park, Gahyun Youn, Heoung-Keun Kang, Hyung Joong Kim, Jeong-Jin Seo, and Soo-Bang Ryu, "Assessment of Cerebrocortical Regions Associated with Sexual Arousal in Premenopausal and Menopausal Women by Using BOLD-Based Functional MRI," *Journal of Sexual Medicine* 2, no. 5 (2005): 645–51, doi:10.1111/j.1743-6109.2005.00134.x.

53. Reviewing research articles and science publications on the biology of female sexuality, and having female informants on this subject matter, I am under the impression that researchers—who are more often male than not—do not really know much about women, or sex, or both. The cited study is a case in point.

I have not met many women who would find watching an 'erotic' clip sexually arousing, least of all in a research setting, lying in a noisy fMRI-machine. "A simple reality—the fact that when it comes to sex, people are different from each other, and can even differ from their own earlier selves—is obscured by people's need to overgeneralize their own desires and discomforts" (Bronski et al., "Is Lesbian Sex 'Real Sex,'" *Slate*, October 3, 2013, http://www.slate.com/blogs/outward/2013/10/03/is_lesbian_sex_real_sex.html (accessed June 20, 2014).

54. It should be noted that a corresponding concept of andropause, which affects men, is a disputed concept. While there is no trouble in finding research on menopause in general, and using medical imaging technologies in particular, I found research on andropause sparse and had so far no success in digging up brain-imaging studies on andropause. This one-sidedness in the menopause/andropause discourse could be seen as an example of the exercise of paternalism and male hegemony that is embedded in cyborg visuality.
55. Nasim Maleki, Clas Linnman, Jennifer Brawn, Rami Burstein, Lino Becerra, and David Borsook, "Her versus His Migraine: Multiple Sex Differences in Brain Function and Structure," *Brain* 135, no. 8 (2012): 2546–59, doi:10.1093/brain/aws175.
56. Joanna Kempner, "Gendering the Migraine Market: Do Representations of Illness Matter?," *Social Science and Medicine* 63, no. 8 (2006): 1986–97.
57. http://www.webmd.com/balance/features/how-male-female-brains-differ (accessed June 28, 2014).
58. Anne Fausto-Sterling, *Sexing the Body: Gender Politics and the Construction of Sexuality* (New York: Basic Books, 2000).
59. Erik H. Chudler, "He Brains, She Brains," http://faculty.washington.edu/chudler/heshe.html.
60. Joyce, *Magnetic Appeal.*
61. Robyn Bluhm, "New Research, Old Problems: Methodological and Ethical Issues in fMRI Research Examining Sex/Gender Differences in Emotion Processing," *Neuroethics* 6, no. 2 (2013): 319–30.
62. Joanna Kempner, "Gendering the Migraine Market: Do Representations of Illness Matter?," *Social Science and Medicine* 63, no. 8 (2006): 1986–97.
63. Evelyn Birge Vitz and Paul Vitz, "Women, Abortion, and the Brain," *Public Discourse*, http://www.thepublicdiscourse.com/2010/09/1657/.
64. Ibid.
65. One may argue here, in the same vein, whether men make good stock traders because they are influenced by higher levels of testosterone, which makes them take more risks. Following a successful experience, they are driven to take riskier decisions than women would. However, in contrast to arguing about women's ability to make their own health decisions, a similarly public and lively discourse on men, their brains, and their hormones cannot be found.
66. Erika Packard, "The Brain in the Voting Booth," hhttp://www.apa.org/monitor/feb08/brain.aspx.
67. http://www.youtube.com/watch?v=CWAR7FeY4pA&feature=related (accessed October 15, 2013).
68. Cited in Brian Greene, "Santorum Says Emotions Too Strong to Allow Women in Front-Line Combat," http://www.usnews.com/news/articles/2012/02/10/santorum-says-emotions-too-strong-to-allow-women-in-front-line-combat.
69. Barbara Tversky, "Narratives of Space, Time, and Life," *Mind and Language* 19, no. 4 (2004): 380–92.
70. Which is why I speak of a *narrative dialectic.*
71. Sung Ho Kim, "Max Weber," in *The Stanford Encyclopedia of Philosophy*, ed. Edward N. Zalta, http://plato.stanford.edu/archives/fall2012/entries/weber/.

72. *See* Timothy Morton, *Ecology without Nature* (Cambridge, MA: Harvard University Press, 2009).

73. For why this imagination, precisely because it is political, cannot be ultimately grounded and, thus, inheres the epistemic gap, and why it is, therefore, inseparably intertwined with ontology, see Oliver Marchart's overview of post-foundationalism and William Connolly's and Jane Bennett's works on becoming and affect in political theory. Oliver Marchart, *Die Politische Differenz* (Berlin: Suhrkamp, 2010); Marchart, *Post-foundational Political Thought: Political Difference in Nancy, Lefort, Badiou and Laclau* (Edinburgh: Edinburgh University Press, 2007); William E. Connolly, *A World of Becoming* (Durham, NC: Duke University Press, 2010).

74. Ernst E. Boesch, "The Myth of Lurking Chaos," in *Between Culture and Biology: Perspectives on Ontogenetic Development*, ed. Heidi Keller (Cambridge: Cambridge University Press, 2002).

75. Alternatively, we could say they result in "over-coding."

76. Boesch, "The Myth."

77. Lisa Feldman Barrett, "Psychological Construction: The Darwinian Approach to the Science of Emotion," *Emotion Review* 5, no. 4 (2013): 379–89.

78. Fritz Breithaupt's (I consider them: temporalizing) cultures of empathy [Fritz Breithaupt, *Kulturen Der Empathie* (Frankfurt: Suhrkamp, 2008)] are complemented by Suzanne Keen's (spatializing) forms of empathy [Suzanne Keen, "Empathetic Hardy: Bounded, Ambassadorial, and Broadcast Strategies of Narrative Empathy," *Poetics Today* 32, no. 2 (2011): 349–89] and Jeffrey Alexander's (discursive) modes of integration [Jeffrey C. Alexander, "Theorizing the 'Modes of Incorporation': Assimilation, Hyphenation, and Multiculturalism as Varieties of Civil Participation," *Sociological Theory* 19, no. 3 (2001): 237–49, doi:10.1111/0735–2751.00139].

79. Weiss et al., *Worlds of ScienceCraft*; Alexander I. Stingl and Sabrina M Weiss, "Mindfulness as/Is Care," in *Wiley-Blackwell Handbook of Mindfulness*, ed. Ellen Langer, Amanda Ie, and Christelle T. Ngnoume, 608–29 (Hoboken, NJ: Wiley-Blackwell, 2014).

80. Suzanne Keen, "Empathetic Hardy: Bounded, Ambassadorial, and Broadcast Strategies of Narrative Empathy," *Poetics Today* 32, no. 2 (2011): 364f.

81. "Inferential distance is a relational measure, so in explicating inferential distance we need to specify the relata. The inferential relata for any scientific program are interest-relative, as dictated by the scientific project. The goal of cognitive neuroscience is to map functional components of mind to neural structures." Adina L. Roskies, "Neuroimaging and Inferential Distance," *Neuroethics* 1, no. 1 (2008): 19–30, doi:10.1007/s12152-007-9003-3.

82. Roskies, "Neuroimaging."

83. Owing to lack of space, a ten-page-long explication of *epistemic gap* had to be dropped from this chapter.

84. Roskies, "Neuroimaging," 30.

85. Bjorn Hofmann, "The Technological Invention of Disease," *Med Humanities* 27, no. 1 (2001): 10–19.

86. Alexander Stingl, "Digital FairGround: The Virtualization of Health and Illness, and the Experience of 'Becoming Patient' as a Problem of Political Ontology and Social Justice," *Current Perspectives of Social Theory* 32 (2015): 53–93.

87. Hofmann, "Technological Invention," 17.

88. Ibid., 10.

89. Ibid., 14.

90. In a similar vein, S. Fredriksen, "Diseases Are Invisible," *Medical Humanities* 28, no. 2 (2002), doi:10.1136/mh.28.2.71, writes,

The success of medial technology has led to an unavoidable distrust of our own senses. Our everyday knowledge is devalued. We know more about diseases today than ever before, but lack confidence in this knowledge. We do not feel sure whether we will perceive any symptoms before it is too late. In despair, we seek medial expertise and technology to interpret and alleviate our worries. Uncertainty prevails because problems often narrow down to a sense transcendent question: is there a test that ought to be taken, is there a question that ought to be asked. Medical success is paid for by a lack of unity and control . . . We have to learn to live with the possibilities opened up by the technology—without being completely seduced by them. Medicine is, at rock bottom, a normative and not a technoscientific enterprise. Values such as care, compassion, and solidarity give medicine direction and legitimation, not sense transcendence, precision or truth as such. Technology is a valuable tool in the pursuit of normative ends, but it is not an end in itself. (72–73)

91. I am not arguing here that this is some sinister conspiracy of the pharmaceutical industry nor any particular group's or individual person's fault. In following Foucault, who understood power not as a concept to describe structural relations of dominance and oppression but as a concept to interrogate relations that are constructive, transformative, and ultimately dialectical conditions for knowledge and for selves. These relations are, therefore, considered governmental: We cannot ever fully exist outside and free of relations of this kind, nor must we despair and think our efforts to make a difference are in vain. Foucault understands the Kantian concept of *critique* to mean a form of resistance to understand the conditions that are necessary (while not sufficient) for a situation to exist that one is enmeshed in as a subjectivity, and which kinds of articulation and practices can be deployed to make difference; in other words, critique is a form of resistance that allows one "not to be governed as much." For the situation of clinical reasoning and interactions involving medical images, as well for communications between researchers, gatekeepers, research commissioners and regulators, as well as implicated parties, such as concerned stakeholders and or side-affected publics, this boils down to understanding the doctor-patient or science-public situation as such:

> It's not about not trusting your doctors or not trusting scientists, it's about how we mutually enable trust by understanding our respective epistemic responsibilities, and engage in our practices with others accordingly.

92. Says Gillian Russel, "Epistemic Viciousness," in *Martial Arts and Philosophy: Beating and Nothingness*, ed. Graham Priest and Damon Young, 129–44 (Chicago: Open Court, 2010):

> *Epistemic* means having to do with beliefs and their justification. *Viciousness* normally suggests deliberate cruelty and violence: *possessing of vices.* (The opposite being a *virtue.*) Vices (such as avarice, alcoholism and nail-biting) are ordinary things, and most of us struggle with a few, but *epistemic* vices are defects with respect to the formation of beliefs. (129).

93. It is obvious that I take Susan Buck-Morss's account of Walter Benjamin a lot further. Susan Buck-Morss, *The Dialectics of Seeing: Walter Benjamin and the Arcades Project* (Cambridge, MA: MIT Press, 1989).

94. Oliver Marchart, *Die Politische Differenz* (Berlin: Suhrkamp, 2010); Chandra Mukerji, "The Territorial State as a Figured World of Power: Strategics, Logistics, and Impersonal Rule*," *Sociological Theory* 28, no. 4 (2010): 402–24; Patrick Carroll, "Water, and Technoscientific State Formation in California,"

*Social Studies of Science*, March 2012; Alexander Stingl and Sabrina M. Weiss, "Beyond and before the Label: The Ecologies and Agencies of ADHD," in *Krankheitskonstruktionen Und Krankheitstreiberei*, ed. Michael Dellwing and Martin Harbusch, 201–31 (Wiesbaden: Springer Fachmedien Wiesbaden, 2013).

95. Maria Lugones, "Heterosexualism and the Colonial/Modern Gender System," *Hypatia* 22, no. 1 (2007): 186–209.
96. Walter D. Mignolo, "The Geopolitics of Knowledge and the Colonial Difference," *South Atlantic Quarterly* 101, no. 1 (2002): 57–96; Walter Mignolo, *The Darker Side of Western Modernity* (Durham, NC: Duke University Press, 2012).
97. Carla Hustak and Natasha Myers, "Involutionary Momentum: Affective Ecologies and the Sciences of Plant/Insect Encounters," *Differences* 23, no. 3 (2012): 74–118.
98. Scott F. Gilbert, Jan Sapp, and Alfred I Tauber, "A Symbiotic View of Life: We Have Never Been Individuals," *Quarterly Review of Biology* 87, no. 4 (2012): 325–41.
99. Joe Henrich, Steven Heine, and Ara Norenzayay, "The Weirdest People in the World?," *The Behavioral and Brain Sciences* 33, nos. 2–3 (2010): 61–135.
100. Joyce, *Magnetic Appeal*.

# Contributors

**Stanley H. Ambrose** received his PhD in anthropology at the University of California, Berkeley, in 1984. Following post-doctoral research at UCLA on isotopic analysis of the evolution of the human diet, he joined the anthropology faculty at the University of Illinois, where he heads the Environmental Isotope Paleobiogeochemistry Laboratory. He conducts archaeological, paleoanthropological, geological, and ecological research in Kenya, Ethiopia, and India and laboratory research on environmental and dietary reconstruction with stable isotopes. His current research focuses on the evolution of modern human capacities for cooperation, planning, and language and the environmental, demographic, and evolutionary impacts of the Toba supereruption.

**Celia Andreu-Sánchez** is associate professor of media, advertising, and journalism at Universitat Autònoma de Barcelona and Universitat de Girona and head of the Neuro-Com Research Group at Universitat Autònoma de Barcelona. She is also a researcher at División de Neurociencias at Universidad Pablo Olavide in Sevilla, headed by Professor José María Delgado-García, and she is an iOS developer. She holds a PhD in communication at the Universidad Rey Juan Carlos in Madrid; a MS in psychobiology and cognitive neuroscience at Universitat Autònoma de Barcelona; a BA in audiovisual communication; a MA in audiovisual communication and in advertising at the Universitat Autònoma de Barcelona; and the Advanced Neuroimaging's Course in Cognitive Sciences and Psychiatry by the Department of Psychiatry and Forensic Medicine at the Universitat Autònoma de Barcelona (Barcelona Biomedical Research Park) (http://www.neuro-com.es).

**Luis Rocha Antunes** was a Harvard University Fellow in 2013–14 and a Visiting Fellow for the Danish Ministry of Science, Technology, and Innovation at the University of Copenhagen in 2009–10. He is PhD candidate and lecturer in film studies at the University of Kent and the Norwegian University of Science and Technology, with funding from the Portuguese Foundation for Science and Technology. His research interests include film perception, experiential film aesthetics, Norwegian cinema, world cinema, and Arctic film. He coined the concept of multisensory film experience, and has published articles on various related topics appearing in Queens University Press, *Essays in Philosophy, Film International and Journal of Scandinavian Cinema.*"

**Andrée E. C. Betancourt** is an adjunct assistant professor of communication studies, theater, and film at Northern Virginia Community College. Dr. Betancourt received her PhD in communication studies from Louisiana State University, and she was awarded a Graduate School Dissertation Fellowship for "Under Construction: Recollecting the Museum of the Moving Image," a study that demonstrates ways in which we recollect our memories and ourselves through museum-going and technologies of reproduction. A freelance writer and editor for a national consulting firm in the D.C. area, Dr. Betancourt has worked in the film industry and for numerous arts and cultural institutions in the United States and Europe. Her research centers on the relationship between popular culture and new communication technology, with a focus on representations of memory and cultural identity located in moving images, cultural institutions, and related virtual communities. Betancourt's work appears in *Television and the Self: Knowledge, Identity and Media Representation* (2013), and http://www.DreBetancourt.net features her portfolio.

**Dana Coester** is an assistant professor in the Reed College of Media at West Virginia University and serves as the creative director for the media innovation center. She helped direct several award-winning interactive campaigns as the assistant vice president for branding and creative direction for WVU's University Relations division, and she designed the award-winning multimedia website "Starting Over: Loss and Renewal in Katrina's Aftermath." She has more that fifteen years of experience in magazine publishing and communication design, working as an art director and contributor with Time, Inc. Her work examines the future of storytelling with special interests in creative direction, multimedia, experimental media co-creation, and new narrative forms at the intersection of digital storytelling and neuroscience. Coester earned her master's degree in journalism from the University of Missouri-Columbia in 1993.

**Steven Gibson** earned a master's degree in communication studies at California State University, Northridge and is working toward a doctorate in education at Northcentral University. His research has focused on questions of cognition and communication. Some of his studies have addressed how people respond to mediated communication and communicate about conflict. He has presented at conferences relating to computer science, artificial intelligence, human communications, and conflict resolution. He has written a series of published newspaper editorials on community issues and given trainings on listening skills and community involvement. Steven also has written articles and chapters in academic collections on the topics of computer science and cognitive research.

**Michael Grabowski** is an associate professor of communication at Manhattan College in New York City. He has won two Emmy Awards and several awards at film festivals for his work on feature films, documentaries, television programs, commercials, music videos, and new media. His work examines how different forms of mediated communication shape the way people think and act within their symbolic environment. His interest in neurocinematics led him to become a scholar-in-residence at NYU's Center for Neural Science in 2009. Currently Grabowski conducts research for clients that include top broadcast and cable television networks, producers, and new media companies. He earned a PhD in culture and communication from New York University in 2006.

**Jenell Johnson** is an assistant professor of communication arts at the University of Wisconsin-Madison, where she is also affiliate faculty in the life sciences communication and the Holtz Center for science and technology studies. She is the author of *American Lobotomy: A Rhetorical History* (2014). With Melissa Littlefield (University of Illinois at Urbana-Champaign), she has published *The Neuroscientific Turn: Transdisciplinarity in the Age of the Brain* (2012), a groundbreaking collection of academic essays that explores the rapid rush to "neuro-fy" academic disciplines (such as neurosociology, neuroeconomics, and neurohistory). She has published essays in Quarterly Journal of Speech, *Rhetoric Society Quarterly, Journal of Advanced Composition, Medicine Studies, Journal of Literary and Cultural Disability Studies*, and *Advances in Medical Sociology: Sociological Perspectives on Neuroscience*.

**Mauri Kaipainen** is professor of media technology at Södertörn University (Sweden). He studied education, musicology, and cognitive science at the University of Helsinki and earned his PhD in 1994 on a computational model of music cognition. His research agenda is built around the concept of interactively explorable multi-perspective media that are based on ontospaces, spatially defined ontologies, associated with content metadata. In addition to interactive and systemic approaches to narrative, the concept has applications in media art, collaborative and community media applications, learning environments, collaborative knowledge management, expert systems, and societal participation.

**Elise E. Labbé** is a professor of psychology and director of clinical training at the University of South Alabama. She also taught at Virginia Polytechnic Institute and State University and the University of Miami. Dr. Labbé received her BA in psychology from Loyola University, New Orleans and her MA and PhD in clinical psychology from Louisiana State University. Dr. Labbé has published more than seventy professional, peer-reviewed publications in clinical and health psychology and has presented at more than ninety regional, national, and international conferences. Dr. Labbé recently published *Psychology Moment by Moment: A Guide to Enhancing Your Clinical Practice with Mindfulness and Meditation* (2011). She teaches undergraduate health psychology and graduate courses in advanced health psychology, and clinical and counseling psychology practicum for the combined clinical/counseling psychology doctoral program. She has developed both clinical and research programs on mindfulness and health.

**Robert C. MacDougall** is professor of communication at Curry College in Massachusetts. He is the author of *Digination: Identity, Organization, and Public Life in the Age of Small Digital Devices and Big Digital Domains* (2011) and the editor of *Drugs and Media: New Perspectives on Communication, Consumption, and Consciousness* (2012). Dr. MacDougall's research centers around the social, political, and cognitive roles communication media have played throughout history. He teaches courses with a special focus on the progressive use of the Internet as a news-gathering apparatus, a venue for social interaction in general and political life in particular. MacDougall earned his PhD from the State University of New York at Albany.

**Miguel Ángel Martín-Pascual** is associate professor of media and journalism in Universitat Autònoma de Barcelona and is head of training at the Spanish Public Television RTVE at Barcelona. He is an iOS developer and a member of the Neuro-Com Research Group at Universitat Autònoma de Barcelona. He also is a researcher at División de Neurociencias at Universidad Pablo Olavide in Sevilla, headed by Professor José María Delgado-García. He holds a DEA in communication at Universitat Autònoma de Barcelona; a MS in psychobiology and cognitive neuroscience at Universitat Autònoma de Barcelona; a BA and MA in politics and sociology at Universidad Complutense de Madrid; and the Advanced Neuroimaging's Course in Cognitive Sciences and Psychiatry by the Department of Psychiatry and Forensic Medicine of the Universitat Autònoma de Barcelona (Barcelona Biomedical Research Park) (http://www.neuro-com.es).

**Emilia Musumeci** is temporary lecturer in criminal justice at the University of Catania, Italy. Her primary research interests are legal history, criminology, and history of medicine. In 2012 she earned a PhD in "Profiles of Citizenship in the Construction of Europe," in the curriculum of history and philosophy of law, with a thesis on the legacy of biological theories of crime that emerged during the second half of the nineteenth century in the current neuroscience and law debate. Among her publications are the book *Cesare Lombroso e le neuroscienze: un parricidio mancato* (2012) and the essays "New Natural Born Killers? The Legacy of Lombroso in Neuroscience and Law," in Paul Knepper and Per Jørgen Ystehede's *The Cesare Lombroso Handbook* (Routledge, 2012), and "The Positivist School of Criminology and the Italian Fascist Criminal Law: A Squandered Legacy?," in Stephen Skinner's *Fascism and Criminal Law: History, Theory, Continuity* (forthcoming).

**Farah Qureshi,** MHS, is a doctoral candidate in social and behavioral sciences at the Harvard School of Public Health, with research interests that focus on social factors that influence the well-being of children and youth. Upon the completion of her training, she looks forward to working across disciplines to promote evidence-based policies and programs that give young people the opportunity to become healthy, educated, and empowered adults. Farah received a master's degree from the Johns Hopkins Bloomberg School of Public Health, where she studied child development and health communications, and a bachelor's degree in writing from the Johns Hopkins University.

**Michael Rich,** MD, MPH, FAAP, FSAHM, is an associate professor at Harvard Medical School and Harvard School of Public Health. Dr. Rich came to medicine after a twelve-year career as a filmmaker (including serving as assistant director to Akira Kurosawa on *Kagemusha*). As the Mediatrician® (http://www.askthemediatrician.org) and director of the Center on Media and Child Health (http://www.cmch.tv) at Boston Children's Hospital, Dr. Rich combines his creative experience with rigorous scientific evidence to advise pediatricians, parents, and other caregivers on how to use media in ways that optimize child health and development. Recipient of the AAP's Holroyd-Sherry Award and the SAHM New Investigator Award, Dr. Rich has developed media-based research methodologies and authored numerous papers and AAP policy statements, has testified to the U.S. Congress, and makes regular national press appearances.

**Bob Schapiro** is a journalist and filmmaker whose current China documentary won an Emmy Award in New York City, where he has written and produced newscasts for WCBS and WNBC. He also reported from El Salvador, Nicaragua, and Lebanon, and, more recently, from Afghanistan. He wrote and directed *Pirates of New York* with Walter Cronkite and *Geisha, Keisha* and *American Pie*. His varied writing career includes credits for several national commercials and an off-Broadway revue. He teaches at Fordham University in the Department of Communication and Media Studies and is completing his PhD dissertation at Drew University. E-mail: bob@newsfilms.org

**Marisa M. Silveri** is a Neuroscientist and Director of the Neurodevelopmental Laboratory on Addictions and Mental Health at McLean Hospital, Associate Professor of Psychiatry, Harvard Medical School and Adjunct Assistant Professor, Boston University School of Medicine. Dr. Silveri has devoted the past two decades to characterizing the development of the adolescent brain, probing the influence of alcohol and drug use and abuse on brain development and function, and identifying neurobiological underpinnings associated with mental illness. She receives funding from the National Institute on Alcohol Abuse and Alcoholism and was awarded the Research Society on Alcoholism's Young Investigator Award. Dr. Silveri also devotes significant effort to community outreach, translating neuroscience into tips for helping teens navigate the second decade of life. These efforts increase public awareness about adolescent brain vulnerabilities, and the importance of discouraging adolescent alcohol and drug use and identifying early indicators of psychiatric illness.

**Jennifer T. Sneider** is an Associate Neuroscientist in the Neurodevelopmental Laboratory on Addictions and Mental Health, McLean Hospital, and Instructor, Department of Psychiatry, Harvard Medical School. She earned a PhD in Psychology from the University of Connecticut. Dr. Sneider's primary area of focus is the hippocampus, and accordingly, has amassed diverse research experiences using rodent and human models of hippocampal-based learning and memory. Dr. Sneider has received funding from the National Institute on Drug Abuse to apply neuroimaging techniques to explore the role of the hippocampus in marijuana dependence. She also collaborates on studies in healthy teens and binge drinking emerging adults. Dr. Sneider has a particular interest in characterizing sex differences and the role of the menstrual cycle on memory function in these populations. She recently received a Young Investigator Award from the Brain & Behavior Research Foundation, which will investigate neurobiological correlates of depression in women.

**Alexander I. Stingl** is a member of the research faculty with the Center for Science, Technology, and Society at Drexel University, Philadelphia. He is also a visiting, collaborating, and consulting researcher with the Social Science Faculty of the University of Kassel, the Center for Logic and Philosophy of Science at the Vrije Universiteit Brussels, the Institute for General Medicine, and University Clinic Erlangen-Nuernberg and is contract instructor at Leuphana University Lueneburg. He has written and co-authored books, chapters, and articles in science and technology studies, sociology, philosophy, media archeology, history of science, and cultural analysis. His most recent publication, co-authored with Sabrina M. Weiss and Sal Restivo, is *Worlds of ScienceCraft* (2014). His new book, *The Digital Coloniality of Power*, is forthcoming in 2015. Under the umbrella frame of the "political and historical ontology of biodigital citizenship," he is presently working on nearly a dozen different research projects on the body, biomedicine, digital culture, decoloniality, radical Otherness, transmediality, nomadic statehood, semantic agency, and radical democracy.

**Pia Tikka** is a filmmaker who has directed features *Daughters of Yemanjá* (Brazil-Finland 1996) and *Sand Bride* (Finland 1998) and has worked in international film productions. She is the author of *Enactive Cinema: Simulatorium Eisensteinense* (2008), Enactive Cinema project *Obsession* (2005) awarded with Möbius Prix Nordic prize and co-author of the interactive film-game *Third Woman*, exhibited in the Galapagos Art Space, New York (2011). She is a founding member of the research project Enactive Media (2009–11), Aalto University, Finland. Currently Tikka is affiliated in the research project aivoAALTO. Her NeuroCine-group combines filmmaking practice with the methods of neuroimaging to study the neural basis of cinematic imagination. She earned a doctor of arts degree from the University of Art and Design in Helsinki.

# Index

For Product Safety Concerns and Information please contact our EU
representative GPSR@taylorandfrancis.com Taylor & Francis Verlag GmbH,
Kaufingerstraße 24, 80331 München, Germany

Printed and bound by CPI Group (UK) Ltd, Croydon, CR0 4YY
08/06/2025
01896991-0011